A Complete Textbook for GNM Internship

Vijay Kumar Gauttam
PhD in Nursing MSN RN RM

JAYPEE

JAYPEE BROTHERS MEDICAL PUBLISHERS
The Health Sciences Publisher
New Delhi | London

Jaypee Brothers Medical Publishers (P) Ltd.

Headquarters

EMCA House, 23/23-B
Ansari Road, Daryaganj
New Delhi 110 002, India
Landline: +91-11-23272143, +91-11-23272703
+91-11-23282021, +91-11-23245672
e-mail: jaypee@jaypeebrothers.com

Corporate Office

4838/24, Ansari Road, Daryaganj
New Delhi 110 002, India
Phone: +91-11-43574357
Fax: +91-11-43574314
e-mail: jaypee@jaypeebrothers.com

Overseas Office

JP Medical Ltd.
83, Victoria Street, London
SW1H 0HW (UK)
Phone: +44-20 3170 8910
e-mail: info@jpmedpub.com

EU GPSR Authorised Representative

Logos Europe, 9 rue Nicolas Poussin
17000, La Rochelle, France
Phone: +33 (0) 6 67 93 73 78
e-mail: contact@logoseurope.eu

Website: www.jaypeebrothers.com
Website: www.jaypeedigital.com

Inquiries for bulk sales may be solicited at: jaypee@jaypeebrothers.com

A Complete Textbook for GNM Internship

First Edition: 2015

Reprint: 2025, **2026**

ISBN 978-93-5152-786-2

Printed in India at Sterling Graphics Pvt. Ltd.

Dedicated
_to_

My Parents and Teachers

Preface

This comprehensive textbook serves as a ready-reference tool for GNM internship students. The contents of this textbook has been arranged as per Indian Nursing Council syllabus and it contains five parts:

Section 1 is designed for nursing students, faculty, and staff educators learning to use technologies effectively and efficiently in their teaching. Based on educational theory and best practices, the text integrates resources from a variety of disciplines. The text begins with broad teaching and learning concepts that have relevance across a variety of technologies. Multimedia uses multiple forms of information content and processing mainly text, audio, graphics, and video for communication to cater the various user demands.

Section 2 is designed to improve one's ability to conceptualize, construct, test, problems solve, and acquire knowledge, all of which are characteristics of scientific inquiry and the creative process required when conducting research. We have discovered, in teaching research methods courses and supervising dissertation committees, that students often have a difficult time conceptualizing the most appropriate research design, en route to collecting the data and answering the stated research questions or hypotheses. Based on this observation, we sought to find the best text that could help resolve this critical issue.

Section 3 covers a range of topics for nursing students and those looking to advance in their nursing career. Topics covered include resilience and leadership, nursing careers and careers success, writing for publication in nursing and successful grant writing, integrated case management, law in nursing, nursing history, spirituality in nursing, and more.

Section 4 is designed for management development of professional nurses in the twenty-first century. The text provides the best management concepts and theories of management available from the field of generic management, as well as from nursing management sources. It also provides theoretical and practical knowledge that will aid clinical nurse managers in meeting the demands of constantly changing patient care services.

Section 5 introduces students to the growing research field of health economics. Rather than offer details about health systems around the world without providing a theoretical context, health economics combines economic concepts with empirical evidence to enhance readers' economic understanding of how health care institutions and markets function. It views the subject in both microeconomic and macroeconomic terms, moving from the individual and firm level to the market level to a macroeconomic view of the role of health and health care within the economy as a whole.

As the authors are truly technology-savvy learners, advance in their professional careers, the authors are often reminded of the important roles that faculty play in helping nursing students to be successful. I hope our readers will gain ideas by using this textbook for promoting success of many future nursing students.

I sincerely welcome constructive criticism from readers that would help me to enrich my knowledge. I greatly appreciate your willingness to share your thought and suggestion with me, and good suggestions will be considered for incorporation in the next edition.

Vijay Kumar Gauttam

Acknowledgments

I am grateful to almighty *God (Lord Shiva)* whose grace, unconditional love and blessing accomplished me.

I wish to thanks my father *Shri Ramswaroop Gauttam* and my mother *Smt Lali Devi* for their constant blessing in this enterprises.

I am deeply indebted to my PhD Guide *Dr (Mrs) Jogindra Vati,* Principal Shri Guru Harikrishan Sahib College of Nursing, Mohali (PB) for her constant inspiration and guidance.

I would like to thank my brother Mr Ajay Gauttam, his wife, Mrs Anju Sharma and his loving son Master Laksh Gauttam.

Special thanks are due to my friends *Mr Ratish Nair, Mr Haromohan Yadav, Mr Arun Jindal, Mr Ashok Bishnoi, Mr Rahul Tiwari, Mr Anil Parashar, Mr Yogesh, Mr Rohitash Yadav,* and *Mr Ram Kumar Garg* for constant source of re-energizing my intellectual potential.

Lastly, I also thank my wife *Mrs Jyoti Sharma* for sparing me out of other pursuits of her time so that I could complete this book.

Special thanks are due to *Shri Pradeep Chaudhary* (Chairman), *Shri Rajesh Sharma* (Secretary), *Teaching and Non-Teaching faculty* members of *RR College of Nursing, Ajmer* (Rajasthan) for constant source of re-energizing my intellectual potential.

Also my sincere thanks to M/s Jaypee Brothers Medical Publishers (P) Ltd, who has played an important part in completing this textbook venture, Ms Shagufta Khan (Project Manager) and all the team members for being so kind, cooperative and positive that working has been a pleasure with her guidance.

From the Publisher's Desk

We request all the readers to provide us their valuable suggestions/errors (if any)

at: ***jppgmee@gmail.com***

so as to help us in further improvement of this book in the subsequent edition.

Contents

Section 4: ADMINISTRATION AND WARD MANAGEMENT

Section 5: HEALTH ECONOMICS

1

Section

Educational Methods and Media for Teaching in Practice of Nursing

COURSE DESCRIPTION

Hrs. 45

This course is designed to introduce the students to the concept of teaching as an integral part of nursing, its relationship to nursing process and also the importance of effective communication in nursing.

Upon completion of this course the students will be able to:

- Explain the concept of teaching in changing the behavior of the client
- Describe techniques used for teaching clients
- Describe the use of different media in teaching and effective communication.

Course Content

Unit I: Introduction

- Meaning aims and purposes of education
- Meaning of teaching and learning
- Principles of teaching and learning
- Teaching responsibilities of a nurse
- Methods of teaching, methods of clinical teaching
- Preparation of teaching plan.

Unit II: Media

- Definition, purposes and types of media.
- Preparation and use of audio-visual aids: graphic aids, printed aids, three dimensional aids, projected aids
- Limitations, advantages and uses of different types of media.

Practical Work

Students will organize teaching in the wards/clinics using nursing process approach and prepare variety of audio-visual aids to implement their teaching either individually or in groups. Students will also submit written teaching plan to the concerned teacher of selected clinical area.

1

Introduction unit

INTRODUCTION

Education is the most important and most noble of human endeavors. All other activities have their foundation in education. Education is so important that it will continue even in eternity. It enables humans to achieve their fullest personal, spiritual, mental, social, and physical potentials. The ability of being educated is what distinguishes humans from animals. Education transforms an individual and allows her to effect change in her environment.

Education involves both the world of ideas and the world of practical activity; good ideas can lead to good practice and good practices reinforce good ideas. In order to behave intelligently in the educational process; education needs direction and guidance which philosophy can provide. Hence, philosophy is not only a professional tool for the educator but also a way of improving the quality of life because it helps us to gain a wider and deeper perspective on human existence and the world around us.

Meaning of Education

Education does not mean mere schooling. To become educated is to learn to become a person. First view of that the word 'education' is derived from the Latin word 'Educatum' which means 'to bring up' or 'to nourish'. Second view is that the word 'education' is derived from 'educare' which means 'to lead out' or 'to draw out'. In a broad sense, education refers to an act or experience that has a formative effect on the mind, character or physical ability of an individual. Education in this sense never ends, we truly learn from experience throughout our lives. Education and philosophy are inseparable because the ends of education are the ends of philosophy, i.e. wisdom; and the means of philosophy is the means of education, i.e. inquiry, which alone can lead to wisdom. Any separation of philosophy and education inhibits inquiry and frustrates wisdom.

Definition of Education

- According to Swami Dayanand, 'Education is a means for character formation and righteous living'.
- According to Mahatma Gandhi, 'By education I mean an all round drawing our of the best in child man-body, mind and spirit'.
- According to Rig Veda, 'Education is something which makes a man self-reliant and selfless'.
- Education according to George Knight (1980) is a lifelong learning process that can take place in an infinite variety of circumstances and contexts.
- According to Kleining (1985), education is 'The range of activities both formal and informal whereby people are initiated into or realigned with the evolving traditions, structures, and social relations which are taken to constitute their education.'
- Peter (1975) wrote: 'Education consists in initiating others into activities, modes of conduct and thoughts which have standards written into them by references to which it is possible to act, think and feel with varying degrees of relevance and taste'.

Aims of Education

Aims of education are related to time and space. They are also changeable. The history of educational development in india stands evidence to this fact:

- *Aims of education in the Brahmanic Period:* The aim of education during this period was an all-sided development of man. Education was regarded as a means of salvation or emancipation. The chief aim of education was to unfold the spiritual and normal power of the individual. Education was thus determined by religious values.
- *Aims of education in the Buddhist Period:* The aim of education during this period was to create a sense of equality among all; 'Satya' and 'Ahinsa' were the directive principles of this system of education. The child was taught to control and suppress his worldly desires in accordance with the eightfold code of conduct enunciated by Lord Buddha.
- *Aims of education in the Muslim Period:* The aim of education during this period was to prepare an individual for the worldly life as well as for the spiritual life. It was education of Islamic culture and scriptures which regulated human behavior accordingly.

- *Aims of education in the British Period:* The aims of education during this period were different. The system of British education was implanted in this country with purely political motives. It aimed at dividing Indians spiritually and intellectually into the English-knowledge class of men and non-English-knowledge masses of people. It was in accordance with Macaulay's 'Downward filtration theory'.

  After the independence of the country Pt. Jawahar Lal Nehru remarked, 'Great changes have taken place in the country and the educational system must be keeping with them. The entire basis of education must be revolutionised'. Social, political and economic conditions of the country are fast changing. It is, therefore, very important that we should assess everything carefully in the light of present situation and fix-up aims of education:
- *Individual aim of education:* It means that education should develop the individuals according to their interests and capabilities. It means free growth of individuality, helping every boy and girl to achieve the hugest degree of individual development. All social institutions exist for the betterment and improvement of the individual. Education aims at training and development of the individual. It is only this type of individual who come out as a good citizen.
- *Social aim of education:* Man is essentially a social animal. He is born into a social heritage. He has become what he is due to the influences upon him of other social beings—parents, teachers, schoolmates, brothers, sisters, friends, and colleagues, etc. therefore, he is only a unit of a larger whole 'society'—usually the state. He can live as an individual only because he is in a society. Man enjoy the facilities of health, housing, food, education, transport, communication and so many other comforts of modern living which cannot be enumerated exhaustively. He enjoys these comforts only because of his membership in an organized society.
- *Vocational aim of education:* Vocation education thus, exercises a liberalizing effect on man. There is no vocation without education. Every vocation has an educational value. Education with the vocational aim in the background will prepare each individual for an occupation. Vocational aim of education is also known as 'Bread and Butter Aim, 'Blue Jacket Aim' and 'White Collar Aim'.
- *Spiritual aim of education:* Education makes a person spiritually sound. A person who is spiritually sound behaves better. He/she is able to do well while being trained for social efficiency, sound morally and physical betterment. It gives strength to human soul and mind.

PURPOSES OF EDUCATION

The one continuing purpose of education, since ancient times, has been to bring people to as full a realization as possible of what it is to be a human being:

- To develop the intellect
- To serve social needs
- To contribute to the economy
- To create an effective work force
- To prepare students for a job or career
- To promote a particular social or political system
- To provide for the fullest possible development of each learner for living morally, creatively, and productively in a democratic society.

FUNCTION OF EDUCATION

Ever since the education system was invented, there have been a lot of ideas and criticisms of how it should work. Most people believe that public education after all is the engine that moves a society toward a common destiny. Basically, there are two functions of education that are to help to socialize the young into becoming 'good citizens' and prepare people for employment and to be generally productive citizen.

In the broadest sense, education includes the formal and informal experiences that train, discipline, and shape the mental and physical potentials of the maturing person. According to Ferrante, there are following functions of education:

- *The function of socialization:* The socialization process has become part of our lives; the family is the primary context within with the child receives initial socialization that differs based on society, social class, and family background. As a result early childhood education takes on special significance because children are developing their self-concept and social awareness. More than half of the nations of the world have some formal early childhood education that starts at age of 3 to 5 years old. Early childhood education provides children valuable learning experience that is not available at home and the fact that young children also need to interact with other children and adults other than their siblings and parents.
- *The function of cultural transmission:* Cultural transmission is not a straight forward process but one that reflects the dynamics and heterogeneous viewpoints of a pluralistic society. Cultural transmission is a universal process, serious thoughts are very much concern on what culture is transmitted and what should be

transmitted. As a consequence, in every society there are expectations concerning ideas about the products that school should produce. These expectations are building into the curriculum that provides for instruction in areas seen as desirable through the planned experiences in line with the concerns and trends in the society. In this way schools are believed to serve the crucial function of preparing young people for society.

- *The function of social control and personal development:* Social control includes social mechanisms that regulate individual and group behavior, leading to conformity and compliances to the rules of a given society or social group. Sociologists identify two basic forms of social controls that are, internalization of norms and values and the use of sanctions, which can be either positive - reward or negative—punishment. Schools are expected to instil values related to social control and personal development.
- *The function of selection and allocation:* The selection and allocation function of schooling, schools tend to act as sorting and sifting mechanism in preparing students for the workforce. As a result the selection and allocation function dominates schooling through assessment, testing, or examinations and credentialing.
- *The function of change and innovation:* As schools provide a link to the future, schools are considered as change agents that play a very critical role in the successful initiation, implementation, and continuation of planned educational change. Depending on the school and classroom context, in particular, teachers are important change agents that must possess knowledge of innovation that can be gained through experience or study, have a positive attitude, show confidence, and encourage student's participation.

MEANING OF TEACHING

Teaching is an essential part of education. Its special function is to impart knowledge, develop understanding and skills. It generally excludes inculcation of values like truth. It is usually associated with the imparting of knowledge of 3 R's-Reading, Writing and Arithmetic representing various school subjects.

Definition of Teaching

- According to Edmund Amidon, 'Teaching is defined as an interactive process, primarily involving classroom talk, which takes place between teacher and pupil and occurs during certain definable activities'.

- According to TF Greens, 'Teaching is a task of a teacher, which is performed for the development of a child'.
- According to HC Morrison, 'Teaching is an intimate contact between a more mature personality and a less mature one which is designed to further the education of the latter'.
- According to J Brubacher, 'Teaching is an arrangement and manipulation of a situation in which there are gaps and obstructions, which an individual will seek to overcome and from in which he will learn in the course of doing so'.
- According to Burton, 'Teaching is the stimulation, guidance, direction and encouragement of learning'.

Characteristics of Good Teaching

- Teaching is both an Art and Science
- Teaching as a relationship
- Teaching is formal social services
- Teaching as a skilled occupation
- Teaching is stimulation and encouragement
- Teaching is guidance
- Teaching is training the emotion of the students
- Teaching is both conscious and unconscious process
- Teaching means of perception
- Teaching is causing to learn
- Teaching is a matter of helping the students to respond to his/her environment in an effective manner.

MEANING OF LEARNING

The term '*learning*' has been interpreted to mean, 'Change in response or behaviour (such as innovation, elimination or modification of responses, involving some degree of performance) caused partly or wholly by experience, such experience being in the main conscious but sometime including significant unconscious components, as is more common in motor learning or in reaction to unrecognized or subliminal stimuli.

Definition of Learning

- According to Daniel Bell, 'Learning is modification due to energies of organism and environment impinging on the organism itself'.
- According to Gates, 'Learning is modification of behavior through experience'.
- According to Crow – Crow, 'Learning involves the acquisition of habits, knowledge and attitude'.

- According to Ruch, 'Learning is a process, which brings about changes in the individual way of responding as a result of contact with aspects of environment'.

Characteristics of Learning

According to *Yoakman and Simpson* have enumerated general characteristics of learning:

- *Learning is active:* Learning does not take place without a purpose and self-activity. In the teaching-learning process, the activity of the learner counts more than the activity of the teacher. The principle of learning by doing is the main principle and it has been recommended by all modern educationists.
- *Learning is intelligent:* Meaningless efforts do not produce permanent result. Any work done mechanically is without any soul. When a child learn something unintelligently, he/she is likely to forget it very soon. He/she does not assimilate but simply commits to memory. Only efforts made intelligently have lasting effects.
- *Learning is purposeful:* Purpose play a big role in learning. According to Ryburn, "This purpose is always connected with the use of some instinctive power, with the use of the energy with which we are endowed with birth". We do not learn anything and everything that comes in our way, in a haphazard, manner. All school activities should be purposeful so that the child should feel real urge for learning.
- *Learning is growth:* The world growth is generally associated with the body which is growing, but through the mental growth of the learner. Although it is latent yet we can perceive it growth. Through his daily activities the child grows both mentally and physically.
- *Learning is organized experience:* Learning is not mere addition to knowledge. It is not mere acquisition of facts and skills through drill and reputation. It is reorganization of experience.
- *Learning is adjustment:* Learning helps the individual to adjust himself adequately to the new situations. Children meet with new situations which demand solution. Repeated efforts are required to react to them effectively. Life is full of experiences, and each experience leaves behind some effects in the mental structure. These effects modify our behavior.
- *Learning is both individual and social:* Learning is more than an individual activity. It is a social activity also. Individual mind is affected by the group mind consciously as well as unconsciously as individual is influenced by his friends, relatives, classmates, parents, etc. social agencies like the family, church, film and gangs of playmates have

a tremendous influence on the child and are always moulding and remoulding him.

Learning depends upon insight: Lasting learning depends upon insight. Insight has sometimes been described as the 'flash of understanding'.

PRINCIPLES OF TEACHING AND LEARNING

Teaching is a complex, multifaceted activity, often requiring us as instructors to juggle multiple tasks and goals simultaneously and flexibly. The following small but powerful set of principles can make teaching both more effective and more efficient, by helping us create the conditions that support student learning and minimize the need for revising materials, content, and policies. While implementing these principles requires a commitment in time and effort, it often saves time and energy later on.

- *Effective teaching and learning involves acquiring relevant knowledge about students and using that knowledge to inform our course design and classroom teaching:* When we teach, we do not just teach the content, we teach students the content. A variety of student characteristics can affect learning. For example, students' cultural and generational backgrounds influence how they see the world; disciplinary backgrounds lead students to approach problems in different ways; and students' prior knowledge (both accurate and inaccurate aspects) shapes new learning. Although we cannot adequately measure all of these characteristics, gathering the most relevant information as early as possible in course planning and continuing to do so during the semester can (a) inform course design (e.g. decisions about objectives, pacing, examples, format), (b) help explain student difficulties (e.g. identification of common misconceptions), and (c) guide instructional adaptations (e.g. recognition of the need for additional practice).
- *Effective teaching and learning involves aligning the three major components of instruction: learning objectives, assessments, and instructional activities:* Taking the time to do this upfront saves time in the end and leads to a better course. Teaching is more effective and student learning is enhanced when (a) we, as instructors, articulate a clear set of learning objectives (i.e. the knowledge and skills that we expect students to demonstrate by the end of a course); (b) the instructional activities (e.g. case studies, labs, discussions, readings) support these learning objectives by providing goal-oriented practice, and (c) the assessments (e.g. tests, papers, problem sets, performances) provide opportunities for students to demonstrate and practice the knowledge and skills articulated in the objectives, and for instructors to offer targeted feedback that can guide further learning.

- *Effective teaching involves articulating explicit expectations regarding learning objectives and policies:* There is amazing variation in what is expected of students across American classrooms and even within a given discipline. For example, what constitutes evidence may differ greatly across courses; what is permissible collaboration in one course could be considered cheating in another. As a result, students' expectations may not match ours. Thus, being clear about our expectations and communicating them explicitly helps students learn more and perform better. Articulating our learning objectives (i.e. the knowledge and skills that we expect students to demonstrate by the end of a course) gives students a clear target to aim for and enables them to monitor their progress along the way. Similarly, being explicit about course policies (e.g. on class participation, laptop use, and late assignment) in the syllabus and in class allows us to resolve differences early and tends to reduce conflicts and tensions that may arise. Altogether, being explicit leads to a more productive learning environment for all students.
- *Effective teaching involves prioritizing the knowledge and skills we choose to focus on: Coverage is the enemy:* Do not try to do too much in a single course. Too many topics work against student learning, so it is necessary for us to make decisions—sometimes difficult ones—about what we will and will not include in a course. This involves (a) recognizing the parameters of the course (e.g. class size, students' backgrounds and experiences, course position in the curriculum sequence, number of course units), (b) setting our priorities for student learning, and (c) determining a set of objectives that can be reasonably accomplished.
- *Effective teaching involves recognizing and overcoming our expert blind spots:* We are not our students! As experts, we tend to access and apply knowledge automatically and unconsciously (e.g. make connections, draw on relevant bodies of knowledge, and choose appropriate strategies) and so we often skip or combine critical steps when we teach. Students, on the other hand, do not yet have sufficient background and experience to make these leaps and can become confused, draw incorrect conclusions, or fail to develop important skills. They need instructors to break tasks into component steps, explain connections explicitly, and model processes in detail. Though it is difficult for experts to do this, we need to identify and explicitly communicate to students the knowledge and skills we take for granted, so that students can see expert thinking in action and practice applying it themselves.
- *Effective teaching involves adopting appropriate teaching roles to support our learning goals:* Even though students are ultimately responsible for their own learning, the roles we assume as instructors are critical in

guiding students' thinking and behavior. We can take on a variety of roles in our teaching (e.g. synthesizer, moderator, challenger, and commentator). These roles should be chosen in service of the learning objectives and in support of the instructional activities. For example, if the objective is for students to be able to analyze arguments from a case or written text, the most productive instructor role might be to frame, guide and moderate a discussion. If the objective is to help students learn to defend their positions or creative choices as they present their work, our role might be to challenge them to explain their decisions and consider alternative perspectives. Such roles maybe constant or variable across the semester depending on the learning objectives.

- *Effective teaching involves progressively refining our courses based on reflection and feedback:* Teaching requires adapting. We need to continually reflect on our teaching and be ready to make changes when appropriate (e.g. something is not working, we want to try something new, the student population has changed, or there are emerging issues in our fields). Knowing what and how to change requires us to examine relevant information on our own teaching effectiveness. Much of this information already exists (e.g. student work, previous semesters' course evaluations, dynamics of class participation), or we may need to seek additional feedback with help from the university teaching center (e.g. interpreting early course evaluations, conducting focus groups, designing pre-and post-tests). Based on such data, we might modify the learning objectives, content, structure, or format of a course, or otherwise adjust our teaching. Small, purposeful changes driven by feedback and our priorities are most likely to be manageable and effective.

ROLE AND RESPONSIBILITIES OF THE NURSES IN TEACHING

- Good nursing teachers see as their most important task to help students learn; they design their teaching to support student learning in the best possible way.
- Nursing teachers display enthusiasm for their subject, and a desire to share it with their students.
- Nursing teachers draw on their knowledge of their subject, their knowledge of their learners, and their general pedagogical knowledge to transform the concepts of the discipline into terms that are understandable to their students.
- Good nursing teachers encourage learning for understanding and are concerned with developing their students' critical-thinking skills, problem-solving skills, and problem-approach behaviors.

- Good nursing teachers show respect for their students; they are interested in both their professional and their personal growth, encourage their independence, and sustain high expectations of them.
- Good nursing teachers set clear goals, use valid and appropriate assessment methods, and provide high quality feedback to their students.
- Nursing teachers recognize the importance of context, and adapt their teaching accordingly. They know how to modify their teaching strategies according to the particular students, subject matter and learning environment.
- Good nursing teachers show versatility and flexibility. They have broad competence both in the use of various teaching methods and teaching at different levels, and in the mastery of varying subject contents.
- Good nursing teachers are prepared to develop their teaching through cooperation with others, within the academic setting as well as in the surrounding society.
- Nursing teachers are also good learners. For example, they learn through their own reading, by participating in a variety of professional development activities, by listening to their students, by sharing ideas with their colleagues, and by reflecting on classroom interaction and students' achievements.

METHODS OF TEACHING

Every teacher should create his/her own teaching method by choosing and adapting available technique in accordance with his/her own personality and the objectives and the content of the course that he/she teaches. Therefore, the general method of teaching used by a teacher would represent a composite of style or quality of teaching, a characteristic mode of teaching behavior which would reflect his/her value and educational philosophy.

A method is not merely a device adopted for communicating certain items of information to students and exclusively the concern of the teacher who is supposed to be at the 'giving end'. A method must link-up the teacher and his pupils into an organic relationship with constant mutual interaction.

Definition

- According to Thut and Gerbersich, 'A method is a well defined pattern of procedures within which a variety of the techniques and devices may appear as circumstances may require.'

- According to M Verma, 'Method is an abstract as logical entities that we can distinguish between manner and methods, in reality, they form an organic whole and matter determines method analogously as objective determines means; content and spirit determine style and form of literature'.
- According to Broudy, 'Method refers to the formal structure of the sequence of acts commonly denoted by instruction. The term 'method' covers both strategies and tactics of teaching and involves the choice of what is to be taught, and in which order is it to be presented.'
- According to Adams, 'The new teaching recognizes the right of the pupil to do things in his own way, within reasonable limits'.

Objectives of Methods of Teaching

- They should develop the capacity for clear thinking
- They should provide adequate opportunities for participation in freely accepted projects and activities in which cooperation and discipline are constantly in demand
- They should aim at developing 'love for work'
- They should expend the student's interest
- They should aim at providing opportunities to students to apply practically the knowledge and skill acquired by them
- They should aim at the quickening of interest and training in efficient technique of learning and study.

LECTURE METHOD

The lecture is still the most frequently used method of instruction. The lecture method is an effective way to introduce new information or concepts to a group of learners. The learners always appreciate a concise, stimulating and well-delivered lecture. Lecture method refers to the teaching procedure involved in clarification or explanation of the students of some major idea.

This method lays emphasis on the penetration of contents. Teacher is more active and students are passive but he also uses question answers to keep them attentive in the class. It is used to motivate, clarify, expand and review the information. By changing Ms Voice, by impersonating characters, by shifting his posing, by using simple devices, a teacher can deliver lessons effectively, while delivering his lecture; a teacher can indicate by her facial expressions, gestures and tones the exact slode of meaning that he wishes to convey. Thus we can say that when teacher takes the help of a lengthy-short explanation in order to clarify his ideas or some fact that explanation is termed as lecture or lecture method.

Purposes of the Lecture Method

- *To motivate:* The teacher can present the chief points and aspects of a study. Topic or new subject-unit more effectively through a lecture. Teacher can point out some of the significant persons, events and problems and in this way arouse the curiosity of the students, who would feel more motivated for later activities, as a result of this method.
- *To clarify:* In the course of the study of a unit, chapter, or a topic, students are generally struck up and are troubled by the same or similar difficulties. A short lecture will, at such stage help in clarifying the doubts and thus results in a lot of saving of the valuable time, of teachers and students.
- *To expand:* As Gandhi pointed out, 'A Teacher is the best Text Book', for the students. Teachers read a lot, consults references, know by experience and can add much more information than supplied by textbooks. So also, lecture method can be utilized to present additional material or the information.
- *To revise:* After the topic or chapter is completed, students need audience regarding the salient points, covered in the lessons. At that stage, a teacher can, in a short talk or lecture, point out the main ideas of the chapter, just covered.

Preparation of the Lecture

- Prepare for the lecture, become very familiar with the subject matter.
- Identify and prepare supporting aids to illustrate the points made.
- Keep chalk and blackboard or flip chart and marker pen ready for noting key points.
- Provide examples to link the subject matter to the lives of the learners.
- Sequence the contents logically, sequentially and systematically, building upon previous content areas.
- Ask questions to check whether the learners are following.
- Provoke the learners to ask questions.
- Maintain eye contact with the learners to assess whether they are following or not, whether they are interested or bored.
- Maintain time stipulations, do not get carried away, but at the same time do not sacrifice essential material for the sake of time.
- Have a seating arrangement in which all can see the aids equally well and hear the lecture. A circular seating arrangement, or if there are too many people, a double circle is useful.

- Be aware of your own body movements, and facial expressions.
- Speak clearly, loudly, and use simple language.
- Avoid being prescriptive, try to be provocative.
- If there is more than one trainer, then the others can supplement, as well as monitor the process of learning.

Techniques of Lecture Method

Every method depends on oral instruction to give information, to arouse attention and interest, and to develop receptive attitudes on the part of the trainees. Therefore, as an instructor, organize oral presentations with the following techniques in mind:

- *Maintain good eye contact:* The teacher should address the students with his/her eyes as well as with his/her voice. The eyes have a unique power to transmit the mood of the teacher to the student.
- *Speak in a natural, conversational voice:* The lecture should be presented in a clear, natural tone of voice. The importance of the voice of the teacher is clearly pointed up in this comment of a student. Clear tone, distinct enunciation, good diction help all students to hear and understand, no matter what part of the room they maybe in.
- *Gestures:* Whatever gesture the lecturer uses should be in a natural part of the total expression of what he/she is communicating. In other words, the teacher's actions should blend with his/her speech; they should be spontaneous and animated and a part of natural style of the individual.
- *Rapport:* The teacher should at the outset of the lecture try to establish rapport with his/her students. This maybe done through an exchange with students in a conversational tone about some event at the school; this will help to foster a sense of ease and give the impression of personal interest.
- *Stimulate trainees to think:* Think, as used here, refers to creative thinking rather than to a mere recall of facts previously learned. Use a number of instructional devices for stimulating trainee thinking. Among those devices are thought-provoking questions, class discussions, problem situations, challenging statements, and rhetorical questions (a question to which no answer is expected). Another device is the use of suggestions, such as 'I want you to think along with me,' and 'Consider your reaction to this situation.'

Advantages of Lecture Method

- Allows the presentation of facts, information and concepts in a relatively short span of time.
- Multiple resource persons, knowledgeable and with different points of view can interact with the learners

- Can be used with illiterate learners
- A diverse range of supportive materials can be used to support the content areas, e.g. slides, charts, posters, etc.
- A large number of learners can be accommodated at one time.

Disadvantages of Lecture Method

- The world view of the speaker dominates
- It does not promote interaction in most cases
- Participants can get carried away by the charisma and personality of the speaker instead of focusing on an analyzing what he/she is saying
- The pace is trainer-controlled.

DEMONSTRATION METHOD

The dictionary meaning of the word 'demonstration' is the outward showing of a feeling, etc. a description and explanation by experiment; so also logically to prove the truth; or a practical display of a piece of equipment to snow its display of a piece of equipment to show its capabilities. In short it is a proof provided by logic, argument, etc.

To define 'it is a physical display of the form, outline or a substance of object or events for the purpose of increasing knowledge of such objects or events. Demonstration involves 'showing what or showing how'. Demonstration is relatively uncomplicated process in that it does not require extensive verbal elaboration.

Requirements of Good Demonstration

The success of any demonstration following points should be kept in mind:

- It should be planned and rehearsed by the teacher beforehand.
- The apparatus used for demonstration should be big enough to be seen by the whole class. If the class maybe disciplined she may allow them to sit on the benches to enable them a better view.
- Adequate lighting arrangements be made on demonstration table and a proper background table need to be provided.
- All the pieces of apparatus are placed in order before starting the demonstration. The apparatus likely to be used should be placed in the left hand side of the table and it should be arranged in the same order in which it is likely to be used.
- Before actually starting the demonstration a clear statement about the purpose of demonstration be made to the students.

- The teacher makes sure that the demonstration lecture method leads to active participation of the students in the process of teaching.
- The demonstration should be quick and slick and should not appear to linger on unnecessarily.
- The demonstration should be interesting so that it captures the attention of the students.
- It would be better if the teacher demonstrates with materials or things the children handle in everyday life.
- For active participation of students the teacher may call individual student in turn to help him in demonstration.
- The teacher should write the summary of the principles arrived at because of demonstration on the blackboard. The blackboard can be also used for drawing the necessary diagrams.

Techniques of Good Demonstration

Use a variety of techniques in presenting background knowledge and in developing proper attitudes. The following techniques relate more to the actual demonstration:

- *Position the trainees and training aids properly:* If you direct trainees to gather around a worktable or a training aid, make sure every trainee has an unobstructed view.
- *Show and explain each operation:* Perform each operation in step-by-step order. Whenever possible, give the instructions while you demonstrate. Do not hurry; do not emphasize speed in performing operations or in moving from one operation to another during the demonstration step. Make certain the trainees understand the first step before you proceed to the second step, and so on. Repeat difficult operations.
- *Observe safety precautions:* By observing safety precautions, you may take a few more seconds to rig a safety line, don a safety mask, or tag an electric cable; but the time is not wasted. You impress the trainees with the importance of exercising extreme care in dealing with potentially dangerous equipment.
- *Give proper attention to terminology:* Call each part of a training aid by its proper name each time you call attention to it. For trainees to remember the correct nomenclature, however, requires more than your use of the proper names of parts. The following suggestions should prove helpful:
  - List the names of parts on the chalkboard
  - Refer trainees to any available chart that shows the parts and names of parts

- Conduct a terminology drill on the parts of the training aid while the aid is in its assembled or disassembled condition.

Advantage of Demonstration Method

- It is an economical method as compared to a purely student centered method
- It is a psychological method and students take active interest in the teaching learning process
- It leads the students from concrete to abstract situations
- It is suitable method if the apparatus to be handled is costly and sensitive. Such apparatus is likely to be handled and damaged by the students
- This method is safe if the experiment is dangerous
- In comparison to Heuristic, Project method it is time saving but purely Lecture method is too lengthy
- It can be successfully used for all types of students
- It improves the observational and reasoning skills of the students.

Disadvantage of Demonstration Method

- It provides no scope for 'Learning by Doing' for the Students as students are only observing the Teacher performing
- Since Teacher performs the experiment at his/her own pace many students may not be able to comprehend the concept being clarified
- Since this method is not child centered it makes no provision for individual differences, all types of students including slow learners and genius have to proceed with the same speed
- It fails to develop laboratory skills in the students
- It fails to impart training in scientific attitude. In this method students many a times fail to observe many finer details of the apparatus used because they observe it from a distance.

GROUP DISCUSSION

This is a commonly used method because a group discussion uses learners' own past experiences in a very deliberate manner. In this method the learners are divided into groups of 5 to 15 and given a real life or relevant subject matter or question to discuss. This discussion is carried on by the learners on the basis of their own past experiences, attitudes and values, from which they arrive at new knowledge and new insights. Discussion cannot be hypothetical or speculative. It is important to realize that the discussion is not an end in itself but rather each small group should then presents its discussions to the large group and on the basis of their presentations, working principles should be developed. It is a common mistake to have the discussions without subsequent presentation and summarization.

Steps of Group Discussion

- Instruct the group clearly about the task, specify time and the form of presentation
- Divide the large group into small groups
- Different groups maybe given different tasks; in this case the groups should be divided first
- Let the groups discuss (through sharing and analysis) the matter under consideration for the stipulated time
- Let all the groups reassemble into a large group
- Let one or two individuals from each group present their discussion to the large group
- Add any relevant points that you feel have been left out and use the group presentations to arrive at a theoretical framework.

Advantages of Group Discussion

- It allows the learners to be in control, in respect of pace, content and focus
- If provides opportunities for the learners to express themselves
- It allows the learners to validate their knowledge and skills
- It allows learners to clarify, reflect and reconfigure their experiences
- It helps in promoting a sense of belonging in a group
- It can be empowering once the learners realize their own ability for critical thinking and change through this medium.

Disadvantages of Group Discussion

- It is time consuming
- It requires facilitation; if facilitation is poor then the process is vitiated
- There is a possibility that dominant or aggressive members may hijack the process
- Members might not be serious and that affects the quality of the discussion
- Requires more space than a lecture
- It is difficult to monitor the progress of many different small groups

- Trainer needs special skills to facilitate, debrief and summarize the discussions.

SEMINAR

The seminar method is the most modern and advanced method of teaching. A seminar is an advanced group technique which is usually used in higher education. The seminar is similar in many ways to small group discussion, except that a seminar always uses the problem-solving approach. The effectiveness of the seminar method is conditioned by the nature and the method of the deliberations which take place, which in turn, are dependent on the selection and preparation of the topic and the leader in charge of the seminar discussion.

Meaning: An instructional technique it involves generating a situation for a group to have guided interaction among themselves on a theme. It refers to a structured group discussion what usually follows a formal lecture or lectures often in the form of an essay or a paper presentation on a theme.

Objectives of Seminar Method

This method is employed to realize the higher objectives of cognitive and affective domains which have been enumerated below:

Cognitive Objectives

- To develop higher cognitive abilities
- To develop the ability of responding in this manner would involve higher cognitive actions
- To develop the ability of keen observation of experience, feelings
- To develop the ability to seek clarification and defend the ideas of others effectively.

Affective Objectives

- To develop the feeling of tolerance to the opposite ideas of others
- To develop the feelings of cooperation with other colleagues and respect of the ideas and feelings of others
- To develop the emotional ability among the participants of the seminar
- To acquire the good manners of putting questions and answering the questions of others effectively. The human interaction under this technique develops the good manners and skills among the participants.

Steps of Seminar Method

The seminar method involves the following steps:

- *Selection of topic:* The topic of seminar should be relevant to the subject of study.
- *Assignment of topic to individual's students or team:* The topic maybe assigned to one student or to a group of students.
- *Collection of relevant information:* Information required for seminar can be collected from various sources namely books, magazines, internet, institutions, place and persons.
- *Preparation of draft paper:* Based on the information collected the student may prepare a draft paper and submit it to the teachers for comments. Revise the draft paper based on the comments of the teachers. The refined draft is submitted for approval.
- *Program scheduling:* The date, time and venue of the seminar is fixed. A seminar leader maybe selected from the students
- *Seminar paper presentation:* The student/students shall present the paper in the seminar. The teacher may function as the moderator during the initial stages.
- *Discussion/interaction:* A number of respondents from the students make comments on the topic. This will be followed by a general discussion. All the group members should actively participate in discussion.
- *Summing-up deliberation:* The moderator sums up the deliberation.
- *Evaluation/feedback:* Both teachers and students evaluate the program.
- *Preparation of final report:* A final seminar report is prepared covering all the additional points discussed and consolidated.

Roles in Seminar Method

- *Role of the organizer:* Planning, selection of topics, speaker selection, date, venue
- *Role of the president:* Directing the program encourages participation, limiting deviations, summing up, and vote of thanks
- *Role of the speaker:* Presentation, question and answer
- *Role of the participants:* Seek clarifications, and appreciate
- *Role of the observer:* Observations.

Types of Seminar Method

- *Mini seminar:* A seminar conducted in classroom by more than two students under the guidance of student leader with well prepared different aspects of topics

- *Main seminar:* A seminar conducted at departmental or institutional level
- *National seminar:* A seminar conducted at national level
- *International seminar:* A seminar conducted at international level.

Advantages of Seminar Method

- Thinking and reasoning power developed
- Attributes like tolerance
- Development of better learning habits
- Makes interaction learner centered
- Work is democratically divided
- Configurationistic type of learning.

Limitations of Seminar Method

- Time consuming
- Cannot be organized on all the content of subject matter
- Cannot be used for all levels of education
- Limited group discussions
- Seminar tends towards debate leading to conflict.

SYMPOSIUM

Symposium is a method of higher learning. It is also an instructional method which is used to achieve higher cognitive and affective objective. The symposium is a method group discussion in which two or more person under the direction of a chairman present separate speech which gives several aspects of one question. Its purpose is to investigate a problem from several points of view—the purpose is not to give a series of arguments in debate.

Meaning: A meeting of persons to discuss a problem or theme. The word has many meanings. Firstly, Plato has used this term for 'good dialogue' to present the views towards God. Another meaning of the term is the intellectual recreation or enjoyment.

Objectives of Symposium

- To identify and understand the various aspects of theme or problems
- To develop the ability to take decision and judgment
- To develop the values and feelings regarding a problem
- To enable the listeners to form policies regarding a theme or problem

- For sharing of information
- For obtaining and gaining respect for various points of views
- It is for inspiring interest.

Characteristics of Symposium Technique

- It provides the broad understanding of a problem or a topic
- The opportunity is provided to the listener to take decision about the problem
- It is used for higher classes to specific themes and problems
- It develops the feeling of cooperation and adjustment
- The objectives as synthesis and evaluation are achieved by employing the symposium.

Precautions/Guidelines for Symposium

DO'S

- The moderator should be sure to prepare the speakers or see that they are prepared
- The moderator should know the rules of procedures sequence of speaking and way in which the forum will be conducted
- They should be aware of the ideas and background of other performers. Like panellists they might benefit from a brief warm-up
- The chairman in the entire forum situation must plan very carefully for the questioning period those followers the prepared speeches, unless he wishes to risk boredom.

DONOT'S

- The chairman or whoever is responsible for preparing the agenda, should not attempt to stack the cards by omitting or ignoring vital phases of the problem as the problem he selects or delegates the speakers.
- The chairperson to face-up to an inadvertent misinterpretation or omission. To distort or omit an important point of view deliberately is to invite disaster.

Role of Teacher in Symposium

- Organizer
- Chairperson
- Leads the follow-up discussion.

Role of Students in Symposium

- Listener
- Directing questions
- Participation in follow-up discussion.

Advantages of Symposium Technique

- It expands mental horizon
- It helps in broad based participation
- It develops free and frank attitude
- It stimulates broad understanding and develops attitude of tolerance and cooperation
- Teacher able to evaluate students creatively
- It provides wide variety of opinion for the listeners.

Limitations of Symposium Technique

- Limited control of chairman over the proceedings
- Speaker may tend to deviate from said agenda causing difficulty in understanding
- Limited listener/audience participation
- Since audience has to form decision this technique is more suitable for a mature audience
- While the higher objective of cognitive domain can be achieved, affective domain is not emphasized properly.

PANEL DISCUSSION

A panel discussion is a type of discussion, where groups of experts ('panels') or other participants address issues from a given topic that emerged during a report that was presented beforehand (in various forms). We can also say that panel is a group of experts or people who have some special knowledge of the chosen topic. They exchange views on the topic, usually in front of an audience who may have a chance to ask questions at some point. Most panels have a chair or other leader.

A panel consists of a small group of six or eight persons, who carry-on a guided and informal discussion before an audience as if the panel were meeting alone. The proceedings of the panel should be the same as for informal discussion: volunteering of facts, asking questions, stating opinions —all expressed with geniality, with respect for the contributions of other members, without speech making, and without making invidious personal references.

Purposes of Panel Discussion

- To spread new pieces of knowledge
- To analyze the current problem from different angle
- To identify the value
- To provide information and facts
- To organize for mental recreation.

Stages of Panel Discussion

There are three stages of panel discussion preparation and implementation:

Stage 1

- Defining discussion aims
- Specifying issue aspects
- Separating disputatious aspects of a particular issue form those that are clear
- Specifying discussion topic
- Scheme of the discussion progress—choosing analysis methods, ways and forms of argumentation, etc.

Stage 2

Actual discussion.

Stage 3

Discussion conclusions, accepting and approving the problem solution.

Members of Panel Discussion

Panel discussion involves the following members:

- *Moderator:* Moderator is the time manager and act as a leader during discussion
- *Panelists:* These are the experts who are the main speaker of the panel. There are four to ten panelists in the discussion
- *Instructor:* The schedule of panel discussion is prepared by instructor and some time has to plan rehearsal of discussion
- *Audience:* After end of the session the audience are allow to put question and seek clarification.

Advantages of Panel Discussion

- It develops the interest and positive attitude towards the problem
- It develops the capacity to respect others ideas and opinions

- It provides the opportunities of assimilation of theme and content
- It develops the ability of problem-solving and logical thinking capacity
- It allows the experts to present different opinions.

Limitation of Panel Discussion

- The experts may not be good speakers
- Personalities may overshadow content
- Some time the subject may not be in logical order.

ROLE-PLAY

Role-playing is the spontaneous acting out of roles in the context of human relations situations. It is part of the two broad methods devised by JL Moreno-Sociodrama and Psychodrama. The term role-playing and Sociodrama or Psychodramas frequently are used interchangeably. Sociodrama deals with the interactions of people with other individuals or groups as represented in some cultural role, such as mother, nurse, leader, etc. on the other hand, Psychodrama is also practiced in a group setting, but is mainly concerned with the unique problems of a particular individual.

Role-play is used in a variety of ways

- Role-play is used to stimulate discussion on complex issues. A brief enactment by trainers or learners or both can be used to stimulate further group discussion on similar issuer and experiences that learners share.
- Develop skill in leadership, interviewing and social interaction, e.g. learning how to put another at ease, how to listen, how to lead discussion, how to be a member of team responsible for patient.
- Develop skill in group problem-solving, e.g. the group works as a whole to develop the problem of concern to the group, to develop the situation, to identify critical issues and to come to some mutual agreement.
- In certain situations, a role-play is also used to practice some skills. For example, the adult education instructor can be trained to practice how to motivate adult learners by enacting different roles. The prime method of learning here is by practicing and receiving feedback from learners and trainers after that practice.
- Role-play is a re-enactment of past experiences. In this sense, all learners are involved to enact an issue or a situation about which they are familiar in their past. For example, a group of 25 illiterate women learners can be divided into 5 sub-groups to prepare and re-enact the experience of being a wife in the family. Since all the learners share

this experience and all of them are involved in re-enactment, learning occurs here through the twin steps of preparation and re-enactment.

Advantages of Role-play

- It is emerging
- It helps the suppressed and illiterate to express their feelings
- It is simple and low cost
- It focuses on problems which are very real in nature
- It presents complex issues simply and in a short while
- It does not need material or advance preparation.

Disadvantages of Role-play

- There is a possibility of it becoming entertainment which vitiates learning
- Participants can get too involved in their roles and later loose objectivity during analysis
- Acting can become an end in itself and participants can overact or distort the roles
- That the observers need to observe must be explained clearly or else the discussion, which occurs later on the basis of this observation, will be inadequate.

PROJECT METHOD

The project method is the outcome of the pragmatic educational philosophy of Dewey, the well known American philosopher-cum-educationist. It was developed and perfected by Dr William Head Kilpatrick of the University of Columbia. Projects and project method have been applied to almost every kind of teaching, new or old and to almost every types of result gained from teaching, until it has become almost impossible to derive a meaning for the term that can be said to be truly its own.

According to Ballard, 'A project is a bit of real life that has been imported into the school'.

According to Burton, 'The problem is a project which results in doing. The motor element is not what makes the activity a project, but the problem-solving of practical nature accompanying the activity'.

According to JA Stevenson, 'A project is a problematic act carried to completion in its natural setting'.

According to Snedden, 'Project is a unit of educative work in which the most prominent feature is some form of positive and concrete achievements'.

According to WW Charters, 'In topical organization principles are learned first while in the projects the problems are proposed which demand in the solution the development of principles by the learner as needed'.

Characteristics of Projected Method

- A project is a purposeful activity
- A project is a wholehearted activity
- A project is an activity in natural setting
- A project is an activity is a social setting
- A project is a bit of real life introduced in school
- A project is a problem-solving of a practical nature
- A project is a positive and concrete achievement
- A project is an activity through which solution of various problems are found out.

Principles of the Project Method

- *The principle of purpose:* Knowledge of purpose is a great stimulus which motivates the child to realize his goal. The child must have an ideal. 'Why is he doing certain things?' Purpose motivates learning. Interest cannot be aroused by aimless and meaningless activities.
- *The principle of activity:* Opportunities should be provided to students that make them active and learn things by doing. Physical as well as mental activities are to be provided to them. They are to be allowed to 'do' and to 'live through doing'.
- *The principle of experience:* Experience is the best teacher. What is learnt must be experienced? The children learn new facts and information through experience.
- *The principle of social experience:* The child is a social being and we have to prepare the student for social life. Training for a corporate life must be given to him. In the project method, the students work in groups.
- *The principle of reality:* Life is real and education to be meaningful must be real. The project method is a method of education the child and therefore, it must also be real. Real life situations should be presented in the life of the school.
- *The principle of freedom:* The desire for an activity must be spontaneous and not forced by the teacher. The student should be free from imposition, restrictions or obstructions so that he may express himself fully and freely. He must be given the freedom to choose an activity, to do an activity according to his interests, needs and capacities.
- *The principle of utility:* Knowledge will be worthwhile only when it is useful and practical. This method develops various attitudes and values which are of great significance from the practical point of view.

Different Types of Project Method

- *The producer type:* In which the emphasis is directed towards actual construction of material object or article.
- *The consumer type:* Where the objective is to obtain either direct or various experience, such a as reading and learning from stories, listening to a musical delectation, etc.
- *The problem type:* In which the chief purpose is to solve a problem involving the intellectual processes.
- *The drill type:* Where the objective is to attain a certain degree of skill in a reaction—as learning a vocabulary.

Steps in a Project Method

- *Providing a situation:* A teacher should arrange a situation, in which some problems are available, and see that the Students have their interest in those problems.
- *Choosing and purposing:* Here also a teacher's help, in selecting and finding out the aim and purposes of the project is available. The project should be of a real need to students.
- *Planning:* Students and teachers both should cooperate in drawing out a blue-print of a project. There should be a few alternate plans. A discussion is quite necessary at this stage and the suggestions of all the students should be critically examined.
- *Executing the plan:* Among the students, duties should be assigned in a way, that all get the activities of their choice. Each student should be contributor. Taste, ability, temperament and sincerity of the pupil should be the contributors. It need to patience of the contributors.
- *Judging:* Self-criticism is training worth giving. The teacher should aim at the realization of the objectives of a project.
- *Recording:* The students should maintain full records of the various steps. Planning, discussions, assignment of duties, criticisms and similar other points are noted down for future reference and guidance.

Essentials of a Good Project

- Timely
- Usefulness
- Interesting
- Challenging
- Economical
- Rich in experiences
- Cooperativeness

Advantages of the Project Method

- It is based on the law of learning: The law of readiness, the law of exercise and the law of effect
- It is elated with life
- It has correlation with all the subjects
- It provide training for a democratic way of life
- It is upholding dignity of labor
- It helps in stressing problem-solving
- It is providing freedom
- It helps in solving the problem of indiscipline.

Disadvantages of the Project Method

- It is neglecting intellectual work
- Haphazard and unconnected teaching
- Difficulty in getting suitable textbooks
- It has artificial correlation
- It is unsuitable for the shirkers and shy
- It is too much reliance on young children
- Lack of competent teachers
- Unsuitable for transfers.

FIELD TRIP

The field trip is probably the oldest visual aid, have been used centuries ago by the early Greek teacher who took their classes to the natural situation for firsthand knowledge. It is most concrete and the most real of the audio-visual procedures. Synonyms for the term 'field trip' are; tour, excursion and education trip. Through the use of field trips, the nursing student can gain firsthand knowledge of the community agencies and their functions and relationship to the hospital in helping the patient.

It maybe defined as 'an educational procedure by which the student studies firsthand objects and materials in their natural environment'.

Steps of Field Trip

The following steps are suggested as a guide in organizing and conducting field trip:

- *Knowledge of resources:* Determine those setting which offer potential education experience for nursing students through field trip and analyze the educational value to be obtained from each possible trip. This requires an exploratory visit by the teacher so that he/she can determine whether or not the field trip planned will contribute to the attainment of desired objectives.

- *Rapport of personnel:* Establish and maintain cordial relations with those incharge of the situation to be visited. This is one of the first steps in the development of a trip. A friendly welcome by the visited authorities is conductive to learning.
- *Objectives:* State objectives for the unit carefully and completely and then select the learning activities which will best contribute to the attainment of the objectives.
- *Time and transportation:* Make the necessary arrangement for the time and the place of meeting and for the length of the visit, with the administrative personnel in the place to be visited. Planning for transportation maybe done with the students, making sure that all students have transportation.
- *Preparation of the students:* The trip should be made in connection with some unit, material or project and therefore, should develop naturally out of the class setting. A good trip assignment not only indicates the objective and its location but also stimulate the student to think about it in terms of importance, purpose, practice and personnel.
- *Supervision:* The trip should proceed in an orderly manner with all the students in an alert and observing frame of mind. It should be supervised carefully in order to protect both the student and the institution. Safety and comfort should be considered.

Advantages of Field Trip

- It serves as an effective means of correlating the subjects of the curriculum
- It provides actual source material for the study
- It creates a situation which helps to develop observation and keenness
- It arouses interest and vitalizes instruction, thereby providing motivation.

Disadvantages of Field Trip

- It may not be correlated with the curriculum at the most effective time
- Bus schedules may not coincide with the time of the trip
- Size of the group
- Students may not have the necessary data to obtain the maximum learning from such experience.

WORKSHOP

The new innovations and practices of education are introduced by organizing workshops, in which persons are trained to use new practices in their teaching-learning process.

'Workshop is defined as assembled group of ten to fifteen people who share a common interest or a problem'.

'A room or a building in which things are made or repaired using tools or machinery'.

'A period of discussion and a practical work on a particular subject in which a group of people share their knowledge and experience'.

Objectives of Workshop

- *Cognitive objectives*
  - To solve the problems of teaching profession
  - To provide the philosophical and sociological background for instructional and teaching situation
  - To identify the educational objectives in the present context
  - To develop an understanding regarding the use of a theme and problem.
- *Psychomotor objectives*
  - To develop the proficiency for planning and organizing teaching and instruction activities
  - To develop the skill to perform a task independently
  - To determine the use of teaching strategies effectively
  - To train the persons for using the different approaches of teaching
  - To seek, explore and identify the solutions to the problems
  - To provide awareness and training of new practices in education in service teachers
  - To encourage a high degree of individual participation.

Procedure/Stages of Workshop

Generally, workshops are organized for 3 to 10 days duration. The period of the workshop maybe 40 days depending on the nature of the task assigned to the workshop. It is organized in the following stages:

Stage I – Presentation of the theme.
Stage II – Practice the approach for its applicability.
Stage III – Evaluate the materials prepared by the participants.
Stage IV – Follow-up.

Advantages of Workshop

- It used to realize higher cognitive and psychomotor objectives
- It helps the instructor to create an environment
- It develops and improves professional efficiency of the teachers and provides opportunities and situations to develop the individual capacities of a teacher

- It gives freedom to the students to test and make changes slowly at their own pace with the help from teacher and one another
- It is used to realize the higher cognitive and psychomotor objectives
- It encourages social, personal development and provides vocational help to the students
- It is unique in its ability to help students see well and write better.

Limitations of Workshop

- Regular teachers do not take much interest to understand and use the new practices in their classroom
- It can be organized only for a small number of persons, so mass training cannot be done
- Teachers show disinterest in practical activity
- It requires a lot of time from both participants and staff
- It demands special facilities or materials
- Technique can be followed for higher classes participants must be given detailed instructions for the easy implementation.

EXHIBITION

Exhibitions are a way for students to demonstrate their learning from a specific project, class, academic year, or the course of a high school career. They give students an opportunity to apply new skills toward a chosen topic, within clearly articulated guidelines, and to reflect on their accomplishments. Exhibitions can inspire students to take more personal responsibility for their work when they design a project, document it, and present it to the public—excellent preparation for college and beyond.

Many times in the school, a department of the school or a class put-up their work for showing it to the people outside the school, and such a show called exhibitions.

Requisites for Exhibition

- The exhibition should have a central theme with a few sub themes to focus attention to a particular concept
- The exhibits should be clean, labelled properly
- The concepts of contrast in color and size should be used for lying out the exhibitions
- The exhibits should be so placed so the most visitors can see them
- The place and exhibits should be well lighted
- To capture attention and interest of visitors, both motion and sound should be utilized

- The exhibition should have some exhibits with operative mechanism such as switches, handles, to be operated by the visitors to observe some happenings
- The exhibition should include lot of demonstrations as they involve deeply the students and the visitors
- The exhibition should be able to relate various subjects' areas to provide integrated learning.

Advantages of Exhibition

- Exhibitions couple information with pleasure
- Exhibitions foster creativity among students
- Exhibitions give students a sense of accomplishment and achievement
- Exhibitions inspire the students to learn by doing things themselves and they get a sense of involvement
- Exhibitions develop social skills of communication, cooperation, coordination
- Exhibitions foster better school community relations and make community members conscious about the school.

Disadvantages of Exhibition

- Requires thorough preparation
- Time consuming
- Require funds or budget.

METHODS OF CLINICAL TEACHING

Teaching in clinical settings presents nurse educators with challenges that are different from those encountered in the classroom. In nursing education the classroom and clinical environments are linked, because students must apply in clinical practice what they have learned in the classroom.

In reality the classroom, laboratory and clinical experiences must be integrated to provide realistic opportunities for the students to attain the overall course objectives.

Elements of Philosophy of Clinical Teaching

- Clinical education should reflect the nature of professional practice
- Clinical teaching is more important than classroom teaching
- Student in the clinical setting is a learner, not a nurse
- Sufficient learning time should be provided before performance is evaluated

- Clinical teaching is supported by a climate of mutual trust and respect
- Clinical teaching and learning should focus on essential knowledge, skills and attitudes.

Process of Clinical Teaching

Clinical teaching is a complex interaction of the student and teacher. It involves a sharing and mutual experience on the part of both teacher and student and is carried out in an environmental of support and trust. This process is not linear, each component influence others:

- Identifying outcomes for learning
- Assessing learning needs
- Planning clinical learning activities
- Guiding learners in clinical practice
- Evaluating clinical learning and performance.

CASE STUDY

Case studies are widely used to complement and enliven didactic educational material and they can be adapted for a variety of teaching situations. Case studies also can be used in other educational formats to complement didactic information. In a small group setting, a presenter can describe a case without any audio-visual tools and can lead the audience to recommend clinical options for discussion, rather than using structured multiple choice responses. In training workshops, case studies can be used for role-playing activities designed to focus on patient/provider interaction. Self-study educational activities, such as web-based interactive programs, also effectively use case studies. Problem based learning, a teaching method that is being more widely used in continuing medical education, involves distributing case studies to learners and having them individually research the relevant clinical information.

Definition

'The case study describes the life history of an individual or all of the factors which affect a situation'. For example, the medical case study center about the patient, his/her disease and the related medical treatment. The nursing case study center around the patient, his problems, his/her needs and nursing care.

Steps for Creating an Effective Case Study

Step 1. Identify the learners and write educational objectives: The development of effective educational material begins with consideration of the learner and his or her learning needs. Needs assessment identifies specific issues that maybe challenging, confusing, or controversial to learners. The focus of the case will depend on learners and on the specific skills relevant to their medical practice. For example, in the case study used to illustrate this guide, a patient with active substance abuse problems is admitted to the hospital through the emergency department with a diagnosis of disease. The actual design of a case begins with the creation of specific learning objectives once the learners and topic are defined. It is often more difficult to design objectives to fit an existing patient case scenario than to start with learning objectives and build a new case around them.

Step 2. Describe the patient and develop sufficient case detail: The first part of a case description provides baseline information on the patient and moves the learner toward the first clinical decision point. Key baseline information may include age, sex, infection status, reported symptoms at presentation, recent medical history, relevant social history, findings from physical examination, results of laboratory studies, and findings of diagnostic work-up.

Step 3. Focus the learner on discrete clinical decision points: The purpose of the decision point is to focus learners' attention on discrete opportunities for informed decision-making. It is important to develop a well-defined question that addresses an educational objective. In the case example, Darrel is being discharged from the hospital after treatment for disease, and the learner is asked to select a recommended discharge plan. The learning objective for this clinical decision point anticipates that the learner will be able to design a care plan that offers treatment and support for patients with any type of disease.

Step 4. Present viable options at decision points: It is important to present a number of relevant, mutually exclusive decision options to the learners. Each choice should be comparable to the others in terms of importance, plausibility, and level of detail. For example, the options to choose from are balanced and most address the key elements of the discharge plan: treatment, care and follow-up.

Step 5. Analyze options and select one course of action: At this point, the case study presentation usually includes a brief lecture segment supporting the relevant clinical issues related to the preferred response. If available, new developments and current data supporting the preferred choice are presented. The current data are discussed in the context of the patient's situation, and the various options are contrasted and weighed.

Step 6. Introduce new information and continue to next clinical decision point: The case study can continue with new information from a follow-up appointment (e.g. ongoing symptoms, adverse effects of medication, or laboratory results), leading the learner to another clinical decision point. These points can be designed to address either the same or different educational objectives.

Advantages of Case Study

- It helps to establish in the student's mind a definite syndrome of various diseases
- It acquaints the student with professional literature which has special bearing on nursing problems
- It stimulates the student to meet his/her problems by critical and reflective thinking, relating knowledge and the specific situation found in the patient being studied
- It helps the student to integrate all her knowledge of the various subjects-bacteriology, pharmacology, pathology, dietetics, physiology and sociology
- It contributes to the building up of a specific body of knowledge in nursing science.

Limitations of Case Study

- Time consuming
- Some time sufficient reference materials are not available in ward library
- Students may not see relevance to own situation.

NURSING ROUND

Nursing rounds is to improve the overall quality of nursing staff and quality of work an effective method, but also a common method of clinical teaching. With the changing pattern of modern nursing, reforming the content and form of nursing rounds, expand the connotation of nursing rounds, is the inevitable trend of development of nursing.

In recent years, specialist nursing staff from nursing department with professional training, continuing education and nursing-job requirements of teaching bedside nursing rounds, not only improved the nursing staff but also analyze and judge their capacities and induction of expression to ensure the overall quality of care in nursing has received good results.

Purposes of Nursing Round

- To illustrate skilful nursing care
- To compare method of meeting nursing needs and to give more purposeful care to the patient
- To demonstrate effect of drugs, i.e. indication, actions and reaction of drugs
- To give opportunity for use of different applications and therapies.

Types of Nursing Round

- *Nurse matrons' rounds:* This round can provide senior nurses with the opportunity to achieve key aspects of their role. These include ensuring professional and clinical nursing standards, improving infection control.
- *Nurse management rounds:* This round involve the nurse incharge of the shift seeing each patient. And it gives the nurse manager an overview of the condition and needs of all the patients on the wards and the ability of staff to meet these needs. Also these rounds have potential benefits for patients, relatives, for the nursing team and for other healthcare professionals.
- *Patient comfort rounds (PCRs):* It is an important part of maintaining and monitoring the fundamental aspects of individual patient care. They should be carried out at 2-hour intervals whenever possible, commencing after lunchtime and continuing for the rest of the day. At night time, PCRs should be carried out before patients go to sleep and again in the early morning. It maybe necessary to carry-out more regular care to some patients. The purpose of PCRs is to maintain a regular review of the patient nursing needs, support the nursing process and evaluate nursing care.
- *Teaching rounds:* Nurses learn in a variety of ways through courses, accredited programs, seminars, conferences, self-directed study and so on. One of the most effective ways, however, is to participate in special clinical teaching rounds. These are aimed at all learners, whether pre-registration students or qualified staff. Teaching round is to learn from direct patient contact with facilitation from an experienced nurse teacher. And also to teach and evaluate nursing care. It is useful in developing clinical practice, evidence-based care.

Methods of Nursing Round

- Nursing rounds by the nurse and the head of the chair to require care and responsibility of team leader, responsibilities of nurses, auxiliary nurses and nursing students to participate.
- Before the rounds pre-selection round of infectious disease cases, in order to expand nursing knowledge, as we choose the symptoms and signs more typical; critically ill and associated complications; disease complex and rare cases of infectious diseases teaching rounds. Such as: severe hepatitis patients complicated with gastrointestinal bleeding cases; measles, chickenpox and so have a rash of infectious diseases; less incidence of kala-azar and other infectious diseases.
- Identify cases of infectious disease the responsibility of team leader to communicate with patients and their families to obtain the consent of patients and their families and coordination.

- The responsibility of head nurses and nursing responsibility for patients should be fully familiar with the basic situation: bed number, name, age, diagnosis, prognosis, and treatment, special check-positive results, dietary requirements, care level, the current state of mind, etc.
- Propose appropriate nursing diagnosis; develop care plans and nursing measures.
- Head nurse, and teaching patients to be more comprehensive understanding of the situation, do a good job on the disease-related symptoms and signs in-depth to explain; on the epidemiological characteristics of infectious diseases, treatment and prevention of disease.
- Rounds generally carried out in the patient's bedside. Involving patient privacy and the protection of medical issues are not discussed in patients with bedside can choose the health care office and ward round time normally should be 30 to 60 minutes.
- The head nurse and nursing education issues will have been prepared to participate in rounds of nurses has always been a question, and demonstrate standardized care operations, the final we discuss it together and head nurse commenting on the care plan has been developed to modify the revised care plan nursing interventions must be implemented as a subsequent content.

Advantages of Nursing Round

- The increased awareness of holistic nursing care to improve the overall quality of care
- Through collective discussion, broadening the idea of nurses
- Rounds process allows patients to have some knowledge and understanding of the disease
- It improve the nurse-patient relationship is conducive to mental and physical health of patients
- Nursing round promote the nursing staff knowledge of the disease have a comprehensive understanding of patient's condition for the development of a reasonable care plan, and implement an effective nursing intervention.

Disadvantages of Nursing Round

- This is difficult if rounds come at the end of a busy morning or at the close of the day
- The patient may overhear the discussion
- If group is large, the head nurse may not be able to speak loudly enough to be heard.

REPORTS

Definition of Report

- 'Reports are the exchange of information or ideas with other colleagues and other professionals of the health system relatively to the care provided to the patient'
- 'A reports are ought to be brief and to include all the relevant information, without further details'.

Types of Report

There are Two Types of Reports

- *Oral report:* Oral reports are given when the information is for immediate use and not for permanency. They maybe based on material included in a written report. An oral report based on the nursing person, who is assigned to patient care, to another nursing person who is planning to relieve to his/her. Staff and student nurses give oral reports to the charge nurse who in turn reports to them new orders, changes in assignments and other information which they need in order to carry to one another. There are different types of oral reports between the nursing personnel and health care workers:
  - Reports between the head nurse and his/her assistant
  - Reports between nurses who are assigned to bedside care
  - Reports of staff members to the charge nurse
  - Charge nurse nurse's report to bedside nurses
  - Reports to the clinical instructors
  - Reports to the head nurse to the director of nursing and his/her assistant.
- *Written report:* Reports are written when the information is to be used by this by several people or is more or less of important value included in this category are day and night reports, census, interdepartmental reports to admitting and interagency reports to the public health nurse, school nurse, clinic head nurse. Other reports which are written are special reports on unusual condition found in patients who may lead to complaints or law suits. Reports on accidents to patients, visitors, and personnel, mistakes in medication, complaints of patients and visitors are other types of written reports.

Criteria for Good Reports

- Good reports are clear, concise and should be complete
- Reports should be written all pertinent, identifying data, i.e. the date and time, the people concerned, the situation, and the signature of the person making the report

- Reports should be clearly stated and well organized for easy understanding
- Good reports should not contain any extraneous materials
- Good oral reports are clearly expressed and presented in an interesting manner.

BEDSIDE CLINIC

The bedside clinic always entails the presence of the patient. Either the group visit the bedside or the patient is brought to the conference room. Bedside clinics are conducted by the head nurse or clinical instructor. In a bedside clinic the patient's medical history and therapy are discussed in briefly. The nursing problems which his/her car presents are described and emphasis is placed on his/her nursing care including its physical, mental and social components.

'Teaching at the bedside' is defined as teaching in the presence of the patient. Sometimes thought to be applicable only to the hospital setting, bedside teaching skills apply to any situation where the teaching occurs in the presence of the patient, including the long-term care facility and the office setting.

Purposes of Bedside Clinic

- To improve the students ability to solve nursing problem regarding care of the patient
- To be able to find out the opportunities for health talk at the bedside
- To understand certain types of apparatus being used on patient
- To realize the need for understanding each patient those require nursing care
- To improve the quality and better nursing care.

Phases of Bedside Clinic

There are three phases of bedside clinics

a. *Patient introduction:* The head nurse or clinical instructor who knows patient describes his/her personal characteristics, family relation condition, home, community background, physical and mental condition. His/her medical history and therapy as they relate to his nursing care are briefly presented also.

b. *Patient centered discussion:* The discussion follows, a few simple questions are asked to obtain the needed information about the patient. The material is summarized and the most important points are emphasis.

c. *Post-clinic evaluation:* The student can be evaluated in terms of their ability to meet the stated purposes of clinic through their observations and ability to use problem-solving technique.

Advantages of Bedside Clinic

- It develops quality of education and decision taking
- It enables to students to develop self-confidence
- It increase strengthen of learning
- It put the student in an actual situation
- It permits comparison between reality and theory.

Limitation of Bedside Clinic

- It takes time
- It potential patient discomfort
- It enquires specific skills and techniques.

INDIVIDUAL CONFERENCES

The individual conferences are designed to help the student explore his/her goals and aspirations as well as reasons that he/she may choose to achieve or underachieve in school. During the individual conferences, teacher and the student will meet individually for 15 to 20 minutes per week.

Purposes of Individual Conference

- To reinforce key concepts
- To foster facility in the application of basic science concepts to clinical problems
- To develop greater facility in problem solving, calculating, and applying quantitative reasoning
- To introduce additional topics selected for their clinical relevance
- To promote cooperative, active learning in an informal small-group setting.

Steps of Individual Conference

- Before each round of conferences, think through your purposes for them. Some of many overlapping possibilities:
  - Establishing a good working relationship with your students
  - Reassuring anxious students
  - Motivating students to get started, persist, or work harder on their writing
  - Helping students generate ideas or arguments or plans for papers
  - Clarifying your expectations for papers
  - Answering questions students have.

- Talk in class and give students a brief handout about what to expect during the conferences. Spell out the logistics: where to meet you, how long the conferences will last, what to bring, what to prepare, how to reschedule.
- At the beginning of each conference, work to establish rapport and to put students at ease (especially early in the semester) and be sure to set an agenda for the conference, one that is realistic given the time you have.
- Keep the conference focused on what most needs work and on what is appropriate for the writer at that stage of working on that particular paper. For example, a student needs to work on developing ideas more fully or on clarifying a main point, concentrate on that.
- To help focus and establish agendas for conferences and to encourage students to think critically about their writing, consider having students write out some questions in advance.
- During conferences, get students talking–generating ideas, articulating plans, experimenting with language, posing questions, responding critically to their own ideas and drafts.
- Encourage students to ask questions.
- Encourage students to write down specifics that emerge from your conversation: ideas, and plans for revisions.
- Make your advice as specific as possible. And check that students understand what your are saying.
- Require follow-up conferences for the few students who need more individual attention from you.
- After a round of conferences is over, spend a small amount of class time talking about them—asking students what was helpful about the conferences, sharing some students' effective ideas and strategies with the whole class.

Advantages of Individual Conference

- It helps to explain answers to questions of individuals
- It helps in supplement instructions
- It can be used as a means of assisting the individual who is having difficulties in keeping up with the classroom situation.

GROUP CONFERENCES

An individual conference involves two people while a group conference includes more than two individuals. The group should be small enough to permit each member to participate. If properly conducted, team conferences, nursing care conferences, initial and evaluation conferences are two-way discussion, they are true conferences. However, the term conference is loosely used to mean any coming together of two or more individuals in an informal meeting for the purpose of giving or exchanging ideas.

The team idea as applied in the field of nursing is a fairly recent origin, but groups of individuals in a loose pattern of organization with undefined relationship has existed in our hospital wards almost ever since inception. The clinical nursing conference has come to be recognized as a pivotal component of total teaching plan in clinical nursing.

Definition

Group conference is 'a group discussion using problem-solving to determine the ways of providing care for the patients to whom students are assigned as a part of their clinical experience.'

Objectives of Group Conference

- Identifies the patient's nursing care problem
- Recognizes the ability and limitation of all students
- Helps to communicate ideas, information related to patient care
- Utilizes scientific information to influence the patient care
- Makes generalization from specific information that is factual
- Helps to report, interpret, channelize and carry-out hospital and health care problem
- Teaches what is required to help team members fulfill their roles
- Helps to plan nursing care cooperatively with other team members
- Brings also maximum creative potential of the team.

Purposes of Group Conference

- To guide in teaching
- To acquire more knowledge
- To discover the interest, needs and problems of the individual student
- To help the student to help himself or herself.

Principles of Group Conference

- Establishment of a definite purpose and specific issues to be covered
- Adequate preparation by the leader for all conferences expedites fulfillment of expectations for the conference
- Knowledge of the student
- Provide sufficient time
- Establish good rapport

- Good listening
- Positive effect
- Recording of data.

Major types of Group Conference

- *Team leader direction conference:* These are held at the beginning of the work shift an hour prior to the ending of the shift. The purpose is to give and receive pertinent, accurate information concerning the care of the patient and to create an atmosphere to encourage collective and cooperative participation.
- *Patient centered conference:* Planned meeting to identify problem and evaluate patient care. These conferences provide means for all team who are directly contributing to the care of a group of patients who have benefit from the experience of others. The clinical nurse coordinator and supervisors are the important member of patient centered conference.
- *Nursing service management conference:* It should be a part of planned scheduled meeting for each unit or section. The supervisor assisted by the clinical coordinator is the leader here.
- *Inter shift and inter departmental conference:* Which is necessary to pass on pertinent information from one individual or group to another.

Phases of Group Conferences

- *Opening phase:* It define as first two minute of the conference. The task here is to make a commitment to work on a problem relating to a particular patient. This often set a tone for the entire session.
- *Working phase:* The task of this phase to arrive at a consensus on problem identification and solution. Once the patient is selected, it is found that a great deal of time during this phase is spent in delineating the problem clearly. The problems are identified and the group can often reach its own solutions. Offering concrete solution to problem allow the student to feel they are getting something from the group. The teacher should ensure the opinion of the students about the validity of his/her suggestion.
- *Closing phase:* Once the group has worked through problem-solving and decided to the solution, the next phase is closing phase. The main task here is to delegate the responsibility to one or more students for acting on the problems continuously.

Advantages of Group Conferences

- It helps the students to collect information in creative a way
- It provides a real practical experiences and involvement to the students

- It fortifies the thinking of students so that the judgment capacity of student increases
- Each member of the conference will actively participate.

Disadvantages of Group Conferences

- It has little use if the students do not accustom the situation
- Conference hours maybe utilized for classroom teaching.

PREPARATION OF TEACHING PLAN

According to GH Green, the teacher who has planned his/her lesson wisely, related to his topic and to his classroom without any anxiety is ready to embark with confidence upon a job he/she understands and is prepared to carry it to a workable conclusion.

A proper planning of the lesson is the key to effective teaching. The teacher must know in advance the subject matter and the mode of its delivery in the classroom. This gives the teacher an idea of how to develop the key concepts and how to correlate them to real-life situations and how to conclude the lesson.

Meaning of Lesson Planning

Planning for a lesson means identification of the sequence and style of presentation and evaluation procedure to be adopted for classroom teaching of a lesson. Hence, it is a proposition in advance which establishes a linkage between the why, what and how of teaching in one period. While attempting to do this the teacher may foresee likely problems in classroom communication and may arrange certain materials and decide about techniques to be adopted to ensure a smooth and effective teaching-learning situation. Thus a lesson plan is a means of taking advance decisions about the selection, sequencing and execution of various activities to be performed in a classroom with a view to ensuring learning of children.

Definition of Lesson Planning

- 'Lesson plan is writing the method of delivery, and the specific goals and timelines associated to the delivery of lesson content'
- 'Lesson plan is written guide for trainer's plan in order to achieve the intended learning outcomes. It provides specific definition and direction on learning objectives, equipment, instructional media material requirements, and conduct of the training'.

Characteristics of a Good Lesson Plan

- It should be written
- It should have clear aims
- It should be linked with the previous knowledge
- It should show technique of teaching
- It should contain suitable organized subject matter
- It should divide into unit
- It should provide for individual differences
- It should be flexible
- It should include assignments for students
- It should refer to reference material
- It should provide for self-evaluation.

Steps of Lesson Planning

The following steps need to be decided for developing a lesson plan.

- *Objectives:* The objectives will be both general as well as specific. In order to achieve the objectives, some subject matter or content is required. This content is to be selected as per the competence with reference to the specific objectives of the lesson as well as the previous knowledge of the learner. The objectives of teaching a particular lesson should be stated as per the competency to be developed amongst children.
- *Content:* The subject matter that is intended to be covered should be limited to the prescribed time. The matter must be interesting and it should be related to the pupils' previous knowledge. It should also be related to daily life situations.
- *Methods:* The most appropriate method is chosen by the teacher. The method selected, should be suitable to the subject matter to be taught. Suitable teaching aids must also be identified by the teacher. The teacher may also use supplementary aids to make his/her lesson more effective.
- *Evaluation:* A teacher must evaluate his/her lesson to find the extent to which he/she has achieved the objectives of his/her lesson. Evaluation can be done even by recapitulation of subject matter through suitable questions.

Methods of Lesson Planning

A lesson maybe planned in various ways. Several methods have, therefore, been evolved. The most commonly used method is the

Herbertian method. The steps followed in Herbertian method of lesson planning are:

- *Introduction:* It pertains to preparing and motivating children to the lesson content by linking it to the previous knowledge of the student, by arousing the curiosity of the children and by making an appeal to their senses. This prepares the child's mind to receive new knowledge. This step, though so important, must be brief. It may involve testing of previous knowledge of the child. Sometimes the curiosity of pupil can be aroused by some experiment, chart, and model study or even by some useful discussion.
- *Presentation:* It involves stating the object of the lesson and exposure of students to new information. The actual lesson begins and both teacher and students participate. A teacher should make use of different teaching aids to make this lesson effective. She/he should draw as much as is possible from the students making use of judicious questions. In mathematics lessons it is desirable that a heuristic atmosphere prevails in the class.
- *Association:* It is always desirable that new ideas or knowledge be associated to the daily life situations by citing suitable examples and by drawing comparisons with the related concepts. This step is all the more important when we are establishing principles or generalizing definitions.
- *Generalization:* In mathematics lessons generally the learning material problem leads to certain generalizations which then lead to the establishment of certain formulae, solving problems, principles and laws. An effort should be made that the students draw the conclusions themselves. A teacher should guide the students only if their generalization is either incomplete or irrelevant.
- *Application:* In this step of a lesson plan the knowledge gained is applied to certain situations. This step is in conformity with the general desire of the students to make use of generalization in order to see for themselves if the generalizations are valid in certain situations or not. This is used for assessing the effectiveness of the lesson by asking students questions on the contents of the lesson.
- *Recapitulation:* Recapitulation can be done by giving a short objective type test/problem-solving method to the class.

Features of a Good Lesson Plan

- Through lesson planning the teacher will be able to pinpoint for him/her the objectives of teaching that particular lesson. The objectives should be such that they are:
  - Attainable during a span of one period only
  - In sequence with the objectives already attained by the learners.

- The teacher will discover whether the subject matter is adequate enough to be transacted during the period.
- He will identify, in advance, the activities to be carried out by the learners.
- He will be able to anticipate the expected answers of the learners.
- A good lesson plan should present good linkage between the objectives, teacher and student activities, on the one hand and the method, the teaching aid and the evaluation items on the other.
- The plan should neither be too short nor too long.
- It should focus on specific piece of content so as to attain the competency in hand.
- The activities planned should be quite interesting to the young learners.
- It should focus on the development of a clear understanding among children instead of rote memorization.

Advantages of Lesson Planning

- It makes teaching systematic and well organized
- It helps teachers to learn to foresee and tackle learning difficulties of children
- It enables teachers to utilize the available time properly
- It helps in developing insights about learning needs and abilities of children
- It helps teachers to develop the habit of undertaking immediate corrective measures
- It gives confidence to teachers during teaching
- It helps teachers in identifying adequate content and its proper sequencing for teaching a lesson.

Limitations of Lesson Planning

- It makes teaching organized but rigid
- If followed strictly, it leaves no room for innovativeness on the part of the teacher
- Too much of emphasis on it may make things routinized
- It is good for beginner teachers. Experienced teachers usually have little faith in structured classroom behaviors
- It is difficult to anticipate all possible kinds of classroom situations in advance and therefore lesson plans lack relevance.

Performa for Lesson Plan

Title of course: ____________________ Name of student: ____________________
Topic: ____________________ Name of teacher: ____________________
Unit: ____________ Date: ____________ Time: ____________
Place: ____
Students: ____
Method of teaching: ____
Audio-visual aids: ____
Previous knowledge of the group: ____
General objective: ____
Specific objective: ____

S. No.	Specific Objectives	Duration/ Time	Content	Teacher/ Learner Activities	AV Aids	Evaluation
			Introduction Content Conclusion Assignment References		Blackboard, Leaflet, Pamphlet, OHP, LCD, etc.	

SUMMARY

This unit has attempted to introduce the philosophical basis of education explaining how the educational system of a nation is influenced by its philosophy and its contribution in the field of education with special reference to the school setting, curriculum, and role of the teacher and nature of discipline. Teaching methods of an ideal teacher needs to be well conversant about using the language. It is indispensable to create awareness and congenial atmosphere on the part of a teacher. In order to develop lecture, group discussion is a vital thing. As a teacher, we have to ensure that group performance will be effective in learning.

2 unit

Media

INTRODUCTION

Educational media have the potential to transform the process of teaching and learning. Audio-visual (AV) material must be seen in their relationship to teaching as a whole and to the learning process as a whole, until the teacher understands the relationship between audio-visual material and teaching learning process. Audio-visual materials are produced, distributed and used as planned components of educational programs. It helps the process of learning that is motivation, classification and stimulation.

Audio-visual aids are multisensory materials which motivate and stimulate the individual. It makes dynamic learning experience more concrete realistic and clarity. It provides significant gains in thinking and reasoning. Audio-visual aids are sensitive tools used in teaching and as avenues for learning. These are planned educational materials that appeal to the senses of the people and quicken learning facilities for clear understanding.

Audio-visual aids, audio-visual material, audio-visual media, communication technology, educational or instructional media and learning resources—all these terms, broadly speaking, means the same things. The use of newer terms 'educational technology' or 'instructional technology' is primarily due to the dynamic expansion of programd learning, computer assisted instruction and educational TV.

Popular saying on AV aids

'I hear, I forget'

'I see, I remember'

'I do, I understand'.

DEFINITIONS OF AV AIDS

- *According to Burton,* 'Audio-visual aids are those sensory objects or images which initiate or stimulate and reinforce learning'.
- *According to Carter V Good,* 'Audio-visual aids are those aids which help in completing the triangular process of learning that is motivation, classification and stimulation'.
- *According to Edger Dale,* 'Audio-visual aids are those devices by the use of which communication of ideas between persons and groups in various teaching and training situations is helped. These are also termed as multi sensory materials'.
- *According to Kinder S James,* 'Audio-visual aids are any device which can be used to make the learning experience more concrete, more realistic and more dynamic'.
- *According to McKean and Roberts,* 'Audio-visual aids are supplementary devices by which the teacher, through the utilization of more than one sensory channel is able to clarify, establish and correlate concepts, interpretations and appreciations'.

PURPOSES OF AV AIDS

- To serve an instructional role in itself
- To create interest among the group
- To make teaching as an effective process
- To enable the audience to look listen and learn
- To quicken the phase of learning
- To economies teachers effort
- To foster or develop the knowledge
- To add variety and newness to the lesson, provide vicarious experiences
- To overcome possible hurdles during the act of teaching
- To bring expected behavioral changes among the learner
- To stimulate curiosity
- To provide a basis for more effective perceptual and conceptual learning
- To initiate and sustain attention and personal involvement of the students in learning
- To provide concreteness, realism, and life likeness in the teaching-learning situation
- To bring the remote events of either space or time into the classroom

- To bring the meaningfulness of abstract concepts
- To gain practical skills
- To introduce opportunity for situational or field types of learning as contrasted with linear - order verbal and written communications
- To provide a basis for more effective perceptual and conceptual learning
- To increase and sustain attention and concentration
- To supplement and enrich teachers own teaching to make teaching-learning more concrete.

FUNCTIONS OF AV AIDS

- It can serve as an open window through which the student can view the world and its phenomena by bringing remote events into the classroom.
- It provides an opportunity for situational type of learning.
- It provision of active participation of the students.
- It facilitates and advances the process of applying what is learned to realistic performance and to the real life situation.
- It facilitates freedom among learners, increases retention as they stimulate responses of the whole organization to the situation in which learning take place.
- It enable the student to learn faster, remember for longer duration, gain more accurate information, understand the concepts with adequate meaning. Thus learning become more meaningful, enjoyable and effective.
- It gives variety to classroom techniques, provides changes in the atmosphere of the classroom and allows some freedom from the formal instruction or traditional type.
- It promotes scientific temper as students observe demonstrations and scientific phenomena.
- Students will get opportunity to handle, touch and feel, operate, manipulate the audio-visual aid. It gives added appeal because it satisfies temporarily at least the nature desire for mastery and ownership.
- It increases the concreteness, clarity, effectiveness, of the ideas and skill being transferred.
- It saves time and energy.
- It stimulates thinking and motivates action.
- It stimulates self-activity on the part of the learner by which it offers reality of experience.
- It develops continuity of thoughts.

PRINCIPLES TO BE FOLLOWED FOR THE EFFECTIVE USE OF AV AIDS

- *Principle of selection:* Teaching aids prove effective only when they suit the teaching objectives and unique characteristics of the learners. The following points maybe kept in view in this regard.
  - They should suit the age-level, grade-level and other characteristics of the learners.
  - They should have specific educational value besides being interesting and motivating.
  - They should be true representatives of real things.
  - They should help in the realization of desired learning objectives.
- *Principle of physical control:* There has to be a proper arrangement of keeping aids safely and also to facilitate their access to and use by teacher.
- *Principle of proper presentation:* Proper presentation of teaching aids is very necessary.
  - Teachers should carefully visualize the use of teaching aids before their actual presentation.
  - They should fully acquaint themselves with the use and manipulation of the aids to be shown in the classroom.
  - Adequate care should be taken to handle an aid in such a way that no damage is done to it.
  - The aid should be displayed properly so that the entire students are able to see it, observe it and derive maximum benefit out of it.
  - As far as possible, distraction of all kinds should be eliminated so that full attention maybe paid to the aid.
- *Principle of response:* Teaching aids will be more effective if teachers guide the students to respond actively to the audio-visual stimuli that they derive the maximum benefit in learning.
- *Principle of evaluation:* There should be continuous evaluation of both the audio-visual material and accompanying techniques in the light of the realization of the desired objectives.

SOURCES OF AV AIDS

Different types of AV media and in many instances, to their sources. Because of temporary nature of the sources, the fluctuations of market prices and the limited space here available.

- Government and Non-governmental organizations
- Educational institutions
- Professional organizations
- Voluntary organizations (national and international)
- Commercial producers of educational material
- Commercial advertisement
- In nursing organizations like TNAI, INC, etc.

PROBLEMS IN THE USE OF TEACHING AIDS

While teaching aids are becoming more and more popular day by day, there are still some problems to be faced and solved. Some of these are:

- *Apathy of the teachers:* Teachers in general are yet to be convinced that teaching with words is not enough. It alone is very tedious, wasteful and ineffective.
- *Indifference of students:* The judicious use of aids arouses interest but when one used without a definite purpose but simply for a show, they lose their significance and importance.
- *Ineffectiveness of the aids:* Due to the absence of proper planning and the lethargy of the teacher and without proper preparation, correct presentation, appropriate application and discussion and the essential follow-up work, the aids do not prove their full usefulness. A film like a good lesson has various steps—preparation, presentation, application and discussion.
- *Financial hurdles:* Governments in some countries, like India, have set-up Bodies for Audio-visual Education and have chalked out interesting programs' for the popularization of teaching aids but the lack of finances, and suitable planned programs is not enabling them to do their best.
- *Irregular power supply:* Most of the projectors, radio and TV cannot work without power. In developing countries particularly, there is an irregular supply of power and that affects the use of teaching aids.
- *Need for training:* Teacher education institutions/colleges or specialized agencies should make special provision for pre-service and in-service training of teachers and workers in the use of these aids.
- *Language difficulty:* Most of the available educational films are in English. This can create a problem in some countries where English is not the main language in use. These films should be dubbed in the local languages and production of films originally in local languages should be encouraged and promoted.
- *Not catering to local needs:* Little attention is paid in the production of audio-visual aids suitable to the local sociological, psychological and pedagogical factors.

- *Improper selection of aids or media:* Teaching aids or media are not selected according to the classroom needs.

CLASSIFICATION OF AV AIDS

Various classifications are given for audio-visual aids according to the type of projection by various authors.

- ***Classification of AV Aids***
  - *Graphic aids:* Chalkboard, chart, graph, poster, flashcards, bulletin board, cartoon, and flannel graph.
  - *Audio aids:* Radio and tape recorder.
  - *Printed aids:* Pamphlets and leaflet.
  - *3-Dimensional aids:* Model, puppets, objects and specimens.
  - *Projected aids:* Slides, over head projector, films, TV, VCR/VCD, camera, microscope, and LCD.
- ***Classification of AV Aids***
  - Simple AV Aids: It includes graphic aids, display boards, 3d-aids, print material, etc.
  - Sophisticated AV Aids: Includes audio-visual aids.

GRAPHIC AIDS

It is a combination of graphic and pictorial material designed for the orderly and logical visualizing of relationships between key facts and ideas, e.g. comparisons, relative amounts developments, processes, classification or organization. It includes the followings:

Chalkboard

The chalkboard, formally known as the blackboard, is not a visual material itself but a vehicle for a variety of visual materials. It is the oldest and the best friend of a teacher. It is a simple and unique device which, in spite of new devices and techniques in teaching, is irreplaceable as well as indispensable. Complex diagrams and other illustrations which take considerable time to transfer to the chalkboard and which have usefulness for several periods. It is the most universally used aid.

Function of Chalkboard

- The teacher can illustrate the main points of the lesson on the blackboard
- A blackboard provides a lot of scope for creative and decorative work
- The teacher can erase writings and drawings and starts afresh

- As a means of making assignments, to state questions, to cite examples of work desired, to pose problems and to list sources for study
- It helps the teacher to focus the attention of his/her students on the lesson
- It is a substitute for dictation of outlines, summaries and directions
- A teacher can review the whole lesson for the benefit of the class with the help of the blackboard.

Types of Blackboard

- *Fixed blackboard:* Fixed in the wall facing the class and normally made of wood or concrete cement.
- *Roller blackboard:* It made of thick canvas wrapped on a roller mostly used for teaching higher classes.
- *Graphic B oard:* It has graphic lines and is used for teaching mathematics, science and statistics.
- *Magna board:* A board which enables teachers to make three dimensional demonstrations with objects on a vertical surface. Small magnets are used to hold suitable objects fixed wherever they are put on this vertical surface.
- *Blackboard on easel:* A portable and adjustable blackboard put on a wooden easel can be taken out of the classroom while taking classes in the open.

Chalkboard of Different Types of Surfaces

- Paint-coated pressed wood
- Dull finished plastic surface
- Ground glass board
- Vitreous-coated steel surface.

Guideline for Effective use of Blackboard

- Blackboard should be kept clean so that writing on it could be easily read by the students from all parts of the room
- Writing should be started from the top left corner
- Writing should be in straight rows
- Letter and drawing should be large enough to be seen from all part of the room
- While writing on the blackboard, the teacher should ensure that the class is attentive
- Duster and handkerchief should be used in cleaning the blackboard
- Writing on the blackboard should be legible

- Teacher should develop the ability to draw freely on the blackboard
- Occasionally students maybe asked to write or draw diagram on the blackboard.

Advantages of Chalkboard

- It can works as a valuable supplementary teaching aid
- It is an economical teaching aid as it can be used over and again
- It is a convenient visual aid for group teaching
- It can works as a good visual aid for drill and revision
- It can be easily used for giving lesson notes to students.

Limitation of Chalkboard

- It makes the lesson a dull routine
- It makes the lesson teacher-paced
- It makes students heavily dependent on the teacher
- Some time chalk powder spread and inhaled by the teacher and students.

Charts

These visual symbols used for summarizing, comparing, contrasting or performing other services in explaining subject matter. A chart is a combination of pictorial, graphic, numerical or vertical material, which presents a clear summary. It is a visual aid which depicts pictorial and written key information in systematic way to summarize, and compare, e.g. figure or diagrams, etc.

The term 'chart 'as a graphical representation of data has multiple meaning:

- A data chart is a type of diagram or graph that organizes and represents a set of numerical or qualitative data.
- Maps that are adorned with extra information for some specific purpose are often known as charts, such as a nautical chart or aeronautical chart.

Purposes of Chart

- To visualize an item, it is otherwise difficult to explain only in words
- To highlight important points
- To provide outline for materials covered in presentation
- To show continuity in process
- To stimulate thinking.

Types of Chart

- *Narrative chart:* Arrangement of facts and ideas for expressing the events in the process or development of a significant issue to its point of resolution or we can show an improvement over a period of years.
- *The chain chart:* Arrangement of facts and ideas for expressing transitions or cycles.
- *The evolution chart:* Facts and ideas for expressing changes in specific items from beginning data and its projections into future.
- *Pull chart:* It consists of written messages which are hidden by strips of thick paper. The message can be shown to the viewer, one after another by 6 pulling out the concealing strips.
- *Flow chart*: Diagrams used to show organizational elements or administrative or functional relationships. In this chart lines, rectangles, circles, are connected by lines showing the directional flow.
- *Tabulation chart:* It shows the schedule of an activity or of an individual, e.g. time-table of a class.
- *Flip chart:* A set of charts related to specific topic have been tagged together and hang on a supporting stand. The individual charts will carry a series of related materials or messages in sequence. The silent points of specific topic will be presented.

Guidelines for Effective use of Charts

- Teacher made charts should be preferred
- Students should be involved in the preparation of charts
- Charts should display information only about one specific area in a subject
- A chart should not contain too much written material
- A chart should not contain too many details
- A chart should give a neat appearance
- When a chart is to be used in the classroom, the teacher should make sure that there is provision for hanging the chart at a vantage point
- The teacher should have a pointer to point out specific factors in the chart
- Charts should be carefully stored and preserved for use in future.

GRAPH

Learners' abilities to recognize concepts such as 'more', 'greater than', 'higher', 'taller', 'smaller', etc. can easily be developed through graphs. Graphs make presentation of quantities data easily interpretable and readily understood.

Definition

'Graphs are the visual teaching aids for presenting statistical data and contrasting the trends or changes of certain attributes'.

Method of preparation of Graphs

- Before making the bar chart makes a rough sketch of it in a notebook
- For drawing the bar graph use the chart paper of 50 × 72 cm size
- Use two different color shades for the two contrasting groups
- The bars should be equi-spaced
- Write the key to the bar graph in a box on the right hand side corner of the chart paper
- Numbers specifying the magnitude of the bars should be on the top on the bars.

Types of Graphs

- *Pie graph:* These are called as circle diagram. The data are presented thorough the sections of portions of a circle.
  - In determining the circumference of a circle we have to take into consideration a quantity known as pie
  - The surface area of a circle is to cover 360 degree
  - The total frequencies or value us equated to 360 degree and then the angles corresponding to component parts are calculated
  - After determining their angle, the required sectors in the circle are drawn.
- *Bar graph:* The graphic presentation extends the scale horizontally along the length of bars. Each bar must be of the same width, height of the bar over a period represents the corresponding time of the variable. Graphs are available in two forms that is vertical and horizontal.
- *Line graph:* To show the trends and relationships, e.g. single line shows the relation and the variation in the quantity. Quantitative data are plotted or when the data is continuous. The concepts are represented with the help of lines drawn either horizontally or vertically. The plotted points are connected to one another, instead of the base thus producing the curve.
- *Pictorial graph:* It is an outstanding method of graphic representation. Pictures are used for the expression of ideal; they are more attractive and easily understood. Vivid pictures will be used to create rapid association with the graphic message; each visual symbol maybe used to indicate quantity.

Advantages of Graph

- It is visually strong
- It can easily compare two or three data sets
- It can compare multiple continuous data sets easily
- Interim data can be inferred from graph line.

Disadvantages of Graph

- It use only with continuous data
- Graph categories can be reordered to emphasize certain effects
- Use only with discrete data.

POSTER

Posters can be used for several purposes. They can be individually constructed to meet the demands of a particular presentation, and maybe used only once, or can be professionally created a printed in large numbers.

'Posters are the graphic aids with short quick and typical messages with attention capturing paintings.'

Purposes of Poster

- To provide general motivation
- To create an aesthetic or atmospheric effect
- To communicate a more general idea
- To thrust the message for leading to action
- For the classroom and community.

Preparation and Rules

- To do a special job
- To promote one point
- To support local demonstration
- Planned for specified people
- Tell the message at single glance
- Use bold letters
- Use pleasing colors
- It should place, where people pass or gather.

Features of a good Poster

- *Brevity:* Message should be concise
- *Simplicity:* Message should be easily understandable

- *Idea:* Should base on single idea and it should be relevant
- *Color:* Suitable color and combination should be used to make the poster attractive and eye catching
- *Display:* While displaying one should be sure to find a place where there is adequate light and where the larger population will see it.

Advantages of Poster

- It attracts attention
- It conveys the message very quickly
- It does not require a detailed study
- Good poster leads to action with good motivation
- It can stand alone and is self-explanatory.

Disadvantages of Poster

- Poster does not always give enough information
- When a poster is seen for longer time it may not attractive. So it should be dynamic.

FLASH CARDS

Flash cards serve a similar purpose to flipcharts. They are smaller than a flipchart and the sheets are not fastened together. They can be prepared on paper or on stiff card—even on old cardboard boxes. They are particularly useful in small groups, where everyone is close enough to see the cards clearly. The user can show each card, to emphasize or illustrate particular points or to stimulate discussion.

'Flash cards are a set of pictured paper cards of varying sizes that are flashed one by one in a logical sequence.'

'Flash cards can be self-made or commercially prepared and are made-up of chart or drawing paper, plain paper using colors or ink on them for drawings'.

Purposes of Flash Card

- To teach the students
- To give health education
- Useful for small group
- Used in group discussions.

Principles of Effective use of Flash card

- The messages can be brief, simple line drawing or photographs, cartoons and the content will be written in few lines at the back of the each card

- 10″ × 12″ or 22″ × 28″ is commonly used size
- 10–12 cards for one talk can be used. It should not be less than 3 and more than 20
- Prepare a picture for each idea which will give visual impact to the idea
- The height of writing on the flash card is to be approximately 5 cm for better visualization.

Guideline for using the Flash Cards

For classroom instruction, the flash cards are to be properly used. The following steps are used while displaying flash cards:

- Give brief introduction about the lesson to students
- Give instructions to students about their actions while you flash the cards
- Flash the card in front of the class by holding it high with both your hands so that all the students can see it
- Let the student respond as per instructions already given
- Review the lesson by selectively using flash cards.

Advantages of Flash Card

- Flash cards can be used to introduce and present topics
- It can be used to apply information already gained by students to new situations
- It can be used to review a topic
- It can be used for drill and practice in elementary classes
- To develop the cognitive abilities of recognition and recall of students
- It can work as a useful supplementary aid and can be effectively used with other material.

Disadvantages of Flash Card

- It cannot be used for a large group
- Prone to get spoiled soon
- Preparation is time consuming.

BULLETIN BOARD

A bulletin board is essential when illustrations have been prepared on thin, flexible paper. It is usually helpful to have an assistant do the mounting, or the planner will have to turn his back to the audience and fumble with the material. A blackboard can be considered a bulletin board, with the aids mounted with tape rather than pins or tacks. Generally, bulletin boards have a blue blazer cloth to work as the back-drop and their most recommended size is 1.5 m × 2 m.

A bulletin board (also called pin board or notice board) is a place where people can leave public messages for example, to advertise things to buy or sell announce events and provide information.

Definition

'It is a soft board which will hold pins or tags almost suitable. Simple device placed either indoor or outdoor. Items generally displayed are photographs, publications, posters, newspaper cut outs'.

Principles of effective use of Bulletin Boards

- The area where the bulletin boards are fixed or placed should be well lighted
- Short out the relevant material specific to the subject or topic
- The height of bulletin board should be one meter above the ground
- On the top center of the bulletin board fix a title for the specific topic of the display material
- Keep the interest of students alive by involving them in collection of material for the bulletin board.

Advantages of Bulletin Boards

- It can be used to introduce a topic and as well to review it
- It arouses the student interest in specific subjects
- It works as a good supplement to normal classroom teaching
- It explains important events and reports special activities.

Disadvantages of Bulletin Boards

- It is not effective for illiterate group
- It takes a lot of preplanning and preparation.

CARTOON

The word cartoon has various meanings, based on several very different forms of visual art and illustration. The term has evolved overtime. The original meaning was in fine art, and there cartoon meant a preparatory drawing for a piece of art such as a painting.

Definition

'A cartoon is humorous caricature which gives a subtle message'. In a cartoon the features of objects and people are exaggerated along with generally recognized symbols.

Principles of effective use of Cartoon

- The quality of the drawing should be high primarily for visual effectiveness
- The symbols used should be familiar and represent a concept or idea to which students can react intellectually.

Advantages of Cartoon

- A cartoon can be effectively used to initiate certain lesson
- It can be used for making a lesson lively and interesting
- It can be used to motivate students to start a discussion.

FLANNEL GRAPH

Flannel graph is a story telling system that uses a board covered with flannel fabric, usually resting on an easel. It is very similar to fuzzy felt, although its primary use is as a storytelling medium, rather than as a toy. Some time also called flannel board. A flannel board of 1.5 m × 1.5 m is most widely used. It can be fixed to next to the chalkboard or can be placed on a stand about one meter above the ground.

Principles of effective use of Flannel Graphs

- The principle involved is the interlooking of fibers of two rough or bairy surfaces, so that the pieces pressed on to a background which is hard and vertical will stay
- It can be illustrated on a larger scale by pressing two tooth brushes or hair brushes together, so the bristle interlook
- The flannel board is usually painted to depict a background scene appropriate to the story being told
- Paper cut outs of characters and objects in the story are then place on the board, and moved around, as the story unfolds
- The cut outs are backed, either with flannel, or with some other substance that adheres lightly to the flannel background, such as coarse sandpaper.

Advantages of Flannel Graph

- It permits numerous and varied arrangements of visual materials
- It permits the use of either chart or small pieces of material can be packed and transported complete notes

- It permits the development of a complete story
- It promotes conscientious planning, which must precede the development of the material in the first place
- It challenges one to develop symbols to portray such things as abstractions
- Easier to construct materials for flannel board than to make slides or movies.

Disadvantages of Flannel Graph

- Time and cost of making material for presentation present a problem
- Cost of boards themselves cannot be overlooked
- Presentation is limited a new idea involves a lapse of time before the new material can be added
- Might tend to deter one from using other more effective methods and techniques when it is evident that other methods might be more appropriate
- To tell a complete story it often takes either too much board space or smaller designs and materials some of which cannot be seen well.

AUDIO AIDS

The learners' auditory senses are involved and then stimulated by materials which are called audio aids. In primary grades, particularly in language learning, it is very essential to strengthen or enrich communication skills among the learners through various listening activities. Further, for accurate pronunciation of alphabets and words it is necessary to give children enough opportunity to listen to their correct pronunciation.

In the classroom situation, the tape recorder, the record player or the gramophone plus radio programs can mainly be used for this purpose, as audio aids help in better learning among learners. Audio aids help in developing the listening skill.

RADIO

Radio is a powerful mass medium used in education for disseminating information, imparting instruction and giving entertainment. It serves with equal ease in both developed and developing countries. It spreads information to a greater group of population thereby saving time, energy, money and manpower in an effective way.

Radio programs are of two types. One type of radio program is called education radio broadcasts—which provide scope for participation of teachers and students. They also supplement school activities. The second category of radio programs are those where a general discussion on social issues, health and diseases, about the universe, etc. is held.

Educational/school broadcasts can be used to great advantage as an aid to teaching learning. The most commonly used modes in educational radio broadcast are talks by individual speakers, panel discussions, interview, radio drama, documentaries and phone in programs.

- *Talks:* Eminent individuals in different fields can be invited to deliver educative radio talks on a given subject/theme. Talks can be very informative for students and aid their learning in the classroom. For instance, a scientist can be called upon to deliver talks on various topics in science to make certain concept clearer to the pupils.
- *Panel discussion:* Panel discussions can be used to provide different point of view on a particular theme. For instance, what steps can be taken to improve the living conditions of the people of a country can be a theme for discussion.
- *Interviews:* Eminent persons in various fields can be interviewed for motivating the pupils to emulate them, their values, their work, their success. For example, eminent, authors, states persons, scientists, etc. can be invited.
- *Radio drama:* Radio drama can be useful for inculcating values as well as for creating interest in literature. Historical plays can help the pupils to understand historical events and characters better. Through radio plays have the limitation of the absence of action, in a way it maybe advantageous as it enables the listeners to concentrate on the content and substance without being carried away by the action.
- *Radio documentaries:* Documentary is a creative of presenting a real story, event or issue. There is no place for fiction in it. Truth and reality are the essence of a documentary. Radio documentary can be a powerful medium to aid learning of facts. Topics in science, history, geography, etc. can be picked up for making radio documentaries.
- *Phone-in programs:* The latest trend in radio programs is phone-in. This makes it interactive and so more participatory and interesting. This enables the listeners to ask questions and get the answers. Phone-in can be used independently as well as in combination with other modes discussed above. Phone-in has rendered radio a very powerful device of learning, as it has made it interactive.

Advantages of Radio Program/School Broadcasting

- It helps in bringing the school into contact with the world around
- It helps in enrichment of school program

- It helps in furnishing up-to-date material
- It helps in developing critical thinking
- It helps in developing leisure time interest and appreciation
- It helps in providing opportunities for student participation
- It helps in popularizing science with a view to developing scientific outlook
- It helps in promoting national as well as international integration, as it has no boundaries.

Limitations of Radio Program/School Broadcasting

- Radio broadcast is one-way communication. Students cannot put questions to the broadcaster
- But it can be and is being done now with the help of two-way telephoning
- The educational value of radio broadcasting depends merely on the use of the sense of hearing
- The students have little opportunity to participate in the instructional activity
- They are passive listeners for most of the time
- In several cases, broadcasting time does not suit all educational institutions
- The number of receiving sets is not adequate in the case of radio broadcasts
- It becomes very difficult to integrate school programs with radio broadcasts
- A continuing listening on the part of the students may make them inattentive and uninterested in the task of gaining learning experiences.

Tape Recorder

A tape recorder is a portable electronic gadget to record, reproduce, erase and re record sound on a magnetic tape. This device can be used without much fuss by anybody by operating the following press buttons attached to the recorder, viz, stop, play, wind, rewind, record, pause, and eject. The tape recorder has two functions in the operation of an AV program: to rehearse a presentation and to record 'live' interviews.

A tape recorder is an excellent device to use for rehearsing a talk, especially when using overhead transparencies, slides or a 35 mm filmstrip. By replaying a tape, the planner becomes aware of how he sounds and can decide where he will want greater or less emphasis.

The planner may want to take a tape recorder out in the field and tape 'live' interviews to learn people's opinions about a current issue. Later on, the taped interviews can be used when projecting the visuals, along with photographs of the person speaking and of the subject of his comments.

Advantages of Tape Recorder

- It provides the flexibility for the teacher to edit and evaluate material
- It can make lesson enjoyable when used along with other subject matter
- It can be easily done from other sources like television, movies, etc. for use in classroom
- It is economical to use as recording can be erases and the tape reused
- It can be recorded on-the-spot event and played at an appropriate time for classroom instruction
- It is easy to operate as it has only a few controls.

PRINTED AIDS

The printed word has a high degree of acceptance, credibility, and prestige. Printed matter is unique in that it can be passed from person to person without distortion. It allows for the reinforcing use of photographs and graphic illustrations which can be understood by illiterates. It is permanent and the message will not change unless it is physically altered.

It can be disseminated and read or viewed by a larger, widespread target audience. It can be reread for reinforcement. Complex and lengthy material can be explained in detail. It can be hidden and read in private. Messages can be printed on almost any surface, including useful items. Printed material can gain prestige by acknowledging authoritative and expert authors. This is particularly important in those societies where the printed word is authoritative.

PAMPHLET

Pamphlet is a piece of small paper that discusses issues related to a particular subject with ample examples and illustrations. Though it is small, yet it can play a vital role in the teaching campaign of an educational organization. A pamphlet may comprise of a single page or more than one page depending upon the requirements of students. If a pamphlet has multiple pages, its pages are usually stapled together for giving it a shape of a small book. It is a small, thin, unbound book made-up of sheets of paper stapled or stitched together and usually having a paper cover.

Preparation of Pamphlet

- Determine the focus and content of your pamphlet project. In most cases, the purpose of pamphlet material will be to educate, to entertain, to enlighten and/or to persuade the target student to take a particular course of action.
- The content might include historical retrospectives, press clippings, photographs, interviews and a call to action for the readers to get involved.
- Determine the size of your pamphlet. The most common sizes are pocket editions (3¾ inches by 5¾ inches) and standard folds (5⅜ inches by 8½ inches).
- Incorporate photographs, graphics and maps to help break-up the text. If the pamphlet contains multiple sections, include a table of contents so material will be easy to find.

Advantages of Pamphlet

- It provides information sometimes available nowhere else, and they are good to supplement a book collection.
- It provides an inexpensive alternative source. Even though there is limited data in some pamphlet, they have the potential of providing valuable resources and data not found elsewhere in the library.
- These are concise with unique data.
- It is cost effective.

LEAFLET

A leaflet is a written or pictorial message on a single sheet of paper. It has no standard size, shape, or format. In selecting the size, shape, and weight of the paper, the primary consideration is that the paper accommodates the message and be easy to distribute. The standard leaflet is A4 size, which is convenient for filing the messages.

Types of Leaflet

- *Single sheet leaflet:* A single-page leaflet gets straight to work. On the front is usually a photograph of the product. The copy is restricted to a headline and perhaps a strap line or slogan. On the reverse is technical information, plus the company's name and address.
- *Four-sided leaflet:* A four-sided leaflet looks a little more generous, and allows conveying more information. Its front page normally has just a headline, photo and logo, leaving the inside spread for text. The back page can be left blank or used for technical information.

- *Stapled brochure:* These brochures provide 8, 12 or 16 pages, or any other multiple of 4. If there is a range of it is time-consuming and costly, requiring the use of special facilities and complex coordination.
- It requires special, extensive, continuing logistical support.
- It requires trained and knowledgeable personnel.

- Products, or if product is complex, it will need the extra room that a stapled brochure provides.
- *Folder:* Use a folder if it has several leaflets, each on a different topic. Folders are ideal when it regularly supply quotations, or when it needs to include technical drawings or data sheets. It can use when the information is likely to change or expand. Use it also when different customers do not need all types' leaflets.

Advantages of Leaflet

- It allows for the reinforcing use of photographs and graphic illustrations which can be understood by illiterates
- It can be disseminated and read or viewed by a larger, widespread target audience
- It can be reread for reinforcement
- Complex and lengthy material can be explained in detail
- It can be hidden and read in private.

THREE-DIMENSIONAL AIDS

Materials that have depth or thickness as well as height, referred to as 3-dimentional, serve as excellent means of providing students with an experience which maybe even better than a direct real-life experience. The 3-dimentional actual objects or their scaled-down or blown-up replicas are called non projected teaching aids.

A variety of 3-dimentional materials, also referred to as realia, are used to provide students with a means of observing reality or an imitation of it, out of its natural setting. These include: model, puppet objects and specimen.

MODEL

Models can be made of plasticine or modelling clay, which is so simple to handle that it, is used in kindergarten. It is true that models provide the knowledge of the internal and external parts of a thing properly which is not possible with other aids like diagrams and charts.

Definition

'A model is a recognizable representation of a real thing three dimensionally, that is height, width, and depth is felt as reality'.

Types of Models

- *Solid models:* It is the replica of an original thing made with some suitable material like clay, plaster of paris, wood, iron, etc. to show the external parts of the things, e.g. globe, clay model of human and animal.
- *Cutaway and X-ray models:* These are the replicas of the original things to show internal parts of a thing. Cross sectional models are difficult to make in the classroom or institutions as they require expertise to construct them. For Example, cross-sectional model of human body.
- *Working models:* These models are either actual working things or their miniature replicas. For illustrating an operation, e.g. a motor, a generator.
- *Sand models:* It is made by using sand, clay, saw dust, and other objects to show trees, buildings, river, etc. For example, a tribal village, a forest area.

Advantages of Models

- It explains the complex and intricate operations in a simplified way and thus makes comprehension easier
- These are lasting and ultimately work out to be cheaper teaching aids
- Still models are easy to make with the help of discarded materials like empty boxes, pins, clips, nails, and clay
- These are to reasonable size and convenient to handle
- It involves the use of all the five senses and thus makes learning effective
- It heightens reality of things and makes learning direct and meaningful as they are three dimensional
- It illustrates the application side of certain principles and laws.

Limitations of Models

- It requires expertise to make
- Time consuming
- Some of the models maybe very expensive.

PUPPETS

One of the old and popular arts in Indian villages is puppetry. Puppetry is an education cum entertaining aid in which puppets manipulated by the performer is a person termed as a characters in a story to be depicted.

Definition

'A puppet is a manipulative doll dressed as a character and the performer is a person termed as a puppeteer. A good puppeteer has to blend his art with dramatization to produce the desired effect'. It is used as an effective teaching aid for languages and social sciences.

Types of Puppets

- *String or marionettes puppets:* Marionettes consist of puppets with hinged body parts which are controlled by nine strings produces required movements in the puppet. These puppets are mainly manipulated by professional puppeteers.
- *Stick puppets:* Stick puppet are the painted cut outs attached by sticks. The actions of these puppets are manipulated by the teacher and students by hiding behind a screen so that only puppets are visible to the audience or the class.
- *Shadow puppets:* Shadow puppets are silhouettes of cardboard which produce shadows on white screen. The motion of these silhouettes is manipulated by the teacher and students.
- *Finger of hand puppet:* Hand puppets are round balls painted as heads with overflowing colorful costumes. These are worn on fingers which operate their movements. These are operated from below the stage.

Selection of Puppet

In writing or selecting a puppet play, the age, background and tastes of the students should be taken into consideration. A short puppet play is always preferable.

Advantages of Puppet

- It creates interest in students
- It gives the knowledge in a brief period
- It is an effective method in teaching
- It motivates the students
- It can easy to carry and operate.

Disadvantages of Puppet

- Needs group cooperation and coordination
- Requires skills in preparation and supply
- Skills needed in presentation.

OBJECTS AND SPECIMEN

An object is the thing in its entirely brought from its natural setting into the classroom to supply the type of sensory experience that will make instruction meaningful. An object might be a thermometer, a splint, a forceps or any such thing which pertains to the subject being taught.

A specimen is a part of an object. It maybe a sample that shows quality of structure: For example, a section of a long bone, a dissected lens from an animal's eye, etc. The education specimen is glittering and translucent, it embedded rich culture specimens and inside story insect, flowers and plants, marine life and so on in order to show the nature vividly. The education specimen enjoys complete insect specimens, good transparency and artificial buffing. It has a distinctive style and numerous in varieties.

Sources of Objects and Specimens

- Local markets
- Manufacturers and factories
- Discarded material from the houses
- Specimen found in the nature can be collected by students from field trips and nature hunt
- Plasters casts can be purchased
- Wild flowers, leaves shells, stones butterflies moths, insects can also be procured.

Mounting the Objects and Specimens

Objects and specimens should be mounted in shallow boxes in an artistic way and the boxes should be covered with cellophane paper. Also label each object or specimen using self adhesive paper.

Advantages of Objects and Specimens

- Collection of objects and specimens become an interesting educational pursuit of the teacher and students alike
- Student's power of observation and first hand experiences is enhanced by collection of objects and specimens
- Student's personal collection of objects and specimens can be good source of doing investigatory projects
- Collection of objects and specimens by students requires interaction with others leading to development of social skills and values
- Students when collect and display objects and specimens derive satisfaction of contributing to the school and teacher something worthwhile

- It arouses some interest among students in learning
- Objects and specimens involve all the five senses in the process of learning
- It makes teaching lively
- It heightens the reality in the classroom.

PROJECTED AIDS

There are many different ways in which a trainer can make the learning experience more interesting and memorable for learners. One technique is to use teaching aids. These are things used in the classroom to aid teaching and training. They fall into two main categories: visual aids such as overheads; and interactive tools such as a video program or resource pack. It is good to bear in mind that too much material and too many different themes can serve to confuse the class.

The three main techniques for this use projection onto a large screen that everyone in the class can see. The oldest is using a photographic slide projector. The more modern and flexible overhead projector enables presenters to design their own text as well as pictorial illustrations. The most high-tech version is the use of a data projector, a computer and presentation software such as Microsoft PowerPoint.

SLIDES PROJECTOR

A slide projector is a specialized projector which has been designed to be used with slides. Slides are small transparencies mounted in sturdy frames which are ideally suited to magnification and projection, since they have a very high resolution and a resulting high image quality. The use of slide projectors is in decline, as other projection methods have become more popular.

There are several different components to a slide projector, starting with a slot where slides can be inserted. Many slide projectors are designed to work with carousels, circular racks of slides which can be rotated to allow a sequential projection of images which maybe automatic, or controlled with a button or remote operated by the user.

The most typical slide, the 2″ x 2″ transparency, is made from a strip of 35 mm film with a width twice that of a filmstrip. After processing, the slides are mounted in cardboard or glass mounts for easy use and for protection.

A slide projector is an opto-mechanical device to view photographic slides. It has four main elements:

a. Electric incandescent light bulb or other light source (usually fan-cooled)

b. Reflector and 'condensing' lens to direct the light to the slide
c. Holder for the slide and
d. Focusing lens.

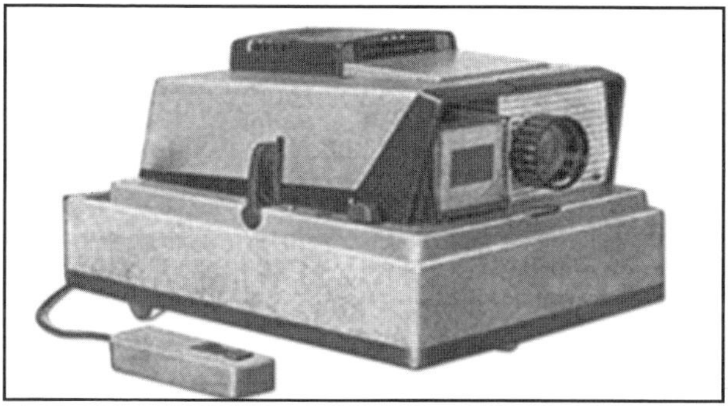

Fig. 2.1: Slide projector

Advantages of Slide Projector

- It is a convenient aid for making classroom teaching interesting
- It can be held on screen as long as needed
- It can be arranged in any order to suit the specific need
- It can be easily revised and updated
- Easily handled, stored and rearranged for various uses
- Increased usefulness with magazine storage and automatic projection
- It can be combined with lapped, and narration for greater effectiveness
- It maybe adopted to group or to individual user
- Disadvantages of slide projector
- Some time the glass slides are breakable
- It requires care in handling and storage.

OVERHEAD PROJECTOR

The overhead projector is the most used in all AV aids. It projects transparencies with brilliant screen images suitable for use in a lighted room. The teacher can write or draw diagrams on the transparency while he teaches; these are projected simultaneously on the screen by the OHP.

Overhead projectors are familiar features in many classrooms and conference rooms. While the LCD projector is becoming more common, many public speaking venues still offer overhead projectors to illustrate key points in presentations. Because this form of technology is readily available, overhead projectors are quite inexpensive to operate.

Many educational institutions have overheads in each classroom because of the low cost and the adaptability of overheads to any discipline. Overheads are also known as OHPs, slides and transparencies. They are pictures or writing printed, written or drawn onto a sheet of acetate. This can be placed on the bed of an overhead projector and via light and magnification technology an image is projected onto a white wall or screen.

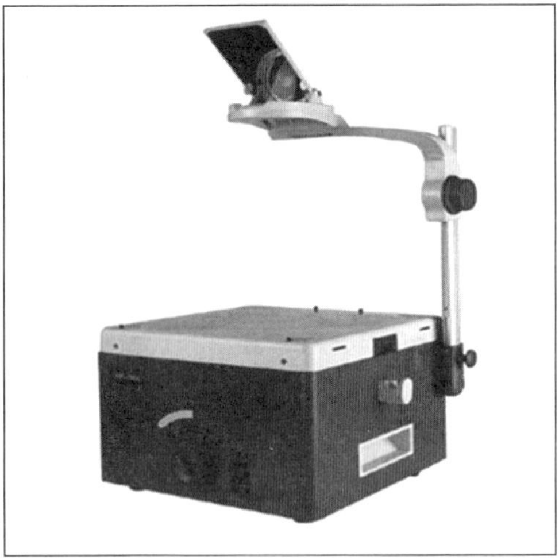

Fig. 2.2: Overhead projector

Purposes of Overhead Projector

- To develop concepts and sequences in a subject matter area
- To make marginal notes on the transparencies for the use of the teacher that can carry without exposing them to the class
- To test students performances, while other classmates observe
- To show relationships by means of transparent overlays in contrasting color
- To give the illusion of motion in the transparency.

Guidelines for Making Effective Transparencies

- Have one main idea an each transparency
- Include only related figures and diagrams
- Use simple lettering style in writing
- Use diagrams in proposition to its lettering

- Keep the message clear and simple
- Emphasize the key messages
- Use color and lettering with discretion.

Precautions of Overhead Projector

- While using the overhead projector do not keep the bulb on for a long time, it can be overheated and damage the acetate transparencies as well as the bulb
- Switch off the bulb after every 5 to 10 minute of use
- While shifting it should be switch off because the bulb may break due to jerks during shifting
- Do not keep the OHP too low, as it will make the image distorted.

Advantages of Overhead Projector

- It permits the teacher to stand in front of the class while using the projector, thus enabling her to point out features appearing on the screen by pointing to the materials at the projector itself and at the same time, to observe the students reactions to his/her discussion.
- Gains attention of the student.
- It is simplest and cheapest of projected aid.
- It can be used in normal classroom light.
- Transparencies can be hand-made or machine made in advance.
- Eye contact is maintained.
- Learning is easier and faster.
- It can be used in variety of ways, i.e. progress of a process, etc. (colors, overlaying, sequencing, movements of objects) Transparencies are re-usable when made from washable colors less strenuous and less pollutant than chalkboard usage.

Disadvantages of Overhead Projector

- It dependence on power
- It mostly one-way nature of communication
- Straining the eye of the learners
- Tendency to proceed faster
- Motion cannot be shown as easily as on film.

FILMS

Film is a multiple communication medium. It presents facts in a realistic way, dramatizes human relations arouses emotions and transmit attitudes. An educational film has been described as the greatest teacher because it teaches not only through the brain but also through the whole body. It has a very powerful influence on the mind of children and in shaping their personality. The main aim of educational films is to elevate and educate them according to the patterns and principles set by the society. For example, there can be a good educational film to help the students to develop a sense of citizenship. A variety of topics: scientific, historical, biographical and current interest can be covered.

Types of Educational Film

- *Entertainment films:* These films aim at emotional rather than intellectual appeal. It may or may not contribute to the building of a broad cultural background.
- *Advertising films:* This type of film is made for the primary purpose of selling services or goods of the advertiser sponsoring the film.
- *Documentary films:* It is one which deals with a social situation. It attempt, in a realistic, undisguised and authentic manner, to interpret the events, the cultures, or the problems of the day for the purpose of assisting man to understand his/her place in society and to stimulate constructive thinking and planning for the future.
- *Text films:* It is one which is made specifically for the purpose of becoming an integral part of a course or courses. The text film may present information, show a process, demonstrate a skill or any other activity.

Advantages of Educational Film

- It increases reading interests of the students.
- A child learns from his/her actual life experience more than he/she learns from the lessons that he/she gets passively in the school. In an educational film, all the learning situations are carefully selected and so have a great educational value.
- The learning situation is quite vivid. Everything is happening in a way as if it is more than living and actual. All the activities are quite clear.
- The film motivates teaching. The interest of the child is aroused and maintained.
- A film show is recreational also. For the child it is play and not works. Thus he/she learns through play way. He/she feels light and happy after the show.
- It develops study habits as children like to know more about the facts they have learnt in the show.

Limitation of Educational Film

- Recapitulation is not possible on the spot. Sometimes the teacher likes and the pupils too wish to dwell longer on a particular shot in the show. But the film does not wait. It goes on. But if needed, it can be rewound and played back.
- Good educational films may not be available.
- The whole process is very costly. All schools cannot afford to have good halls, the projectors and other equipment for the purpose. However, an active teacher can improvise.
- It may have some bad effect on eyesight.

EDUCATIONAL TELEVISION (ETV)

Television is the instrument with the most potential in educating the masses and thereby narrowing don the gap of progress between the developing and developed countries of the world. It is the through television that all can share stimulating and thought-provoking views of renowned advertisers, scientists, educationists, artists and teachers. Television helps in enforcing the public understanding of social, political and scientific advancement of the country.

Kinds of Education TV

- *Open circuit television:* It is the usual type of telecast by commercial or non-commercial stations.
- *Closed circuit television (CCTV):* It is the selective telecast that can be used only by specially equipped receivers. Its range is limited to the length of the cable. CCTV can be used to great advantage in educational institution. Its capabilities are as under:
  - It increases the range of instruction to one or more locations beyond the classroom.
  - It enables institutions to present televised instruction in accordance with their specific needs and schedules
  - It provides opportunities for the exchange of teacher one institution and another linked to a circuit.

Advantages of Education TV

- It permits the use of the best available teacher to teach a subject for a large number of student viewers. It preserves the expert teaching skills of such teachers on videotape or film for later use.
- It provides the teacher an opportunity to observe the instructional methods and ideas of their experts and to increase his/her own knowledge of teaching methods and stimulate new ideas.

- It provides technical advantages not readily available in normal classroom for illustration or demonstration.
- It directs the attention of the student to the exact detail of the object that he/she should see by eliminating distracting surroundings.
- It makes quick and lasting visual as well as aural impressions that can often reduce the time necessary to teach an idea or technique.
- It makes it possible to bring large, scarce, new or confined equipment 'into the classroom' electronically.
- It incorporates useful film sequences, slides, graphic art, etc. and makes available teaching aids within a television presentation, tailored to meet the needs of a particular course or subject.
- It saves time, effort and cost of setting up classroom projection equipment.
- It brings instructional films into classrooms as needed with no special classroom preparation, no darkening of rooms or use of special ventilation in the room.
- It provides more 'immediacy' than instructional films.
- It brings live demonstrations, videotape or film presentations to the classroom instantaneously or immediately after they occur.
- It permits inclusion of up-to-date information, modifications, new equipment or techniques into the classroom instruction.
- It allows the teacher time to observe individual students or to assist them during the television presentation, or to determine what needs further application after the presentation.

Limitations of Education TV

- The medium is limited to one-way communication from teacher to students.
- Students cannot get their doubts clarified.
- The total cost of teaching by television is more than normal classroom instruction, unless television is used to reach a large number of students at one time or sequentially over a period of time.
- Television has special and unique techniques and requires occasional re-arrangement of subject sequence.
- Individual differences of the students are not attended to in a TV lesson.
- TV lessons may not suit school timings.
- TV lessons are not flexible.

VCR/VCD

VCR/VCD is valuable training aids. These aids are excellent tools for illustrating a variety of things under classroom conditions. The use of

VCR/VCD in a course can add variety to the instruction and helps to reinforce or better explain key concepts. VCR/VCD requires as much of the instructor's time and attention as any other teaching aid. A VCR/VCD should not just be 'shown' and should never be used to replace actual instruction. Very little information will be absorbed as a result of the instructor who uses a VCR/VCD as a 'crutch' or as an opportunity to take a rest.

While the VCR/VCD is being shown, the light level in the room should be just dark enough for the picture to be seen, but light enough so the instructor and class will still be in full view of one another. The sound level should be low enough for the instructor to be heard over the audio portion of the film at appropriate places, but loud enough for all to hear.

Suggestions for using VCR/VCD

- Know how to operate the equipment and make sure outlets are available and working. Set up equipment prior to the class
- Set the TV screen where everyone in the audience can see. A corner of a room is usually more desirable than the center
- Make sure the TV screen is large enough to be seen clearly by the farthest student
- Make certain you have the correct film. Preview the film prior to showing it
- You may want to prepare a list of important points the students should observe and list them on a chart. You should also list the questions you plan to ask the students afterwards
- When the lights are dim, start the VCR/VCD. Bring the lights up before the equipment is turned off. Do not allow the room to go completely dark
- Delay rewinding VCR/VCD until the close of the class
- Remember to remove the VCR/VCD from the machine at the end of class and return VCR/VCD as soon as possible after use.

Advantages of VCR/VCD

- Easy to use
- Combine sight, sound, and motion
- Maybe used repeatedly
- Maybe used with groups of all sizes
- Maybe presented in a short time
- Add drama and action to the training
- Make key teaching points as well as demonstrate activities and techniques.

LIMITATIONS OF VCR/VCD

- Need special equipment
- Require previewing before showing
- Sometimes used as a crutch or substitute for preparation.

CAMERA

There are a huge range of uses of digital cameras in the classroom or elsewhere in the education community. Whether used to enhance learning, provide motivation or as a convenient tool—digital cameras can empower both students and teachers. The freedom to experiment with photos encourages a willingness to learn. Visual literacy: the ability to understand and produce visual messages—can be improved.

Advantages of Camera

- It encourages faster learning, more fun and greater creativity with photography
- Images enhance communication (adding photos helps to share experiences—especially for visual learners, it is also much faster than trying to explain everything in words)
- Frees potential photographers of their inhibitions, encourages experimentation
- Learning is enhanced in many situations by use of images in addition to words
- Images can be rapidly added to emails, documents, web sites, etc . there are many possible uses.
- Taking photos or recording information on excursions or field trips
- Preparation of photo sheets to introduce staff or students
- It is great for a quick video clip for a slide show, website or multimedia production.

Disadvantages of Camera

- It can result in poor transfer or streaming of the video
- It can be very troublesome if it is very important that everyone sees the presentation at the same time.

MICROSCOPE

Microscopes are not just for laboratory uses or for researches, it also plays a significant role inside the classroom, in the teaching learning

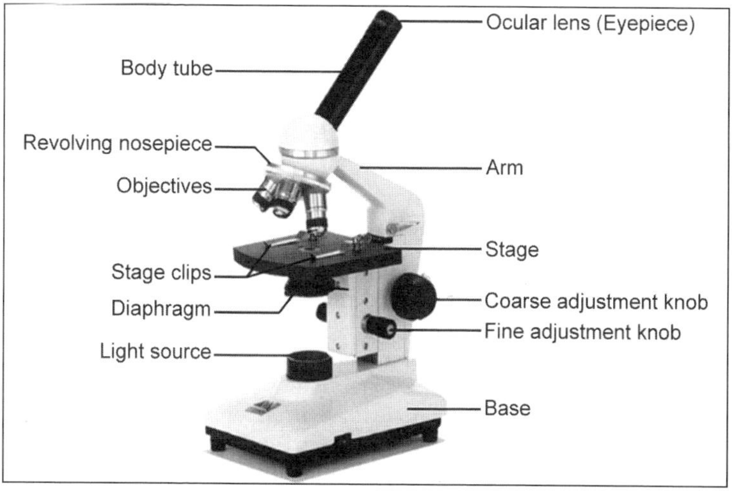

Fig. 2.3: Microscope

process that takes place virtually everywhere. Today, microscope for education has great potential in teaching students about the dynamic and fascinating world of science and technology.

When microscopes are used to teach to children, they can easily grasp the idea presented to them by the teacher, thus, creating a very potent motivational factor. The part of using microscopes inside the schools as a teaching tool is now widely recognized and is emphasized to acquire much desirable results in education.

Purposes of Microscope

In health care, a microscope is used in a laboratory to determine the amount or number of analytes (measured substances) present in a specimen, such as blood, urine, or stool. Laboratory tests maybe ordered for various reasons:

- To detect disease or to quantify the risk of future disease
- To establish or exclude a diagnosis
- To assess the severity of a disease
- To direct the selection of interventions
- To monitor the progress of a disorder
- To monitor the effectiveness of a treatment.

Types of Microscope

- *Dark field microscope:* A dark field microscope uses a special condenser that directs the light away from the objective unless it passes through the cell or object from the side. The background appears dark and the object light. The dark field scope is used when examining unstained cells or objects. The most frequent clinical application is the examination of fluid from a genital chancre for the characteristic corkscrew shaped organism that causes syphilis, treponema pallidum.

- *Fluorescence microscope:* Fluorescence is the emission of long wavelength light (visible light of a specific color) by compounds when excited by short wavelength (higher energy) light. Fluorescence microscopes are used to examine cells or objects stained with fluorescent dyes. They use an ultraviolet light source (mercury vapor lamp) to transmit short wavelength light through the specimen.
- *Inverted microscope:* It is one in which the light source is above the stage and the objectives are beneath the specimen rather than above it. This type of microscope is ideal for examining cells in tissue culture and for manipulating cells as is done in artificial reproductive procedures. The cell culture can be placed on the stage and the technologist can manipulate the cells because access to them is unobstructed.
- *Phase contrast microscope:* This type of microscope uses a condenser with a diaphragm inside that contains an annulus (ring cut out) in the center. The objective is constructed so that it diffracts the light transmitted through the annulus. When this light passes through the specimen, dense objects such as nuclei enhance this effect. Light from dense objects seem to reach the eye a fraction of a second later and the objects appears darker. Phase contrast makes it easier to distinguish different types of unstained cells and is preferred for urinalysis.
- *Interference-contrast microscope:* One disadvantage of phase contrast is that light is refracted from the edge of objects giving cells a halo. Interference-contrast microscopy uses polarizing filters and prisms to achieve the same effect as the annulus without the halo effect.
- *Polarizing microscope:* Some objects, such as certain crystals or minerals are able to change the direction (rotate) of light. This property is called birefringence and the object is said to be anisotropic. The polarizing microscope uses a polarizing filter beneath the stage. This transmits all the light from the lamp through the specimen in the same plane.
- *Transmission electron microscope:* A transmission electron microscope directs a beam of electrons through a specimen. Only a small piece of a cell can be observed in anyone section. Generally, an electron microscope cannot be used to study live cells because they are too vulnerable to the required conditions and preparatory techniques.

Uses of Microscope in Clinical

- *Biopsy:* Tissue examined for cancer or other abnormalities.
- *Blood cell:* Identification of abnormal red and white blood cells, immature cells, and the different types of white cells.

- *Bone marrow aspiration:* Examination of marrow from hipbone or breastbone under a microscope for abnormalities of blood cell precursors and bone marrow tissue.
- *Chorionic villus sampling:* Examination of chromosomes of fetal cells under the microscope to determine if an abnormal number are present of if there is structural damage.
- *Papanicolaou (Pap) test:* Microscopic examination of cells scraped from the cervix to detect cancer.
- *Microbiological exam:* Microscopic examination of specimens (some normally sterile) for the presence of bacteria, parasites, yeast, and fungi. Most often this involves use of the gram stain or acid-fast stain.
- *Cytological exam of body fluids:* Examination of urine, cerebrospinal fluid, pleural, pericardial, and synovial fluid for blood cells, malignant cells, crystals, bacteria, and other cells.
- *Seminal fluid exam:* The determination of sperm concentration, viability, and morphology (appearance).

LCD

Teaching has come a long way from classroom lectures to interactive sessions. Presentations and workshops have made classroom sessions livelier. Teaching today focuses on visuals, which makes learning more fun oriented. Most schools these days' use projectors for their classroom sessions. Projectors are mostly LCD (liquid crystal display) and DLP (digital light processing) type. Such systems allow users to make animated, interactive presentations with movement and video, typically using software like Microsoft PowerPoint.

Advantages of LCD

- Using LCD projectors allows educators to reach students with multiple approaches
- Students enjoy seeing, hearing and interacting with technology rather than simply reading a textbook or listening to a lecture
- Projectors are small enough to be mounted in classrooms or placed on carts to move easily from room to room
- Anything available on an individual computer can be projected onto a large classroom screen or wall
- Internet sites, PowerPoint projects, music videos, science lab instructions and math tutorials come to life at the press of a button
- The use of LCD saves a lot of time.

Disadvantages of LCD

- A digital LCD projector is pixilation. These projectors produce images using individual pixels which can become visible on large screens. This will give the appearance of looking through a screened door when using digital LCD projectors on large screens.
- A digital LCD projector is that the pixels on the chip can burn out. When one pixel burns out, you will not be able to repair it. This will cause digital LCD projectors to show a white or black dot on the screen where the pixel has burned out. In order to fix the problem, you will have to replace the whole chip.

SUMMARY

In this unit, we have learnt about teaching aids. We stared with the changing terminology in the context of teaching aids. In the process, we learnt that there are various terms that have been used synonymously with teaching aids, e.g. audio-visual aids, educational communication technology, and media, etc. we went onto discuss the need and importance of teaching aids. The various types of teaching aids were listed under different ways of classification. The nest sub-unit was devoted to mass media, where different forms of mass media were discussed—Radio, television, films, and computer, etc.

2

Section

Introduction to Research

Unit 3: Introduction
Unit 4: Introduction to Research Process
Unit 5: Introduction to Research Approaches
Unit 6: Introduction to Sampling and Data Collection Process
Unit 7: Introduction to Analysis of Data
Unit 8: Writing of Research Report
Unit 9: Introduction to Research Statistics
Unit 10: Application and Utilization of Research in Nursing Practices

COURSE DESCRIPTION

Hrs. 45

This course is intended to develop fundamental abilities and attitude in the students towards scientific methods of investigation and utilization of research finding so as to improve practice of nursing.

General Objectives

Upon completion of the course the students will be able to :

- Describe the need of research in the practice of nursing
- Describe scientific methods of investigation used in nursing.
- Participate in small and large research activities of the hospital/unit/ward/community.

Course Content

Unit 3: Introduction

- Definition/meaning of research
- Steps in scientific methods
- Need for nursing research
- Characteristics of good research.

Unit 4: Introduction to Research Process

- Statement of research problem
- Statement of purposes and objectives
- Definition of research terms
- Review of literature.

Unit 5: Introduction to Research Approaches

- Types, methods, advantage and disadvantages of each method.

Unit 6: Introduction to Data Collection Process

- Data collection
- Instruments of data collection
- Characteristics of data collection
- Techniques of data collection.

Unit 7: Introduction to Analysis of Data

- Tabulation
- Classification and summarization
- Presentation and interpretation of data using descriptive statistics.

Unit 8: Writing of Report
Unit 9: Introduction to Statistics
Unit 10: Application and Utilization of Research in Nursing Practices

Practical work

Students are to read research literature in the library of the school and participate in or assist in conduction scientific investigation in any health bare setting with the help of the teacher and submit a written report of the investigation in group of five of six, to respective teacher of selected clinical area.

3

Introduction unit

INTRODUCTION

Nursing research is a process of finding out the solution to a problem. It is a sequence of activities which when followed enables the investigator to achieve his/her aim. Research follows the scientific method which is why it can stand the test of time. A scientific practice based on nursing practice, i.e. guided by nursing theory or empirical clinical research findings. Nursing research involves scientific inquiry and so would require knowledge of the characteristics of scientific methods. Research in nursing evolved predominantly when nursing education became a part of higher education and was seeking its own body of knowledge, different from that of medicine. Nursing's first researchers were being prepared in fields other than nursing and have brought to nursing the various paradigms from those fields (Munhall, 2001).

Nursing research refers to the use of systematic, controlled, empirical, and critical investigation in attempting to discover or confirm facts that relate to specific problem or question about the practice of nursing.

MEANING OF RESEARCH

In fact, research is an art of scientific investigation. The Advanced Learner's Dictionary of Current English lays down the meaning of research as 'a careful investigation or inquiry especially through search for new facts in any branch of knowledge'.

- Research is a derivative of the French word; Researche means quest, search, pursuit and search for truth.
- Research in common parlance refers to a search for knowledge.
- It is a careful investigation or inquiry especially through search for new facts in any branch of knowledge.

- It is systematized effort to gain new knowledge.
- According to Clifford Woody research comprises defining and redefining problems, formulating hypothesis or suggested solutions; collecting, organizing and evaluating data; making deductions and reaching conclusions; and at last carefully testing the conclusions to determine whether they fit the formulating hypothesis.

Definition of Research

- It is a systematic enquiry, which is reported in a form that allows the research methods and outcomes to be accessible to others.
- *According to polit and hungler,* 'A systematic search for knowledge about issues of important to nursing'.
- *According to Schotfetdt (1977),* 'Nursing research is defined as the application of scientific inquiry to the phenomena of concern to nursing. The systematic investigation of patients and their health experience is the primary concern of nursing'.
- *According to Polit and Beck (2004)* have broadly defined nursing research as 'systematic inquiry designed to develop knowledge about issues of importance to the nursing profession, including nursing practice, education, administration, and informatics'.
- *According to burns and grove (2005)* have more narrowly defined nursing research as 'a scientific process that validates and refines existing knowledge and generates new knowledge that directly and indirectly influences clinical nursing practice'.

STEPS IN SCIENTIFIC METHODS

Traditional scientific research is characterized by several features. The researcher uses systematic, orderly, and objective methods of seeking information. The scientific method uses empirical data, which are data gathered through the sense organs. Information is gained in the form of data or facts that are obtained in an unbiased manner from some aspect of the real world. The researcher tries to exercise as much control as possible over the research situation, to minimize biased results.

The scientific method is a step-by-step procedure for solving problems on the basis of empirical observations. The major elements are:

- *Begin with a "felt difficulty":* What is your interest? What questions do you want answered? How might a theory be applied in a specific ministry situation? What conflicting theories have you found? The felt difficulty is the beginning point for any study.
- *Write a formal "problem statement":* The Problem establishes the focus of the study by stating the necessary variables in the study and what you plan to do with them.

- *Gather literature information:* What is known? Before you plan to do a study of your own, you must learn all you can about what is already known. This is done through a literature search and results in a synthesis of recent findings on the topic.
- *State hypothesis:* On the basis of the literature search, write a hypothesis statement that reflects your best tentative solution to the problem.
- *Select a target group (population):* Who will provide your data? How will you find subjects for your study? Are they accessible to you?
- Draw one or more samples, as needed. How many samples will you need? What kind of sampling will you use?
- *Collect data:* What procedure will you use to actually collect data from the subjects? Develop a step-by-step plan to obtain all the data you need to answer your questions.
- *Analyze data:* What statistics will you use to analyze the data? Develop a step-by-step plan to analyze the data and interpret the results.
- *Test the null, or statistical, hypothesis:* On the basis of the statistical results, what decision do you make concerning your hypothesis?
- *Interpret the results:* What does the statistical decision mean in terms of your study?

The scientific method provides a clear procedure for empirically solving problems.

NEED FOR NURSING RESEARCH

Research is important to nursing in the following ways:

- It is necessary for the improvement of patient care, through development of new products, procedures and methods of care.
- It could promote better administrative methods in nursing, and more effective use for staff of all cadres.
- Nurse administrators find research useful particularly in the aspect of skill mix and staffing levels.
- As in all other fields, research could form the basis for extension of knowledge in nursing, and provision of scientific knowledge that could enhance the professional status.
- Research also contributes to better teaching methods, better curriculum, and enhances nursing education.
- By continuing research and exposing nursing students to clinical settings where research is conducted, nurse educators help the students to become aware of the changing nature of knowledge and the importance of life-long learning, and inquiry.

- Research encourages scientific accountability in nursing practice, and enables nurses to evaluate the efficacy of their care, and modify/abandon those practices shown to have no effect on the health status of the patients.
- Nursing professionalism is also enhanced through research as more nurses with wide range of knowledge and intellectual ability add to the professional ideals. Practice oriented research is also a great avenue for improving professional practice in nursing.

CHARACTERISTICS OF RESEARCH

The scientific research has the following characteristics (Singh, 2002)

- Research is always directed towards the solution of a problem
- Research is always based on empirical and observational evidence
- Research involves precise observation and accurate description
- Research emphasize to the development of theories, principles, and generalizations
- Research is characterized by systematic, objective and logical procedures
- Research is marked by patience, courage and unhurried activities
- Research requires that the researcher has full experience of the problem being studied
- Research is replicable
- Research uses systematic method of problem-solving
- In research the factors which are not under study are controlled
- Research requires full skill of writing report.

TYPES OF RESEARCH

The basic types of research are as follows:

- *Descriptive vs analytical:* Descriptive research includes surveys and fact-finding enquiries of different kinds. The major purpose of descriptive research is description of the state of affairs as it exists at present. In social science and business research we quite often use the term *Ex post facto research* for descriptive research studies. The main characteristic of this method is that the researcher has no control over the variables; he can only report what has happened or what is happening. Most *ex post facto research* projects are used for descriptive studies in which the researcher seeks to measure such items as, e.g. frequency of shopping, preferences of people, or similar data. *Ex post facto studies* also include attempts by researchers to discover causes even when they cannot control the variables. The methods of research utilized in descriptive research are survey methods of all kinds, including comparative and corelational methods. In analytical research, on the other hand, the researcher has to use facts or information already available, and analyze these to make a critical evaluation of the material.

- *Applied vs fundamental:* Research can either be applied (or action) research or fundamental (to basic or pure) research. Applied research aims at finding a solution for an immediate problem facing a society or an industrial/business organisation, whereas fundamental research is mainly concerned with generalizations and with the formulation of a theory.

  'Gathering knowledge for knowledge's sake is termed 'pure' or 'basic' research'. Four Research concerning some natural phenomenon or relating to pure mathematics are examples of fundamental research. Similarly, research studies, concerning human behavior carried on with a view to make generalizations about human behavior, are also examples of fundamental research, but research aimed at certain conclusions (say, a solution) facing a concrete social or business problem is an example of applied research. Research to identify social, economic or political trends that may affect a particular institution or the copy research (research to find out whether certain communications will be read and understood) or the marketing research or evaluation research are examples of applied research. Thus, the central aim of applied research is to discover a solution for some pressing practical problem, whereas basic research is directed towards finding information that has a broad base of applications and thus, adds to the already existing organized body of scientific knowledge.

- *Quantitative vs qualitative:* Quantitative research is based on the measurement of quantity or amount. It is applicable to phenomena that can be expressed in terms of quantity. Qualitative research, on the other hand, is concerned with qualitative phenomenon, i.e. phenomena relating to or involving quality or kind. For instance, when we are interested in investigating the reasons for human behavior (i.e. why people think or do certain things), we quite often talk of 'Motivation Research', an important type of qualitative research. This type of research aims at discovering the underlying motives and desires, using in-depth interviews for the purpose. Other techniques of such research are word association tests, sentence completion tests, story completion tests and similar other projective techniques. Attitude or opinion research, i.e. research designed to find out how people feel or what they think about a particular subject or institution is also qualitative research. Qualitative research is especially important in the behavioral sciences where the aim is to discover the underlying motives of human behavior. Through such research we can analyse the various factors which motivate people to behave in a particular manner or which make people like or dislike a particular thing. It maybe stated, however, that to apply qualitative research in practice is relatively a difficult job and therefore, while doing such research, one should seek guidance from experimental psychologists.

- *Conceptual vs empirical:* Conceptual research is that related to some abstract idea(s) or theory. It is generally used by philosophers and thinkers to develop new concepts or to reinterpret existing ones. On the other hand, empirical research relies on experience or observation alone, often without due regard for system and theory. It is databased research, coming-up with conclusions which are capable of being verified by observation or experiment.

  We can also call it as experimental type of research. In such a research it is necessary to get at facts firsthand, at their source, and actively to go about doing certain things to stimulate the production of desired information. In such a research, the researcher must first provide himself with a working hypothesis or guess as to the probable results. He then works to get enough facts (data) to prove or disprove his hypothesis. He then sets up experimental designs which he thinks will manipulate the persons or the materials concerned so as to bring forth the desired information. Such research is thus characterized by the experimenter's control over the variables under study and his deliberate manipulation of one of them to study its effects. Empirical research is appropriate when proof is sought that certain variables affect other variables in some way. Evidence gathered through experiments or empirical studies is today considered to be the most powerful support possible for a given hypothesis.

- *Some other types of research:* All other types of research are variations of one or more of the above stated approaches, based on either the purpose of research, or the time required to accomplish research, on the environment in which research is done, or on the basis of some other similar factor. Form the point of view of time, we can think of research either as one-time research or longitudinal research. In the former case the research is confined to a single time-period, whereas in the latter case the research is carried on over several time-periods. Research can be field-setting research or laboratory research or simulation research, depending upon the environment in which it is to be carried out.

  Research can as well be understood as clinical or diagnostic research. Such research follows case-study methods or in-depth approaches to reach the basic causal relations. Such studies usually go deep into the causes of things or events that interest us, using very small samples and very deep probing data gathering devices. The research maybe exploratory or it maybe formalized. The objective of exploratory research is the development of hypotheses rather than their testing, whereas formalized research studies are those with substantial structure and with specific hypotheses to be tested. Historical research is that which utilizes historical sources like documents, remains, etc. to study events or ideas of the past, including the philosophy of persons and groups at any remote point of time. Research can also be classified as conclusion-oriented and decision-oriented. While doing conclusion oriented research, a researcher is free to pick-up a problem, redesign the enquiry as he proceeds and is prepared to conceptualize as he wishes. Decision-oriented research is always for the need of a decision maker and the researcher in this case is not free to embark upon research according to his own inclination. Operations research is an example of decision oriented research since it is a scientific method of providing executive departments with a quantitative basis for decisions regarding operations under their control.

SUMMARY

In this unit, we discuss that research is a planned and systematic application of the scientific method to the study of problems. The scientific method provides the basis for research in all fields including nursing. Knowledge of the characteristics and types of research would enable researchers to establish the nature of research they are interested in.

Introduction to Research Process

4 unit

INTRODUCTION

Research is a careful investigation leading to the discovery and interpretation of information. There are many different types of research that discover or reinterpret information collected by experimentation or observation and suggest practical applications or theoretical implications of that information. In scientific fields, research often involves experimentation which tests a researcher's hypothesis. Research is a process because in some sense it is never finished. The process begins with interest sparked by an observation or question, the desire to discover and learn more, and to come to a new understanding because of what has been discovered. The steps in the research process are identification and definition of the problem or opportunity, planning the research design, selecting a research method, selecting a sampling procedure, data collection, evaluating the data and finally preparing and presenting the research report.

STEPS OF RESEARCH PROCESS

Research process consists of series of actions or steps necessary to effectively carry-out research and the desired sequencing of these steps.

The research process consists of a number of closely related activities. The following order concerning various steps provides a useful procedural guideline regarding the research process:

- Formulating the research problem
- Extensive literature survey
- Developing the hypothesis
- Preparing the research design
- Determining sample design

- Collecting the data
- Execution of the project
- Analysis of data
- Hypothesis testing
- Generalizations and interpretation
- Preparation of the report or presentation of the results, i.e. formal write-up of conclusions reached.

A brief description of the above stated steps will be helpful

- *Formulating the research problem:* There are two types of research problems, viz., those which relate to states of nature and those which relate to relationships between variables. At the very outset the researcher must single out the problem he wants to study, i.e. he must decide the general area of interest or aspect of a subject-matter that he would like to inquire into. Initially the problem maybe stated in a broad general way and then the ambiguities, if any, relating to the problem be resolved. Then, the feasibility of a particular solution has to be considered before a working formulation of the problem can be set-up. The formulation of a general topic into a specific research problem, thus, constitutes the first step in a scientific enquiry. Essentially two steps are involved in formulating the research problem, viz., understanding the problem thoroughly, and rephrasing the same into meaningful terms from an analytical point of view.

  The best way of understanding the problem is to discuss it with ones own colleagues or with those having some expertise in the matter. In an academic institution the researcher can seek the help from a guide who is usually an experienced man and has several research problems in mind. Often, the guide puts forth the problem in general terms and it is up to the researcher to narrow it down and phrase the problem in operational terms. In private business units or in governmental organizations, the problem is usually earmarked by the administrative agencies with which the researcher can discuss as to how the problem originally came about and what considerations are involved in its possible solutions.

  The researcher must at the same time examine all available literature to get himself acquainted with the selected problem. He may review two types of literature—the conceptual literature concerning the concepts and theories, and the empirical literature consisting of studies made earlier which are similar to the one proposed. The basic outcome of this review will be the knowledge as to what data and other materials are available for operational purposes which will enable the researcher to specify his own research problem in a meaningful context. After this the researcher rephrases the problem into analytical or operational terms, i.e. to put the problem in as specific terms as possible. This task of formulating, or defining, a research problem is a step of greatest importance in the entire research process. The problem to be investigated must be defined unambiguously for that will help discriminating relevant data from irrelevant ones. Care must: however, be taken to verify the objectivity and validity of the background facts concerning the problem.

The statement of the objective is of basic importance because it determines the data which are to be collected, the characteristics of the data which are relevant, relations which are to be explored, the choice of techniques to be used in these explorations and the form of the final report. If there are certain pertinent terms, the same should be clearly defined along with the task of formulating the problem. In fact, formulation of the problem often follows a sequential pattern where a number of formulations are set-up, each formulation more specific than the proceeding one, each one phrased in more analytical terms, and each more realistic in terms of the available data and resources.

Flow chart 4.1: Research process

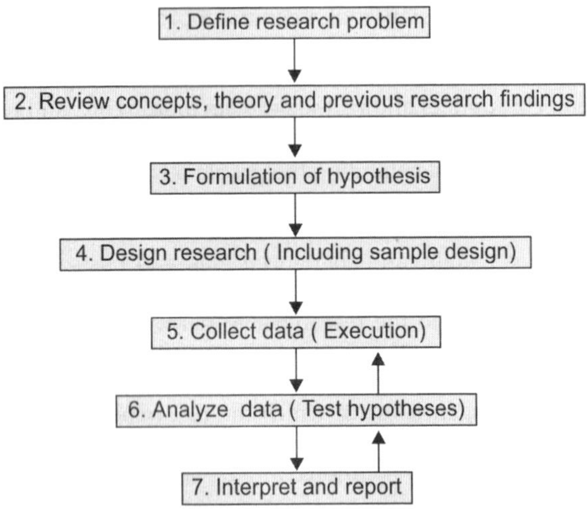

- *Extensive literature survey:* Once the problem is formulated, a brief summary of it should be written down. It is compulsory for a research worker writing a thesis for a PhD degree to write a synopsis of the topic and submit it to the necessary Committee or the Research Board for approval. At this juncture the researcher should undertake extensive literature survey connected with the problem. For this purpose, the abstracting and indexing journals and published or unpublished bibliographies are the first place to go to. Academic journals, conference proceedings, government reports, books, etc. must be tapped depending on the nature of the problem. In this process, it should be remembered that one source will lead to another. The earlier studies, if any, which are similar to the study in hand, should be carefully studied. A good library will be a great help to the researcher at this stage.

- *Development of working hypotheses:* After extensive literature survey, researcher should state in clear terms the working hypothesis or hypotheses. Working hypothesis is tentative assumption made in order to draw out and test its logical or empirical consequences. As such the manner in which research hypotheses are developed is particularly important since they provide the focal point for research. They also affect the manner in which tests must be conducted in the analysis of data and indirectly the quality of data which is required for the analysis. In most types of research, the development of working hypothesis plays an important role. Hypothesis should be very specific and limited to the piece of research in hand because it has to be tested. The role of the hypothesis is to guide the researcher by delimiting the area of research and to keep him on the right track. It sharpens his thinking and focuses attention on the more important facets of the problem. It also indicates the type of data required and the type of methods of data analysis to be used.

  How does one go about developing working hypotheses? The answer is by using the following approach:

  - Discussions with colleagues and experts about the problem, its origin and the objectives in seeking a solution.
  - Examination of data and records, if available, concerning the problem for possible trends, peculiarities and other clues.
  - Review of similar studies in the area or of the studies on similar problems.
  - Exploratory personal investigation which involves original field interviews on a limited scale with interested parties and individuals with a view to secure greater insight into the practical aspects of the problem.

  Thus, working hypotheses arise as a result of a priori thinking about the subject, examination of the available data and material including related studies and the counsel of experts and interested parties. Working hypotheses are more useful when stated in precise and clearly defined terms. It may as well be remembered that occasionally we may encounter a problem where we do not need working hypotheses, especially in the case of exploratory or formulative researches which do not aim at testing the hypothesis. But as a general rule, specification of working hypotheses in another basic step of the research process in most research problems.

- *Preparing the research design:* The research problem having been formulated in clear-cut terms, the researcher will be required to prepare a research design, i.e. he will have to state the conceptual structure within which research would be conducted. The preparation of such a design facilitates research to be as efficient as possible yielding maximal information. In other words, the function of research design is to provide for the collection of relevant evidence with minimal expenditure of effort, time and money. But how all these can be achieved depends mainly on the research purpose. Research purposes maybe grouped into four categories, viz. (i) Exploration, (ii) Description, (iii) Diagnosis, and (iv) Experimentation. A flexible research design which provides opportunity for considering many different aspects of a problem is considered appropriate if the purpose of the research study is that of exploration. But when the purpose happens to be an accurate description of a situation or of an association between variables, the suitable design will be one that minimizes bias and maximizes the reliability of the data collected and analyzed.

  There are several research designs, such as, experimental and non-experimental hypothesis testing. Experimental designs can be either informal designs (such as before-and-after without control, after-only with control, before-and-after with control) or formal designs (such as completely randomized design, randomized block design, Latin square design, simple and complex factorial designs), out of which the researcher must select one for his own project.

  The preparation of the research design, appropriate for a particular research problem, involves usually the consideration of the following:
  - The means of obtaining the information.
  - The availability and skills of the researcher and his staff (if any).
  - Explanation of the way in which selected means of obtaining information will be organized and the reasoning leading to the selection.
  - The time available for research.
  - The cost factor relating to research, i.e. the finance available for the purpose.
- *Determining sample design:* Sampling is the process of selecting units (e.g. people, organizations) from a population of interest so that by studying the sample we may fairly generalize our results back to the population from which they were chosen. Population is the set of individuals, items, or data from which a statistical sample is taken it is also called universe. Sample is representative part of the population which contains each characterizes that entire population possesses.

  Researchers rarely survey the entire population for two reasons. The cost is too high, and the population is dynamic in that the individuals making up the population may change overtime. The three main advantages of sampling are that the cost is lower, data collection is faster, and since the data set is smaller it is possible to ensure homogeneity and to improve the accuracy and quality of the data.

All the items under consideration in any field of inquiry constitute a universe or population. A complete enumeration of all the items in the population is known as a census inquiry. It can be presumed that in such an inquiry when all the items are covered no element of chance is left and highest accuracy is obtained. But in practice this may not be true. Even the slightest element of bias in such an inquiry will get larger and larger as the number of observations increases. Moreover, there is no way of checking the element of bias or its extent except through a resurvey or use of sample checks. Besides, this type of inquiry involves a great deal of time, money and energy, not only this; census inquiry is not possible in practice under many circumstances. For instance, blood testing is done only on sample basis. Hence, quite often we select only a few items from the universe for our study purposes. The items so selected constitute what is technically called a sample.

The researcher must decide the way of selecting a sample or what is popularly known as the sample design. In other words, a sample design is a definite plan determined before any data are actually collected for obtaining a sample from a given population. Thus, the plan to select 12 of a city's 200 drugstores in a certain way constitutes a sample design. Samples can be either probability samples or non-probability samples. With probability samples each element has a known probability of being included in the sample but the non-probability samples do not allow the researcher to determine this probability.

Probability samples are those based on simple random sampling, systematic sampling, stratified sampling, cluster/area sampling whereas non-probability samples are those based on convenience sampling, judgment sampling and quota sampling techniques.

A brief mention of the important sample designs is as follows:

- *Deliberate sampling/purposive sampling:* Deliberate sampling is also known as purposive or non-probability sampling. This sampling method involves purposive or deliberate selection of particular units of the universe for constituting a sample which represents the universe. When population elements are selected for inclusion in the sample based on the ease of access, it can be called convenience sampling. If a researcher wishes to secure data from, say, gasoline buyers, he may select a fixed number of petrol stations and may conduct interviews at these stations. This would be an example of convenience sample of gasoline buyers. At times such a procedure may give very biased results particularly when the population is not homogeneous. On the other hand, in judgment sampling the researcher's judgment is used for selecting items which he considers as representative of the population. For example, a judgment sample of college students might be taken to secure reactions to a new method of teaching. Judgment sampling is used quite frequently in qualitative research where the desire happens to be to develop hypotheses rather than to generalize to larger populations.

- *Simple random sampling:* This type of sampling is also known as chance sampling or probability sampling where each and every item in the population has an equal chance of inclusion in the sample and each one of the possible samples, in case of finite universe, has the same probability of being selected. For example, if we have to select a sample of 300 items from a universe of 15,000 items, then we can put the names or numbers of all the 15,000 items on slips of paper and conduct a lottery. Using the random number tables is another method of random sampling. To select the sample, each item is assigned a number from 1 to 15,000. Then, 300 five digits random numbers are selected from the table. To do this we select some random starting point and then a systematic pattern is used in proceeding through the table. We might start in the 4th row, second column and proceed down the column to the bottom of the table and then move to the top of the next column to the right. When a number exceeds the limit of the numbers in the frame, in our case over 15,000, it is simply passed over and the next number selected that does fall within the relevant range. Since the numbers were placed in the table in a completely random fashion, the resulting sample is random. This procedure gives each item an equal probability of being selected. In case of infinite population, the selection of each item in a random sample is controlled by the same probability and that successive selections are independent of one another.
- *Systematic sampling:* In some instances the most practical way of sampling is to select every 15th name on a list, every 10th house on one side of a street and so on. Sampling of this type is known as systematic sampling. An element of randomness is usually introduced into this kind of sampling by using random numbers to pick-up the unit with which to start. This procedure is useful when sampling frame is available in the form of a list. In such a design the selection process starts by picking some random point in the list and then every nth element is selected until the desired number is secured.
- *Stratified sampling:* If the population from which a sample is to be drawn does not constitute a homogeneous group, then stratified sampling technique is applied so as to obtain a representative sample.

In this technique, the population is stratified into a number of non-overlapping subpopulations or strata and sample items are selected from each stratum. If the items selected from each stratum is based on simple random sampling the entire procedure, first stratification and then simple random sampling, is known as stratified random sampling.

- *Quota sampling:* In stratified sampling the cost of taking random samples from individual strata is often so expensive that interviewers are simply given quota to be filled from different strata, the actual selection of items for sample being left to the interviewer's judgment. This is called quota sampling. The size of the quota for each stratum is generally proportionate to the size of that stratum in the population. Quota sampling is thus an important form of non-probability sampling. Quota samples generally happen to be judgment samples rather than random samples.
- *Cluster sampling and area sampling:* Cluster sampling involves grouping the population and then selecting the groups or the clusters rather than individual elements for inclusion in the sample. Suppose some departmental store wishes to sample its credit card holders. It has issued its cards to 15,000 customers. The sample size is to be kept say 450. For cluster sampling this list of 15,000 card holders could be formed into 100 clusters of 150 card holders each. Three clusters might then be selected for the sample randomly. The sample size must often be larger than the simple random sample to ensure the same level of accuracy because is cluster sampling procedural potential for order bias and other sources of error are usually accentuated. The clustering approach can, however, make the sampling procedure relatively easier and increase the efficiency of field work, especially in the case of personal interviews.
- Area sampling is quite close to cluster sampling and is often talked about when the total geographical area of interest happens to be big one. Under area sampling we first divide the total area into a number of smaller non-overlapping areas, generally called geographical clusters, then a number of these smaller areas are randomly selected, and all units in these small areas are included in the sample. Area sampling is especially helpful where we do not have the list of the population concerned. It also makes the field interviewing more efficient since interviewer can do many interviews at each location.
- *Multi-stage sampling:* This is a further development of the idea of cluster sampling. This technique is meant for big inquiries extending to a considerably large geographical area like an entire country. Under multi-stage sampling the first stage maybe to select large primary sampling units such as states, then districts, then towns and finally certain families within towns. If the technique of random-sampling

is applied at all stages, the sampling procedure is described as multi-stage random sampling.

- *Sequential sampling:* This is somewhat a complex sample design where the ultimate size of the sample is not fixed in advance but is determined according to mathematical decisions on the basis of information yielded as survey progresses. This design is usually adopted under acceptance sampling plan in the context of statistical quality control.
- In practice, several of the methods of sampling described above may well be used in the same study in which case it can be called mixed sampling. It maybe pointed out here that normally one should resort to random sampling so that bias can be eliminated and sampling error can be estimated. But purposive sampling is considered desirable when the universe happens to be small and a known characteristic of it is to be studied intensively. Also, there are conditions under which sample designs other than random sampling maybe considered better for reasons like convenience and low costs.

The sample design to be used must be decided by the researcher taking into consideration the nature of the inquiry and other related factors.

Collecting the Data

In dealing with any real life problem it is often found that data at hand are inadequate, and hence, it becomes necessary to collect data that are appropriate. There are several ways of collecting the appropriate data which differ considerably in context of money costs, time and other resources at the disposal of the researcher. Primary data can be collected either through experiment or through survey. If the researcher conducts an experiment, he observes some quantitative measurements, or the data, with the help of which he examines the truth contained in his hypothesis. But in the case of a survey, data can be collected by anyone or more of the following ways:

- *By observation:* This method implies the collection of information by way of investigators own observation, without interviewing the respondents. The information obtained relates to what is currently happening and is not complicated by either the past behavior or future intentions or attitudes of respondents. This method is no doubt an expensive method and the information provided by this method is also very limited. As such this method is not suitable in inquiries where large samples are concerned.
- *Through personal interview:* The investigator follows a rigid procedure and seeks answers to a set of pre-conceived questions through personal interviews. This method of collecting data is usually carried out in a structured way where output depends upon the ability of the interviewer to a large extent.

- *Through telephone interviews:* This method of collecting information involves contacting the respondents on telephone itself. This is not a very widely used method but it plays an important role in industrial surveys in developed regions, particularly, when the survey has to be accomplished in a very limited time.
- *By mailing of questionnaires:* The researcher and the respondents do come in contact with each other if this method of survey is adopted. Questionnaires are mailed to the respondents with a request to return after completing the same. It is the most extensively used method in various economic and business surveys. Before applying this method, usually a Pilot Study for testing the questionnaire is conduced which reveals the weaknesses, if any, of the questionnaire? Questionnaire to be used must be prepared very carefully so that it may prove to be effective in collecting the relevant information.
- *Through schedules:* Under this method the enumerators are appointed and given training. They are provided with schedules containing relevant questions. These enumerators go to respondents with these schedules. Data are collected by filling up the schedules by enumerators on the basis of replies given by respondents. Much depends upon the capability of enumerators so far as this method is concerned. Some occasional field checks on the work of the enumerators may ensure sincere work.
- The researcher should select one of these methods of collecting the data taking into consideration the nature of investigation, objective and scope of the inquiry, financial resources, available time and the desired degree of accuracy. Though he should pay attention to all these factors but much depends upon the ability and experience of the researcher. In collection of statistical data common sense is the chief requisite and experience the chief teacher.

Execution of the Project

Execution of the project is a very important step in the research process. If the execution of the project proceeds on correct lines, the data to be collected would be adequate and dependable. The researcher should see that the project is executed in a systematic manner and in time. If the survey is to be conducted by means of structured questionnaires, data can be readily machine-processed. In such a situation, questions as well as the possible answers maybe coded. If the data are to be collected through interviewers, arrangements should be made for proper selection and training of the interviewers. The training maybe given with the help of instruction manuals which explain clearly the job of the interviewers at each step. Occasional field checks should be made to ensure that the interviewers are doing their assigned job sincerely and efficiently.

A careful watch should be kept for unanticipated factors in order to keep the survey as much realistic as possible. This, in other words, means that steps should be taken to ensure that the survey is under statistical control so that the collected information is in accordance with the pre-defined standard of accuracy. If some of the respondents do not cooperate, some suitable methods should be designed to tackle this problem. One method of dealing with the non-response problem is to make a list of the non-respondents and take a small sub-sample of them, and then with the help of experts vigorous efforts can be made for securing response.

Analysis of Data

After the data have been collected, the researcher turns to the task of analyzing them. The analysis of data requires a number of closely related operations such as establishment of categories, the application of these categories to raw data through coding, tabulation and then drawing statistical inferences. The unwieldy data should necessarily be condensed into a few manageable groups and tables for further analysis. Thus, researcher should classify the raw data into some purposeful and usable categories. **Coding** operation is usually done at this stage through which the categories of data are transformed into symbols that maybe tabulated and counted. **Editing** is the procedure that improves the quality of the data for coding. With coding the stage is ready for tabulation. **Tabulation** is a part of the technical procedure wherein the classified data are put in the form of tables. The mechanical devices can be made use of at this juncture. A great deal of data, especially in large inquiries, is tabulated by computers. Computers not only save time but also make it possible to study large number of variables affecting a problem simultaneously.

Analysis work after tabulation is generally based on the computation of various percentages, coefficients, etc. by applying various well defined statistical formulae. In the process of analysis, relationships or differences supporting or conflicting with original or new hypotheses should be subjected to tests of significance to determine with what validity data can be said to indicate any conclusion(s). For instance, if there are two samples of weekly wages, each sample being drawn from factories in different parts of the same city, giving two different mean values, then our problem maybe whether the two mean values are significantly different or the difference is just a matter of chance. Through the use of statistical tests we can establish whether such a difference is a real one or is the result of random fluctuations. If the difference happens to be real, the inference will be that the two samples come from different universes and if the difference is due to chance, the conclusion would be that the two samples belong to the same universe. Similarly, the technique of analysis of variance can help us in analyzing whether three or more varieties of seeds grown on certain fields yield significantly different results or not.

In brief, the researcher can analyze the collected data with the help of various statistical measures.

Hypothesis-testing

After analyzing the data as stated above, the researcher is in a position to test the hypotheses, if any, he had formulated earlier. Do the facts support the hypotheses or they happen to be contrary? This is the usual question which should be answered while testing hypotheses. Various tests, such as Chi square test, t-test, F-test, have been developed by statisticians for the purpose. The hypotheses maybe tested through the use of one or more of such tests, depending upon the nature and object of research inquiry. Hypothesis-testing will result in either accepting the hypothesis or in rejecting it. If the researcher had no hypotheses to start with, generalizations established on the basis of data maybe stated as hypotheses to be tested by subsequent researches in times to come.

Generalizations and Interpretation

If a hypothesis is tested and upheld several times, it maybe possible for the researcher to arrive at generalization, i.e. to build a theory. As a matter of fact, the real value of research lies in its ability to arrive at certain generalizations. If the researcher had no hypothesis to start with, he might seek to explain his findings on the basis of some theory. It is known as interpretation. The process of interpretation may quite often trigger off new questions which in turn may lead to further researches.

Preparation of the Report or the Thesis

Finally, the researcher has to prepare the report of what has been done by him. Writing of report must be done with great care keeping in view the following:

- *The layout of the report should be as follows:* (i) The preliminary pages; (ii) the main text, and (iii) the end matter. In its preliminary pages the report should carry title and date followed by acknowledgments and foreword. Then there should be a table of contents followed by a list of tables and list of graphs and charts, if any, given in the report.
  - The main text of the report should have the following parts:
  - *Introduction:* It should contain a clear statement of the objective of the research and an explanation of the methodology adopted in accomplishing the research. The scope of the study along with various limitations should as well be stated in this part.
  - *Summary of findings:* After introduction there would appear a statement of findings and recommendations in non-technical language. If the findings are extensive, they should be summarized.

- *Main report:* The main body of the report should be presented in logical sequence and broken-down into readily identifiable sections.
- *Conclusion:* Towards the end of the main text, researcher should again put down the results of his research clearly and precisely. In fact, it is the final summing-up.
- At the end of the report, appendices should be enlisted in respect of all technical data. Bibliography, i.e. list of books, journals, reports, etc. consulted, should also be given in the end. Index should also be given specially in a published research report.

- Report should be written in a concise and objective style in simple language avoiding vague expressions such as it seems, there maybe, and the like.
- Charts and illustrations in the main report should be used only if they present the information more clearly and forcibly.
- Calculated, confidence limits must be mentioned and the various constraints experienced in conducting research operations may as well be stated.

Definition of Research Terms

- *Analysis of covariance (ancova):* A statistical procedure used to test mean differences among groups on a dependent variable, while controlling for one or more extraneous variables.
- *Analysis of variance (anova):* A statistical procedure for testing mean differences among three or more groups by comparing variability between groups to variability within groups.
- *Between subjects design:* A research design in which there are separate groups of people being compared (smoker vs non-smoker).
- *Case-control design:* A non-experimental research design involving the comparison of a case and a matched control.
- *Confidence level:* The estimated probability that a population parameter lies within a given confidence interval.
- *Control group:* Subjects in an experiment who do not receive the experimental treatment and whose performance provides a baseline against which the effects of the treatment can be measured.
- *Crossover design:* An experimental design in which one group of subjects is exposed to more than one condition or treatment in random order; sometimes called a repeated measures design.
- *Cross-sectional design:* A study design in which data are collected at one point in time; sometimes used to infer change overtime when data are collected from different age or development groups.
- *Deductive reasoning:* The process of developing specific predictions from general populations.

- *Dependent variable:* The variable hypothesized to depend on or be caused by another variable.
- *Double-blind experiment:* An experiment in which neither the subjects not those who administer the treatment know who is in the experimental or control group.
- *External validity:* The degree to which study results can be generalized to settings or samples other than the one studied.
- *Factorial design:* An experimental design in which two or more independent variable are simultaneously manipulated, permitting a separate analysis of the main effects of the independent variables, plus the interaction effects of those variables.
- *Generalizability:* The degree to which the research methods justify the inference that the findings are true for a broader group than study participants; in particular, the inference that the finds can be generalized from the sample to the population.
- *Independent variable:* The variable that is believed to cause or influence the dependent variable; in experimental research, the manipulated variable.
- *Inductive reasoning:* The process of reasoning from specific observations to more general rules.
- *Internal validity:* The degree to which it can be inferred that the experimental treatment, rather than uncontrolled, extraneous factors, is responsible for observed effects.
- *Meta-analysis:* A technique for quantitatively combining and thus integrating the results of multiple studies on a given topic.
- *Null hypothesis:* A hypothesis stating no relationship between variables under study.
- *Observational research:* Studies in which data are collected by observing and recording behaviors or activities relating to a phenomenon of interest.
- *Prospective design:* A study design that begins with an examination of presumed causes and then goes forward in time to observe presumed effects.
- *Qualitative analysis:* The organization and interpretation of nonnumeric data for the purpose of discovering important underlying dimensions and patterns of relationships.
- *Quantitative analysis:* The manipulation of numeric data through statistical procedures for the purpose of describing phenomena or assessing the magnitude and reliability of relationships among them.
- *Quasi-experimental:* An intervention study in which subjects are not randomly assigned to treatment conditions, but the researcher exercises certain controls to enhance the study's internal validity.

- *Randomization:* The assignment of subjects to treatment conditions in a random manner.
- *Reliability:* The degree of consistency or dependability with which an instrument measures the attribute it is designed to measure.
- *Research hypothesis:* The actual hypothesis a researcher wishes to test, stating the anticipated relationship between two or more variables.
- *Research question:* A statement of the specific query the researcher wants to answer to address a research problem.
- *Retrospective design:* A study design that begins with the manifestation of the dependent variable in the present and searches for the presumed cause occurring in the past.
- *Sensitivity:* The ability of screening instruments to correctly identify a case.
- *Transferability:* The extent to which findings can be transferred to other settings or groups.
- *Validity:* The degree to which an instrument measures what it is intended to measure.

REVIEW OF LITERATURE

Definition

'Literature review is the reading and organization of material that represents current knowledge as available in previous studies for the direction of a research study'.

Purposes of Literature Review

Literature review is carried out to:

- Find out what has already been written about the chosen area of interest
- Describe the characteristics of previous studies in the area
- Identify gaps existing in the area of interest
- Establish whether it is feasible to conduct research in that area, or such a research would be duplication
- Identify how other researchers connected their works to theories
- Reveal how previous researchers measured their variables and collected their data
- Identify deficiencies of methodology in previous studies in order to avoid them
- Relate findings of planned studies with the ones that have been done previously.

Sources of Literature Review

These include primary and secondary sources:

- A primary source is the description of a research written by the original researcher. Journals are the best primary source for literature. They are also most current, and available in print and electronic forms.
- A secondary source is a description of a study prepared by someone other than the original researcher. Secondary sources are often interpretations of the original work, and so may not serve all the needs of another researcher. For example, a research article cited by another person in a journal is a secondary source, but that author's own report in the same journal is a primary source. These literature materials could be held in libraries as hard copies, abstracts, indexes, or available as Internet based literature. The librarians, particularly the reference librarians are a key resource to researchers as they are of great assistance with literature. They could direct, provide guidance and even assist with procurement of the needed material.

Searching Nursing Literature on the Internet

- The internet possesses an enormous number of medical and nursing databases, which are very useful for nursing professionals.
- It is quiet impossible to calculate the quantity of medical information on the Internet. So many new resources are created each day that nobody could possibly keep abreast of them and present an exhaustive analysis of all existing medical resources.
- MEDLINE is a comprehensive database for health literature which is managed by National Library of Medicine, USA. International nursing index and Index Medicus are included in MEDLINE.
- Cochrane Review (http://www.cochrane.org/) is another database which gives extensive search options. Cumulative Index to Nursing and Allied Health Literature (http://www.ebscohost.com/cinahl/) is a database of exclusive nursing articles
- Internet search engine Google has developed Google Scholar (http://scholar.google.com), which helps to confine search options to academic papers only.
- Open access journals (http://www.doaj.org) are another source of searching literature. These journals are access free and can be used without restriction provided the policies are accepted. Many standard journals provide their archives for free online access search after a period of time to developing countries.
- Elsevier publications' internet database for nursing journals is accessible athttp://sciencedirect.com/.
- The Nursing Center (http://nursingcenter.com) is the online access site for Lippincott Williams & Wilkins' nursing journals.

- These journals are to be subscribed and most of them are indexed in MEDLINE and CINAHL.
- Many of the journals are published by the organization themselves. The Indian Medlars Centre of National Informatics Centre, New Delhi, has designed two databases.
- IndMED, a bibliographic database of peer reviewed Indian biomedical journals and medIND, full-text of selected IndMED journals.
- These are accessible free of cost from the Center's site <http://indmed.nic.in/> (Ameen, 2004).

SUMMARY

In this unit, we discuss that formulating a research problem; the problem is explored in its broadest form, and then narrowed to the specific area of focus, and ends in problem statement, purpose of the study, objectives, scope and significance of the study. The research problem is therefore the basis of any research activity and needs to be properly understood so that the other steps of the research process would be meaningful. It is important that the researcher shows how the reviewed studies are related to the present study. What more still needs to be done in the area should be identified and suggestions made as to how the present study will provide for that the study problem, purpose and variables should be reflected in the written review, and the interpretations of the study findings also. The length of time spent in review could vary from days to weeks or months depending on the researcher and the type of search in use.

Introduction to Research Approaches

5 unit

INTRODUCTION

Research approach and research design are two terms that are frequently used interchangeably. However research design is a broader plan to conduct a study, and research approach is an important element of the research design, which governs.

The research design spells out the basic strategies that the researcher adopts and incorporates some of the most important methodological decisions that the researcher makes in conducting a research study.

The types of research brings to light the fact that there are two basic approaches to research, viz., quantitative approach and the qualitative approach.

Quantitative research involves "the systematic collection of numeric information, usually under conditions of considerable control and the analysis of that information using statistical procedures".

Qualitative research approach involves the systematic collection and analysis of more subjective narrative materials, using procedures in which there tends to be a minimum of research imposed control. It tends to emphasize the dynamic, holistic and individual aspects of human experience and attempts to capture those aspects in the entirely (fully) within the context of those who are experiencing them.

Difference between quantitative and qualitative approach

Quantitative	Qualitative
• It is a formal objective, systematic process in which numerical data are utilized to get information about the phenomena.	• It is a systematic interactive subjective approach used to describe life experiences and give them meaning.

Contd...

Contd...

Quantitative	Qualitative
• It describes variables, examine relationships among variables and determine cause and effect relationships between variables.	• Describe and promotes understanding of human experiences such as pain, caring, powerlessness and comfort, etc. it focuses on understanding the whole.
• It produces "hard" science that is based on rigor, objective and control. Quantitative researchers believe all human behavior is objective, measureable and purposeful. Only right instrument needed to measure variables.	• "Qualitative research is an artistic and philosophical approach that produces "soft science". It lacks objectivity and control that is necessary to produce "hard science".
• Focus is concise and reductionistic. Reductionism involves breaking the whole into parts that can be examined.	• Focus is usually broad and attempts to give meaning to the whole (holistic).
• It is down to describe, examine relationships and determine causality among variables (cause-effect). Useful in testing theory. It involves logistic, deductive, reasoning to make generalizations about the universe.	• Conducted to generate knowledge concerned with meaning and discovery. It incorporates inductive and dialectic reasoning. Identifies relationships among variables and relational statements are used in theory development.
• Required control (Extraneous variable)	• It uses structured and unstructured observation and communication as means of gathering data.
• Requires use of instruments to collect data that will generate numerical data.	• Data are in form of words and analyzed in terms of individual response, descriptive summarizes or both.
• Required statistical analysis	• Analyzed to organize data into meaningful individualized interpretations that describes one phenomenon under study. • Qualitative analysis is a challenging, labor-intensive activity, guided by few standardized rules.

RESEARCH DESIGN

A research design is a strategy to get the information the researcher wants in a study. It is the overall plan for answering the research questions of testing the hypotheses. The research design incorporates the data collection plan, the sampling plan and the analysis plan. There is no hard rule for specific designs, but the decision of which one to use rests on the researcher and the nature of the research. Each researcher could choose the design deemed most suitable for the specific research. A wide variety of approaches are available to nurse researchers.

The research design, which could also be called methodology, maybe described as qualitative when the data to be collected will be in words and quantitative, when the data would be in numbers (numeric). They could generally be grouped under experimental and non-experimental designs, though in your reading, you may come across other classifications.

Purposes of the Research Design

The major purposes include these:

- To enable the researcher focus on the key variables under investigation
- To facilitate adequate sampling methods
- To ensure that the appropriate data collection method is applied.

Types of Research Design

- Experimental design
- Non-experimental design
- *Experimental design:* Experiments broadly defined are tests that involve at least one treatment (independent variable), units (subjects) to be analyzed by assignment or non-assignment to a treatment and a comparison for inferring effects that maybe attributed to the treatment.

Essential Characteristics of Experimental Designs

To test a relationship and most confidently infer this result, experimental designs must be characterized by three essential elements: randomization, manipulation and control.

- *Randomization:* Randomization refers to participants being assigned by chance to either receive or not receive the treatment condition or intervention. A number of procedures exist for assigning individuals to groups such as coin toss, a random numbers table or computerized random number generators. The key characteristic of all these procedures is that each participant has an equal and known probability of being assigned to either the control or the experimental group. Randomization helps eliminate bias by spreading variability due to extraneous variables equally across the groups under study. The advantage of assigning participants to groups in a random manner is that this should result in the group's initially being similar to one another prior to the intervention. Random assignment to condition does not guarantee that the two groups will be similar to one another. Based on sampling theory, significant difference ($p < 0.05$) between the two groups will occur in 1:20 cases of assigning participants to groups. The sample size should be large enough or else researcher may wish to consider some additional methods of distributing important variables such as matching or use of more homogeneous population. In some research, it is necessary to randomly assign treatment conditions, to units other than the individual participants. Randomization maybe cluster, stratified, fixed or by random assignment.

- *Manipulation:* Manipulation is the process of maneuvering the independent variable so that its effect on the dependent variable can be observed. The causative variable must be amenable to manipulation by the investigator, i.e. the researcher does something to subjects in the experimental condition. It is essential that researchers conduct manipulation checks to see whether the manipulation had its intended effect or perhaps resulted in an unintended effect that could compromise the validity of an experiment. In working to avoid unintended effects researchers should be cautious of the use of reactive measures which can influence participants' responses to the dependent variable. Even though researcher does not actively manipulate the control group, it is important that he or she be aware of what maybe happening to them control group should experience all the same things as participants in the experimental group, except the independent variable. Ethical considerations, organizational policy or some variables like attitudes, age, disease, etc. which cannot be manipulated may disallow manipulation. The ability of the researcher to manipulate the independent variable is a major source of control in experimental studies.
- *Control:* Cook and Campbell identify three uses of the term control in relation to research designs, all of which involve elimination of threats to valid inference namely the researchers control over the research environment; control over the experimental variable; the ability to identify and rule out threats to internal validity. The last type of control is typically achieved through the use of a comparison or control group and through attention to sources of variance. In many nursing studies control groups receive the usual or traditional methods of care rather than no treatment against which effects of the experimental intervention are measured.

Kerlinger discusses the merits of experimental designs in terms of their ability to control variance or to take into account factors that may contribute to differences in the dependent variable. To provide valid answers to research questions, three kinds of variance must be considered: systematic or experimental variance which refers to the systematic effect of independent variable on the dependent variable and is a type of variance which should be enhanced; extraneous variance which refers to the effects of extraneous variables on the dependent variables, which is to be controlled by the design by building the extraneous variable into the design as an independent variable, eliminating or holding constant an extraneous variable by selecting participants as homogeneous as possible on that variable, matching participants and using statistical control; error variance which refers to the variability of measures due to random fluctuations including errors of measurement, which can be controlled by standardizing the instrument/measurement conditions (keeping the time of the day, place instructions, personnel constant) or using sensitive, reliable instruments. Internal validity is the primary objective of experimental methodology.

Types of Experimental Designs

There are of two major types of experimental designs, true experiments and quasi experiments. True experiments include the random assignment of units to comparison groups for inferring a change that has been caused by treatment. Random assignment is an essential component of true experiments that is designed to achieve comparability of comparison groups. Quasi experiments have a treatment, outcomes and units to be analyzed, but random assignment of units to comparison groups is not included for determining the groups of units to be compared. An important assumption underlying all true experimental designs is that equivalence of groups is maintained throughout the course of the experiment and is not compromised by things such as differential attritions, i.e. variable drop out rates may make experimental and control subjects different on critical factors at the time of the analysis. If experimental and control groups become nonequivalent, the design then becomes quasi experimental.

True Experimental Design/Randomized Clinical Trials/Controlled Trials

Overview of True Experimental Design

- The experimental level of research is designed to test theory in laboratory settings or in controlled clinical trials, thus the purpose is to test theory. The greater the degree of control in the research setting, the greater the confidence, that the research findings are accurate. The experimental design the most controlled of all research designs entails manipulation of the independent variables and requires control of all intervening variables. On the basis of theory developed from previous research, each step in the experiment requires a predictive hypothesis regarding the effect of the independent on the dependent variables.

- Cause and effect is always predicted based on theory, thus predictive hypotheses are written at the beginning of the study stating the precise nature of both the manipulation of the independent variable and its effects on the independent variables. All assumptions are spelled out or are either verified by previous research or tested by the current research. All logical steps between cause and effect are specified. Although causal laws can never be proved researchers in experimental designs should be aware of three criteria for causality: a temporal relationship: cause must precede the effect in time; an empirical relationship—there must be an evidence that the independent variable and the dependent variable are associated; a spurious relationship: the relationship cannot be explained by the influence of a third variable. The key issue of the design is internal validity or the assumptions that changes in the dependent variable are actually due to the independent variable.
- Experimental and control groups are created by random assignment. Ethical concerns for the protection of human and animal subjects are the most restrictive. Experimenters more than any kind of researchers, are required to establish that all subjects rights are protected to the greatest degree possible and potential harmful effects are counterbalanced by potential benefits. Data collection is quantitative and prospective. Data analysis is designed to discriminate between and among experimental and control groups. Although experimental studies are the most directly applicable to nursing practice because of their controlled samples, they are the least widely generalizable in and of themselves. This is simply due to the controlled narrowness of the study and sample. Experiments are deigned to be repeated on many samples with small variations in the independent variable overtime.

  A single experiment on a single small sample adds to the test of a part of the theory but not of the entire theory. Many experiments with different samples maybe required to increase generalizability to the point where findings can be widely applied in practice. Thus, the true experiment is regarded as the cornerstone of scientific research, the most powerful strategy for testing causal hypothesis and achieving the four criteria namely: establishing causal relationships; manipulating independent variable; measuring the impact of independent variable on the dependent variable; minimizing or accounting for the effects of factors other than the independent variable on the dependent variable.

Types of True Experimental Designs

A number of different experimental designs meet the criteria for true experiments. These include but are not limited to the classical experimental designs, the factorial design, the multiple treatment groups-repeated measures design and the Solomon four group design.

(a) *The classical experimental design: Kothari* describes them as formal designs either with or without a control group namely before and after without control design, before and after with control design. Similarly post test only design with control group.

- *Pretest-post-test design/before-after design:* All experimental groups are variations on the basic classical experimental designs which consist of two groups, an experimental and control group and two variables, an independent and dependent variable. Units to be analyzed are randomly assigned to each of the experimental and control groups. Units in the experimental groups receive the independent variable that the investigator has manipulated and participants in the control group do not receive the independent variable treatment. Pretest and post-test measures are taken on the independent variables and the control group participants are measured at the same time as the experimental group although no planned change or manipulation has taken place with regard to the independent variable in the control group. Researchers use this design when they are interested in assessing the change from the pretest to the post-test as a result of a treatment or intervention.

$$\frac{\text{R O1 X O2}}{\text{R O1 X O2}}$$

- (R: Random assignment, X: Treatment, O: Observation)
- *Post-test only design:* One group receives a treatment whereas the other group receives no treatment and serves as control. The key difference in the post-test only design is that, neither group are pretested and only at the end of the study are both groups measured on the dependent variable. Some researchers favor this design because they are concerned that the pre-test measures will sensitize participants or that a learning effect might take place that influences individuals' performance on the post-test.

$$\frac{\text{R X O2}}{\text{R \quad O2}}$$

R: Random assignment, X: Treatment, O: Observation)

- *N = 1 True experiments or single subject design:* The sample is one subject, who is exposed to two or more treatments on various occasion. It may involve before and after designs. The design gives the researcher opportunity to focus on an individual and therefore pay more attention to details. It is particularly suitable to the principle of patient centered care, since the interaction between the individual and the treatment is unique, although lessons learned can be applied to other cases as well. But findings cannot be generalized.

(b) *Factorial designs:* Classical experimental designs allow the manipulation of a single variable at a time, holding all other conditions constant. Factorial designs permit the manipulation of more than one independent variable at a time. Furthermore, interaction effects between variables are revealed and the simultaneous testing of multiple hypotheses is thus allowed. The researcher can study the effects of each of the variables (known as main effects) and the interactions between them or their joint effects on the independent variable.
   - Though commonly used design is 2 × 2 factorial design, experiments can be conducted with any number of categories and independent variables. Each factor must have two or more levels thus when new factors are added the analysis becomes more complex. For example, 4 × 5 design means that one of the factors has four categories and the other has five. These designs can also be extended to have more than two factors as in 3 × 2 × 4 factorial design, which means that there are three factors consisting of three, two and four categories respectively.
   - Factorial designs are also referred to as 'levels of treatment' designs. When one of the factors cannot be manipulated, such as sex or race it is referred to as blocking variable. The design that incorporates the blocking variable is known as the randomized block design. Stratified randomization is often used in this case to ensure that approximately equal numbers of participants within categories are randomly assigned to the various groups.

(c) *Multiple treatment groups-repeated measures design:* This design uses several experimental groups each of which receives a different treatment. Control is achieved through comparison among groups and from measures taken on the dependent variable for all groups at time 1 and time 2. It is always not true that a control group will be used that has no treatment at all. There can also be more than one pretest and post-test measure for the dependent variable for all groups.

(d) *Solomon four group design:* This is a rigorous design by controlling effects on the dependent variable that maybe due to factors other than the independent variable. It is essentially a combination of pretest-post-test and post-test only designs. This design requires a large group of homogeneous subjects to make-up the four groups, thus is used less often than other designs. It is difficult to introduce the treatment simultaneously for all groups, in order to avoid extraneous temporal effects and statistical analysis complex. The design consists of four groups of which two are control and two are experimental. Pretest and post-test are carried out with one control and one experimental group only and post-tests only for the other control and experimental group.

Exp. Group 1	O1	X	O2
Control Group 1	O2	–	O4
Exp. Group 2	–	X	O5
Control Group 2	–	–	O6

Strengths and Weaknesses of the Design

- *Strengths:* Ability to diminish bias; permit the researcher to maximize systematic variance and to control the extraneous and error variance; control the threats to validity; degree of confidence they allow the researcher in inferring causal relationships, because of high internal validity.
- *Limitations:* The number of potentially interesting research variables that are not within researcher's purview to manipulate; ethical concerns; organizational prohibitions; human characteristics often interfere with the researcher's ability to control a number of variables experimentally; sample representativeness/homogeneous sample; many cases population is unknown; requires many replications to achieve generalizations; artificiality in laboratory testing; Hawthorne effect; many of the phenomena to be tested lack theoretical background which could be either exploratory or descriptive studies than experimental; issues related to the outcome measure like relevant outcome variables, validity, reliability and systematic bias.

Quasi Experimental Designs

Overview of Quasi Experimental Designs

- This design is distinguished from the true experiment by the lack of random assignment of participants to groups. This lack of control limits confidence in the internal validity of the study. Otherwise the design is exactly same as the experimental design. Data are predominantly quantitative, data analysis distinguishes between and among treatments and among treatment groups. Many field experiments actually use a quasi experimental design when the assignment of participants to the various experimental and control groups cannot be controlled by the researcher. For example, the nurse may want to use an inpatient hospital population in an experiment but physician's control who is admitted to the hospital. A nurse therefore may not have control over extraneous or intervening variables in the available population.

- The researcher is often not allowed control of the treatment variable and cannot achieve randomization because of ethical considerations, institutional policies or other situational factors. In such circumstances, the researcher chooses quasi experimental studies. Quasi experiments do not have equivalence created by random assignment or that do not have control groups for comparison, rather comparisons are made with non-equivalent groups or with periodic measurement of the same group that maybe different due to a number of variables extraneous to the causal variable of interest.

Types of Quasi Experimental Designs

- *Non-equivalent Group Designs:* These designs are those in which dependent variable measures are obtained for an experimental and a comparison group (no randomly assigned) before and after introduction of the independent variable to the experimental group. When non equivalent group designs are employed, the control group may also receive a treatment, usually traditional. The threat to validity are selection-maturation, selection-history and regression.
  - *Basic non-equivalent group design/untreated control group design with pre-test and posttest:* One group of individuals is designed to receive a program, service or treatment and a second group of individuals is designated as a control group. Similar to classical experimental before after design except that participants are not randomly assigned to either groups. The design is used in field research in which variable relationships characterizing human subjects are tested.

    O1 X O2

    O1 O2

    (X: Treatment, O: Observation)
  - There are several threats to internal and external validity; selection bias is an especially relevant threat. Others are related to measurement of the outcome variable namely instrumentation.
  - *Untreated control group design with pre-test measures at more than one time interval:* There are advantages of administering pretests more than one time that strengthen the basic non-equivalent groups design. Multiple pretests permit assessment of whether the groups are becoming disparate at different rates from O1 to O2 when the effect could not be due to the treatment and also allow assessment of spurious treatment effects due to statistical regression. However it is often problematic to obtain pretest measures when the field researcher is unable to delay implementation of treatment moreover funding sources are often unwilling to expend monies for pretest, however researcher

should strive to achieve at least one more pretest measure to the basic non-equivalent groups design.

O1 O2 X O3

O1 O2 O3

(X: Treatment, O: Observation)

- *Post-test only designs:*
  - *Non-equivalent post-test only design:* Here no pretest is held

    X O2 (X: Treatment, O: Observation)

    O2
  - *Multiple control groups:* Use of multiple control groups for comparison

    X O1 (X: Treatment, O: Observation)
    O2
    O3
    O4
- *Other designs:* These designs are useful when a non-equivalent control group cannot be obtained and are applicable when the researcher must create circumstances that are conceptually similar to the no-treatment control group or in other words when only a single group of participants is available for the research.

Removed Treatment Design with Pretest and Post-test

A single pretest-post-test is fundamental. A third post-test is added which is followedby removal of the treatment and one more post-test.

O1 X O2 O3 X– O4

(X: Treatment, O: Observation, X–: Treatment removed)

Subjects often remove themselves from the intervention or are removed by factors that cannot be controlled. The O3-O4 data collections serve as the no treatment control for the O1-O2 data collections. One group participates throughout the course of the study when the treatment is effective there are expected differences between O1 and O2 and between O3 and O4. These differences must be in opposite directions with a clear change following removal of the treatment variable. This latter effect is needed to distinguish differences between the experimental and control conditions that are due to removal of the treatment rather than to the treatment simply having no long term effect.

It is important that observations be made at equal time intervals to assess any spontaneous changes that maybe occurring with the passage of time irrespective of the introduction and removal of treatment. The disadvantages of the design are that it is hard to demonstrate a pattern of effects on which a valid statistical conclusion can be based, i.e. the differences between O1, O2 and O3, O4 as well as between O2, O3 and O3, O4 must not be equal. Because treatment is deliberately removed participants maybecome frustrated and agitated, which may obscure the effect of removed treatment. This design is not suitable for the researcher when he/she has to deliberately remove the treatment.

Repeated Treatment Design

Participants are exposed to the treatment, removed from treatment and then exposed again to the treatment. The design is best employed when the treatment effects are expected to dissipate rapidly or when the effects are expected to be cumulative.

O1 X O2 X O3 X O4

(X: Treatment, O: Observation)

To interpret the effects of treatment the O3, O4 difference must be in the same direction as the O1, O2 difference. This design is useful for testing many nursing interventions that are not especially conspicuous or invasive to the patient such as interaction or psychosocial modalities or touch or reflective techniques. The design is vulnerable to regularly occurring extraneous sources of variance due to participant maturation or history. The frustration as in removed treatment design may confound the O3, O4 difference which could be inferred to be due to replication of the treatments when in fact it was due to reduction in frustration when the treatment was again introduced. The design is particularly vulnerable to the reactive effects of experimental procedures. To enhance external and statistical validity, large sample should be used. The design is best when the treatment being tested is unobtrusive and there is long time interval before reintroduction of the treatment. To prevent the effects of extraneous cyclic rival causes (e.g. seasonal influences) it is best to distribute reintroductions of the treatment randomly.

The Reversed Treatment Nonequivalent Control Group Design with Pretest and post-test

O1 X + O2 (X +, X–: Reversed treatment, O: Observation)

O1 X – O2

X + represents an expected effect in one direction and X–represents an expected effect in the opposite direction. The design is resistant to selection-maturation threats because maturation rarely occurs at the same time in opposite directions in the two groups. It is stronger design in terms of construct validity because it necessitates a carefully specified causal theory to hypothesize an effect in one direction in one group and an opposite effect in the other group. Cook and Campbell emphasize that to be maximally interpretable the reversed treatment design requires a placebo control group that receives a treatment—not expected to influence the outcome measure except through a reactive effect of experimental procedures and a control group that receives no treatment for a baseline of no cause. The design is often difficult to implement because treatments that produce negative effects are considered unethical and deliberate designing of these experimental conditions is questionable.

The Cohort Design with Cyclical Turnover

This design can be useful for studies in which some participants are exposed to a treatment because they cycle through an organization but others are not; cohorts differ minimally; archival records can be used to compare cohorts on specific characteristics.

O1

X O1

Interrupted Time Series Designs

These designs are those in which the independent variable effects are inferred by comparing measures of the dependent variable obtained at multiple time intervals with multiple dependent variable measures obtained after introduction of the independent variable.

Basic Interrupted Time Series Design

- It uses a single group of participants and can use different but similar units of analysis. The design is relevant for quality assurance studies and also can be convenient for conducting pure research. It can supplement information gathered using non-equivalent group designs. When the interrupted time series design is used, the researcher must know exactly when the participants were exposed to the treatment variable in order to infer its effects. If a treatment effect occurs the outcome measures taken after to the treatment should be different from those taken before exposure to the treatment. Hence the time series measures are interrupted. At least 30 time periods should be available when the researcher considers using interrupted time series design without a comparison group. This allows sufficient data to be gathered for an evaluation of a trend overtime following the intervention. The design which has an adequate number of time period observations has a distinct advantage for generalization of results over a variety of time periods. The advantage is the opportunity to examine results within subgroups of participants, thus external validity is strengthened. The study participants can be stratified according to individual and setting characteristics to determine if effects hold across subgroup. Multiple observations after the treatment decrease the potential for measurement error.

O1 O2 O3 O4 O5 X O6 O7 O8 O9 O10

- Cook and Campbell describe several types of interruption effects that can occur. The first is sharp change in mean scores when the interruption occurs, indicating different levels or intercepts of the slopes of pre and post treatment scores. The second interruption effect that can be observed is a change in slope of the mean scores before and after treatment. The interruption effect can also be characterized as continuous or discontinuous and as instantaneous or delayed. Different effects can occur simultaneously in various combinations. The major strength of the basic time series design is that it allows the assessment of outcome effects that are due to maturation prior to the introduction of the treatment. Multiple observations also make it possible to examine the trend of pretest scores for an effect that is due to statistical regression. Furthermore with a large number of time period observations, extraneous effects due to history or cyclic influences can also be evaluated. The major threat is history thus, the researcher must collect data frequently and record carefully all possible events or circumstances that could reasonably influence outcomes. The other threats are instrumentation, selection bias and reactive effects of experimental procedures.

Interrupted Time Series Designs with a Non-equivalent no Treatment Group Time Series

O1 O2 O3 O4 O5 X O6 O7 O8 O9 O10

O1 O2 O3 O4 O5 O6 O7 O8 O9 O10

- The addition of a no treatment control group time series to the basic time series design makes it strong in terms of threat of history because the effects of history can be tested. The design is still be subject to the threat of selection-history interaction if one group is influenced by an event at the time that it is also exposed to the treatment and the threat be enhanced by the addition of factors that increase the non-equivalence of the groups.

The Interrupted Time Series Design with Non-equivalent Dependent Variables

Oa1 Oa2 Oa3 Oa4 Oa5 X Oa6 Oa7 Oa8 Oa9 Oa10

Ob1 Ob2 Ob3 Ob4 Ob5 Ob6 Ob7 Ob8 Ob9 Ob10

The subscripts refers to different measures.

This design has enhanced construct validity. The effects of history can be assessed and the construct validity strengthened by collecting data for some variables that should show treatment effects and for others that should not. Sufficient theory should exist to establish the conceptual relationship of the dependent variables with the treatment.

Interrupted Time Series Design with Removed Treatment

O1 O2 O3 O4 X O5 O6 O7 O8 O9 X– O10 O11 O12 O13

Here two interrupted time series are joined together, i.e. O1 to O9 represents one time series that allows assessment of a treatment effect; O5 to O13 allows assessment of the removal of the treatment. For maximum inference researcher would expect one form of change between O4 and O5 and an opposing change between O9 and O10. However, the second series adds protection from the threat of history to internal validity. Regardless of the effects of resentful demoralization, the design is quite strong because two alternative explanations are required to negate results that occur in a different direction after removal of a treatment.

Interrupted Time Series Design with Switching Replications

O1 O2 O3 O4 O5 O6 O7 O8 X O9 O10 O11

O1 O2 O3 X O4 O5 O6 O7 O8 O9 O10 O11

In this group two non-equivalent groups are exposed to a treatment and serve as control groups_for each other. There are two important reasons for including this design: firstly the design has a strong internal and external validity and secondly it is a practical design that nurse researchers should consider whenever the non-equivalent control group is available. The replication built into the design makes it possible to extend the findings beyond a single population.

Interrupted Time Series Design with Multiple Replications

O1 O2 X O3 O4 X– O5 O6 X O7 O8 X– O9 O10 X O11 O12 X– O13 O14

The design is powerful in testing the causal hypothesis and has the added advantages of modifications that allow the testing of more than one treatment in single study as well as testing interaction effects of treatments. Two treatments can be tested by substituting X1 for X and X2 for X–. The design is however vulnerable to the extraneous effects of cyclical maturation, so random scheduling of treatments and their removal is suggested, while preserving the alternating treatment and removal unless cyclic effects can be ruled out by a strong theoretical base. The weakness of the design is that it is possible only when the effects of a treatment are expected to extinguish rapidly. Also the design ordinarily requires that the researcher have the ability to control the circumstances of the experiment, which is usually not possible with the nursing phenomena. It maybe a useful design for testing forms of behavior modification interventions.

Non-Experimental Design

- The non-experimental design involves those studies without deliberate manipulation of the variables or control over the research setting. There maybe random sampling of subjects, but the researcher does not employ randomization to assign subjects to groups. The non-experimental design includes those studies with the characteristic questions of 'What is/ what are/identify'. They include:
  - *Descriptive studies:* A non-experimental research where the researcher may utilize self report measures that looks at many cases across a few variables, relates one to another but does not demonstrate causality. They are most often used for research that has to do with beliefs, attitudes, or emotions. The researcher is concerned with determining and reporting subjects or objects the way they are. They could also take the form of exploratory studies, surveys, and case studies.
  - *Historical research:* A non-experimental design that describes causes, effects or trends that may help explain present events and anticipate future events. They seek to answer why, and the data sources are original correspondences, diaries, artefacts, witnesses and paper accounts of events.
  - *Cross-sectional designs:* The observations are taken at one time, like a snapshot of participants, especially where the aim is to determine prevalence. Cross-sectional design has the advantage of being economical in time and cost.
  - *Longitudinal studies:* Longitudinal studies are the ones where one or more participants are studied at several points in time. The sample is followed overtime to see how they change. All the variables are measured within a narrow span of time with data collected for each variable at each age level. The aim is to describe patterns of change, the direction and magnitude of causal relationships between the variables.
  - *Prospective designs:* It provides the researcher the opportunity to study a phenomenon overtime as a developmental process unfolds.

- *Retrospective designs:* These are employed when an event or phenomenon in the present is linked to a previous event to determine the antecedents.

Differences between Experimental and Non-experimental Designs

- Experimental designs are characterized by randomization, control and manipulation of subjects; while in non-experimental designs subjects are studied as they are, with much less control, though there maybe random selection of subjects.
- The experimental design is able to determine a cause and effect relationship, which is not possible by the non-experimental design.
- In terms of cost, the experimental design is often more expensive, since the researcher may need to create conditions that may not be possible normally for the purpose of the study.
- Subject availability maybe more with none experimental, but attrition rate is also higher.
- Experimental designs are not suitable for researches that have to do with emotions.
- Experimental studies are amenable to replication while it may not be possible with non-experimental designs.
- Prediction of future occurrences is possible with only experimental design.

SUMMARY

In this unit we discuss about the research approaches and design is the blue print of research, and the implementation of the research depends on the design hence the need for every researcher to understand the different designs in order to effectively implement research. A major purpose of the design is to ensure that the adequate data collection method is applied. The experimental and non-experimental designs were identified as two main types of research designs. The experimental design varieties were mentioned as true experimental, quasi experimental and ex post facto designs. The non-experimental designs described include the descriptive, under which were listed surveys, exploratory studies, cross-sectional, longitudinal, retrospective, prospective and historical studies.

Introduction to Sampling and Data Collection Process

6 unit

INTRODUCTION

Sampling plays a vital role in carrying out any of the research study. For the actual implementation of the research design, certain actions must be undertaken. The whole group or the entire universe on which the research would be conducted, and who will provide the data require special mention and understanding that would facilitate the research effort.

Data collection is the step of the research process where the researcher has contact with the sample selected, in order to collect the needed data from them to answer the research questions and test the hypotheses. Various methods are used to collect data and you will learn about them in this unit.

Population

Population is the total membership of a group, universe or objects in a state or geographical location. It can also be defined as the totality of the universe from which the subjects for a study could be selected, and to whom the results of the study would be generalized.

Sampling

Sampling maybe defined as the selection of some part of an aggregate or totality on the basis of which a judgment or inference about the aggregate or totality is made. In other words it is the process of obtaining information about an entire population by examining only a part of it. In most of the research work and surveys the usual approach happens to be make generalization or to draw inferences based on samples about the parameters of population from which the population are taken.

So we can now define a *sample* is any number of persons, units or objects selected to represent the population according to some rule or plan. The census method is the enumeration of all the numbers or units of the population to get the idea of the population whereas sampling is the method of selecting a fraction of the population in such a way that it represents the whole population.

Sampling is used in practice for a variety of reasons such as:

- Sampling is cheaper than census method. It is economical too.
- As the magnitude of operations is small in case of sampling, so data collection and analysis can be carried out accurately and efficiently.
- Sampling is the only way when the population is as large as the population of a country.
- Sampling enables the researcher to make a precise estimate of the standard error which helps in obtaining information concerning some characteristic of the population.

Sampling methods

Sampling methods are broadly categorized into two groups:

1. Probability sampling methods
2. Non probability sampling methods

Probability Sampling Methods

In probability sampling methods the universe from which the sample is drawn should be known to the researcher. Under this sampling design every item of the universe has an equal chance of inclusion in the sample. Lottery methods or selecting a student from the complete student's names from a box with blind or folded eyes is the best example of random sampling; it is the best technique and unbiased method. It is the best process of selecting representative sample. But the major disadvantage is that for this technique we need the complete sampling frame, i.e. the list of the complete items or population which is not always available.

Probability sampling methods are of *three* types:

(a) *Simple random sampling:* In this method each element has the equal probability to be selected as a sample. It is bias free. Here an element cannot come twice as sample.

(b) *Stratified random sampling:* In stratified random sampling the population is first divided into different homogeneous group or strata which maybe based upon a single criterion such as male or female. Or upon combination of more criteria like sex, caste, level of education and so on. This method is generally applied when different category of individuals constitutes the population viz general. OBC, SC, ST or upper caste, middle caste, backward caste or small farmers, big farmers, marginal farmers landless farmers, etc. To have an actual picture of a particular population about the standard of living, in case of India it is advisable to categorized the population on the basis of caste, religion or land holding otherwise some section maybe under-represented or not represented at all.

Stratified random sampling maybe of two types:

(i) *Proportionate stratified random sampling:* In case of proportionate random sampling method, the researcher stratifies the population according to known characteristics and subsequently, randomly draws the sample in a similar proportion from each stratum of the population according to its proportion. That is, the population is divided into several sub-populations depending upon some known characteristics, this sub population is called strata and they are homogeneous. Suppose, a Gaon Panchayat consists of 1000 voters among which 60% is Hindus, 30% is Muslims and 10% is schedule tribes. Now the investigator wants to draw a sample of 150 voters from the population as per their proportion. That can be done by multiplying the sample number with their proportion; as per this method the sample size of Hindu voter will be 150 × 60% = 90, Muslims will be 150 × 30% = 45 and ST will be 150 × 10% = 15. So the investigator has to collect the complete voter list of the GP and randomly select the sample from each category as calculated above. In this method the sampling error is minimized and the sample possesses all the required characteristics of the population.

(ii) *Disproportionate stratified random sampling:* In this method the sampling unit in each stratum is not necessarily be as per their population. Suppose for the said GP the investigator wants to the know the voting pattern of male and female of Hindu, Muslim and ST voters; in that case he must take equal number of male and female voter from each category. Here the investigator has to give equal weightage to each stratum. This is a biased type of sampling and in this case some stratum is over-represented and some are less-represented; these are not truly representative sampling, still this to be used in some special cases.

(c) *Cluster sampling:* This is another type of probability sampling method, in which the sampling units are not individual elements of the population, but group of elements or group of individuals are selected as sample. In cluster sampling the total population is divided into a number of relatively small sub-divisions or groups which are themselves clusters and then some of these cluster are randomly selected for inclusion in the sample. Suppose an investigator wants to study the functioning of midday meal service in a district in that case he can use some schools clustering in a block or two without selecting the schools scattering all over the district. Cluster sampling reduces the cost and labor of collecting the data of the investigator but less precise than random sampling.

Non-probability Sampling Methods

In this type of sampling, items for the sample are selected deliberately by the researcher instead of using the techniques of random sampling. It is also known as purposive or judgment sampling. For instance an investigator wants to verify the profit making and self dependency of the self-help groups in their chosen enterprises assisted by the central government fund in a state; then the investigator may select one or two districts having more number of SHG, getting comparatively more fund, and researcher having long-term experience in that locality. This is a biased type of sampling bears large sampling errors. This type of sampling is rarely adopted in large and important purposes. However for research purpose this maybe taken by the research scholar.

Some important techniques of non-probability sampling methods are:

- *Quota sampling*
- *Purposive sampling*
- *Systematic sampling*
- *Snow ball sampling and*
- *Double sampling*
- *Quota sampling:* This method of sampling is almost same with that of stratified random sampling as stated above, the only difference is that here in selecting the elements randomization is not done instead quota is taken into consideration. In the above example the GP consists of 60% Hindu voters; for a sample size 150 the proportion is 90 individual, this number of individual is selected from the voter list of Hindu voters not observing the rule of randomization but as quota, so 90 number voters are selected as per convenience of the investigator. As quota sampling is not random so sampling method is biased and lead to large sampling errors.
- *Purposive sampling:* this is also non random sampling method; here the investigator selected the sample arbitrarily which he considers important for the research and believes it as typical and representative of the population. Say, an investigator wants to forecast the chance of coming into the power of a political party in general election; for that purpose he selected some reporters, some teachers and some elite people of the territory and collect their opinions. He considers those are the leading persons and their view are relevant for the chance of coming into the power of the party. As it is a purposive method it has big sampling errors and carry misleading conclusion.

- *Systematic sampling:* In this method every *nth* element is selected from a list of population having serial number. For a large population (say, one lakh) is taken into study and the sample size is 100, so the investigator is to select every *nth* name means 1000th name; the starting name maybe anyone within 1000, so selecting a particular element/person taking the 1000th name cannot represent the different strata or groups that may exist in that big population. Moreover once the starting number is decided and collected data it cannot be changed or switched over the other category as per its definition (systemic). Moreover the list may have the chance to repeat the same category of element by passing the other. It is biased and misleading but useful in homogeneous population.
- *Snow ball sampling:* This is a sociometric sampling technique generally used to study the small group. All the persons in a group identify their friends who in turn know their friends and colleagues, until the informal relationships converge into some type of a definite social pattern. It is just like the snow ball go on increasing its size when rolling in a ice-field. In case of drug addict people it is difficult to find out who are the drug user but when one person is identified he can tell the names of his partner then each of his partner can tell another 2 or 3 whom he knows uses drug . This way the required number of element/person is identified and collects data. This method is suitable for diffusion of innovation, network analysis, decision-making.
- *Double sampling:* In this method sampling is drawn twice. For the first time a large size of sample is selected and send the mailed questionnaire to the respondents (say 500) after receiving back the answered questionnaire (say 300, as all mailed questionnaire do not come back,) the investigator again randomly draws the required number of sample (say 100) and send the modified questionnaire to the respondents. This method is time consuming and expensive.

DATA COLLECTION

Data collection is the process of getting the information (data) that is useful to the study, and which will enable the researcher to answer the research questions and/or test the hypotheses. It is an important step in the research process because those samples selected from the population will now have the opportunity of contributing to the research by providing the data.

INSTRUMENTS OF DATA COLLECTION

For checking new, unknown data required for the study of any problem you may use various devices, instruments, apparatus and appliances. For each and every type of research we need certain instruments to gather new facts or to explore new fields. The instruments thus employed as means for collecting data are called tools.

The selection of suitable instruments or tools is of vital importance for successful research. Different tools are suitable for collecting various kinds of information for various purposes. The research worker may use one or more of the tools in combination for his/her purpose. Research students should therefore familiarize themselves with the varieties of tools with their nature, merits and limitations. They should also know how to construct and use them effectively. The systematic way and procedure by which a complex or scientific task is accomplished is known as the technique. Techniques are the practical method, skill or art applied to a particulate task. So, as a researcher we should aware of both the tools and techniques of research.

The major tools of research in education can be classified broadly into the following categories.

RATING SCALE

Rating scale is one of the enquiry forms. That is a term applied to expression or judgment regarding some situation, object or character. Opinions are usually expressed on a scale of values.

Rating techniques are devices by which such judgments maybe quantified. Rating scale is a very useful device in assessing quality, especially when quality is difficult to measure objectively. For example, 'How good was the performance?' is a question which can hardly be answered objectively.

Rating scales record judgment or opinions and indicates the degree or amount of different degrees of quality which are arranged along a line is the scale. For example, how good was the performance?

Excellent Very good Good Average Below Average Poor Very poor

___|________|_______|_____|_________|_________|_____|____

This is the most commonly used instrument for making appraisals. It has a large variety of forms and uses. Typically, they direct attention to a number of aspects or traits of the thing to be rated and provide a scale for assigning values to each of the aspects selected. They try to measure the nature or degree of certain aspects or characteristics of a person or phenomenon through the use of a series of numbers, qualitative terms or verbal descriptions.

Ratings can be obtained through one of three major approaches:

a. Paired comparison
b. Ranking and
c. Rating scales

The first attempt at rating personality characteristics was the man to man technique devised curing World-war-I. This technique calls for a panel of raters to rate every individual in comparison to a standard person. This is known as the paired comparison approach.

In the ranking approach every single individual in a group is compared with every other individual and to arrange the judgment in the form of a scale.

In the rating scale approach which is the more common and practical method rating is based on the rating scales, a procedure which consists of assigning to each trait being rated a scale value giving a valid estimate of its status and then comparing the separate ratings into an overall score.

Purpose of Rating Scale

Rating scales have been successfully utilized for measuring the following:

- Teacher Performance/effectiveness.
- Personality, anxiety, stress, emotional intelligence, etc.
- School appraisal including appraisal of courses, practices and programs.

Useful Hints on Construction of Rating Scale

A rating scale includes three factors like:

a. The subjects or the phenomena to be rated
b. The continuum along which they will be rated
c. The judges who will do the rating.

All taken three factors should be carefully take care by you when you construct the rating scale.

1. The subjects or phenomena to be rated are usually a limited number of aspects of a thing or of a traits of a person. Only the most significant aspects for the purpose of the study should be chosen. The usual may to get judgment is on five to seven point scales as we have already discussed.
2. The rating scale is always composed of two parts:
   a. An instruction which names the subject and defines the continuum
   b. A scale which defines the points to be used in rating.
3. Anyone can serve as a rater where non-technical opinions, likes and dislikes and matters of easy observation are to be rated. But only well informed and experienced persons should be selected for rating where technical competence is required. Therefore, you should select experts in the field as rater or a person who form a sample of the population in which the scale will subsequently be applied. Pooled judgments increase the reliability of any rating scale. So employ

several judges, depending on the rating situation to obtain desirable reliability.

Advantages

- Rating scales are used for testing the validity of many objective instruments like paper pencil inventories of personality
- Helpful in writing reports to parents
- Helpful in filling out admission blanks for colleges
- Helpful in finding out student needs
- Making recommendations to employers
- Supplementing other sources of understanding about the child
- Stimulating effect upon the individuals who are rated.

Limitations

As it knows that the raters would not like to run down their own people by giving them low ratings. So in that case they give high ratings to almost all cases. Sometimes also the raters are included to be unduly generous in rating aspects which they had to opportunity to observe. It the raters rate in higher side due to those factors, then it is called as the generosity error of rating.

- *The errors of central tendency:* Some observes wants to keep them in safe position. Therefore, they rate near the midpoint of the scale. They rate almost all as average.
- *Stringency error:* Stringency error is just the opposite of generosity of error. These types of raters are very strict, cautions and hesitant in rating in average and higher side. They have a tendency to rate all individuals low.
- *The hallo error:* When a rater rates one aspect influenced by other is called hallo effect. For if a person will be rated in higher side on his achievement because of his punctually or sincerely irrespective of his perfect answer it called as hallo effect. The biasedness of the rater affects from one quality to other.
- *The logical error:* It is difficult to convey to the rater just what quality one wishes him to evaluate. An adjective or adverb may have no universal meaning. It the terms are not properly understood by the rater and he rates, then it is called as the logical error. Therefore, brief behavioral statements having clear objectives should be used.

ATTITUDE SCALE

Attitude scale is a form of appraisal procedure and it is also one of the enquiry term. Attitude scales have been designed to measure attitude of a subject of group of subjects towards issues, institutions and group of peoples.

The term attitude is defined in various ways:

- According to *LL Bernard* 'the behavior which we define as attitudinal or attitude is a certain observable set organism or relative tendency preparatory to and indicative of more complete adjustment'.
- According to *Barr David Johnson* 'An attitude maybe defined as a learned emotional response, set for or against something'.

An attitude is spoken of as a tendency of an individual to read in a certain way towards a phenomenon. It is what a person feels or believes in. It is the inner feeling of an individual. It maybe positive, negative or neutral.

Opinion and attitude are used sometimes in a synonymous manner but there is a difference between two. You will be able to know when we will discuss about opinionnaire. An opinion may not lead to any kind of activity in a particular direction. But an attitude compels one to act either favorably or unfavorably according to what they perceive to be correct. We can evaluate attitude through questionnaire. But it is ill adapted for scaling accurately the intensity of an attitude. Therefore, attitude scale is essential as it attempts to minimize the difficulty of opinionnaire and questionnaire by defining the attitude in terms of a single attitude object. All items, therefore, maybe constructed with graduations of favor or disfavor.

Purpose of Attitude Scale

In educational research, these scales are used especially for finding the attitudes of persons on different issues like:

- Co-education
- Religious education
- Corporal punishment
- Democracy in schools
- Linguistic prejudices
- International cooperation, etc.

Characteristics of Attitude Scale

Attitude scale should have the following characteristics:

- It provides for quantitative measure on a uni-dimensional scale of continuum
- It uses statements from the extreme positive to extreme negative position
- It generally uses a five point scale as we have discussed in rating scale
- It could be standardized and norms are worked out

- It disguises the attitude object rather than directly asking about the attitude on the subject.

Examples of Some Attitude Scale

Two popular and useful methods of measuring attitudes indirectly, commonly used for research purposes are:

a. Thurstone techniques of scaled values.

b. Likert's method of summated ratings.

Thurstone Technique

Thurstone Technique is used when attitude is accepted as a uni-dimensional linear Continuum. The procedure is simple. A large number of statements of various shades of favorable and unfavorable opinion on slips of paper, which a large number of judges exercising complete detachment sort out into eleven plies ranging from the most hostile statements to the most favorable ones. The opinions are carefully worded so as to be clear and unequivocal. The judges are asked not express tier opinion but to sort them at their face value. The items which bring out a marked disagreement between the judges un assigning a position are discarded. Tabulations are made which indicate the number of judges who placed each item in each category. The next step consists of calculating cumulated proportions for each item and Ogives are constructed. Scale values of each item are read from the Ogives, the values of each item being that point along the baseline in terms of scale value units above and below which 50% of the judges placed the item. It we will be the median of the frequency distribution in which the score ranges from 0 to 11.

The respondent is to give his/her reaction to each statement by endorsing or rejecting it. The median values of the statements that he/she checks establishes his/her score, or quantifies his/her opinion. He/she wins a score as an average of the sum of the values of the statements he/she endores.

Thurstone technique is also known as the technique equal appearing intervals.

Sample Items from Thurstone Type Scales

Statement	Scaled Value
I think this company treats its employees.	10.4
Better than any other company does.	9.5
It I had to do it over again I would still work for this company.	5.1
The workers put as much over on the company as the company puts over on them.	2.1
You have got to have pulled with certain people around here to get ahead. An honest man fails in this company.	0.8

Likert Scale

- The Likert scale uses items worded for or against the proposition, with five point rating response indicating the strength of the respondent's approval or disapproval of the statement. This method removes the necessity of submitting items to the judges for working out scaled values for each item. It yields scores very similar to those obtained from the Thurstone scale. It is an important over the Thurstone method.
- The first step is the collection of a member of statements about the subject in question. Statements may or may not be correct but they must be representative of opinion held by a substantial number of people. They must express definite favorableness or unfavorableness to a particular point of view. The number of favorable and unfavorable statements should be approximately equal. A trial test maybe administered to a number of subjects.
- Only those items that correlate with the total test should be retained. The Likerts calling techniques assigns a scale value to each of the five responses. All favorable statements are scored from maximum to minimum, i. e. from a score of 5 to a score of one or 5 for strongly agree and so on 1 for strongly disagree. The negative statement or statement opposing the proposition would be scored in the opposite order, i.e. from a score of 1 to a score of 5 or 1 for strongly agree and so on 5 for strongly disagree.
- The total of these scores on all the items measures a respondent's favorableness towards the subject in question. It a scale consists of 30 items, say, the following score values will be of interest.

30 × 5 = 150 Most favorable response possible
30 × 3 = 90 A neutral attitude
30 × 1 = 30 Most unfavorable attitude

It is thus known as a method of summated ratings. The summed-up score of any individual would fall between 30 and 150. Scores above 50 will indicate a favorable and scores below go an unfavorable attitude.

Sample Items from Likert Type Minnesota Scale on Morale

Responses	Items
SA A U D SD	Times are getting better.
SA A U D SD	Any man with ability and willingness to work hard has a good chance of being successful.
SA A U D SD	Life is just a series of disappointments.
SA A U D SD	It is great to be living in those exciting times.
SA A U D SD	Success is more dependent on lack than on real ability.

Limitations of Attitude Scale

- An individual may express socially acceptable opinion conceal his real attitude
- An individual may not be a good judge of him and may not be clearly aware of his real attitude
- He may not have been controlled with a real situation to discover what his real attitude towards a specific phenomenon was
- There is no basis for believing that the five positions indicated in the Likert's scale are equally spaced
- It is unlikely that the statements are of equal value in 'forness' or 'againstness'
- It is doubtful whether equal scores obtained by several individuals would indicate equal favorableness towards again position
- It is unlikely that respondent can validity react to a short statement on a printed form in the absence of real like qualifying situation
- In spite of anonymity of response, individuals tend to respond according to what they should feel rather than what they really feel.

OPINIONNAIRE

According to Anna Anastusi that 'Opinion polling or opinion gauging is represents a single question approach. The answers are usually in the form of 'yes' or 'no'. An undecided category is often included. Sometimes large number of response alternatives if provided'.

The terms opinion and attitude are not synonymous, through sometimes we used it synonymously. We have till now discussed that attitudes scale. We have also discussed that attitudes are impressed opinions. You can now understand the difference between opinionnaire and attitude scale, when we discuss of out opinionnaire, it is characteristics and purposes.

Opinion is what a person says on certain aspects of the issue under considerations. It is an outward expression of an attitude held by an individual. Attitudes of an individual can be inferred or estimated from his statements of opinions.

An opinionnaire is defined as a special form of inquiry. It is used by the researcher to collect the opinions of a sample of population on certain facts or factors the problem under investigation. These opinions on different facts of the problem under study are further quantified, analyzed and interpreted.

Purpose

Opinionnaire are usually used in researches of the descriptive type which demands survey of opinions of the concerned individuals. Public opinion research is an example of opinion survey. Opinion polling enables the researcher to forecast the coming happenings in successful manner.

Characteristics

- The opinionnaire makes use of statements or questions on different aspects of the problem under investigation
- Responses are expected either on three point or five point scales
- It uses favorable or unfavorable statements
- It maybe sub-divided into sections
- The gally poll ballots generally make use of questions instead of statements
- The public opinion polls generally rely on personal contacts rather than mail ballots.

Sample Items of Opinionnaire

The following statements are from the opinionnaire on the reforms in educational administration introduced:

S.No.	Items	Agree	Undecided	Disagree
1.	Democratic decentralization has helped to develop democratic values and practices in rural people.			
2.	It has been consequent improvements of educational standards.			
3.	Specified subject inspectorate is better than panel type of inspectorate.			
4.	Inspection stripped of administrative powers does not help much.			
5.	Primary education should be brought under a separate directorate as was done in some status.			

QUESTIONNAIRE

A questionnaire is a form prepared and distributed to secure responses to certain questions. It is a device for securing answers to questions by using a form which the respondent fills by himself. It is a systematic compilation of questions that are submitted to a sampling of population from which information is desired.

Questionnaire really on written information supplied directly by people in response to questions. The information from questionnaires tends to fall into two broad categories: 'facts' and 'opinions'. It is worth stressing that, in practice, questionnaires are very likely to include questions about both facts and opinions.

Purpose

The purpose of the questionnaire is to gather information from widely scattered sources. It is mostly used in uses in cases where one cannot readily see personally all of the people from whom he desires responses. It is also used where there is no particular reason to see them personality.

Types

Questionnaire can be of various type on the basis of its preparation. They are like:

- Structured vs Nonstructured
- Closed vs Open
- Fact vs Opinion
- *Structured vs Non-structured questionnaire:* The structured questionnaire contains definite, concrete and directed questions, whereas nonstructured questionnaire is often used in interview and guide. It may consist of partially completed questions.
- *Closed vs open questionnaire:* The question that call for short check responses are known as restricted or closed form type. For example, they provide for marking a yes or no, a short response or checking an item from a list of responses. Here the respondent is not free to write of his/her own, he/she was to select from the selected from the supplied responses. On the other hand, increase of open ended questionnaire, the respondent is free to response in his/her own words. Many questionnaires also included both close and open type questions. The researcher selects the type of questionnaire according to his/her need of the study.
- *Fact and opinion:* In case of fact questionnaire, the respondent is expected to give information of facts without any reference to his opinion or attitude about them. But in case of opinion questionnaire

the respondent gives the information about the facts with his/her own opinion and attitude.

Characteristics of a Good Questionnaire

- Questionnaire should deal with important or significant topic to create interest among respondents
- It should seek only that data which cannot be obtained from other sources
- It should be as short as possible but should be comprehensive
- It should be attractive
- Directions should be clear and complete
- It should be represented in good psychological order proceeding from general to more specific responses
- Double negatives in questions should be avoided
- Putting two questions in one question also should be avoided
- It should avoid annoying or embarrassing questions
- It should be designed to collect information which can be used subsequently as data for analysis
- It should consist of a written list of questions
- The questionnaire should also be used appropriately.

When is it Appropriate to Use a Questionnaire for Research?

Different methods are better suited to different circumstances and questionnaires are no exception to it. Questionnaires are used at their most productive:

- When used with large numbers of respondents
- When what is required tends to be fairly straight forward information
- When there is a need for standardize data from identical information
- When time is allows for delays
- When resources allow for the cast of printing and postage
- When respondents can be expected to be able to read and understand the questions.

Designs of Questionnaire

After construction of questions on the basis of its characteristics it should be designed with some essential routines like:

- Background information about the questionnaire
- Instructions to the respondent
- The allocation of serial numbers
- Coding boxes.

Background Information about the Questionnaire

Both from ethical and practical point of view, the researcher needs to provide sufficient background information about the research and the questionnaire. Each questionnaire should have a cover page, on which some information appears about:

- The sponsor
- The purpose
- Return address and date
- Confidentiality
- Voluntary responses
- Thanks.

Instructions to the respondent: It is very important that respondents are instructed to go presented at the start of the questionnaire which indicate what is expected from the respondents. Specific instructions should be given for each question where the style of questions varies throughout the questionnaire. For example, Put a tick mark in the appropriate box and circle the relevant number, etc.

The allocation of serial numbers: Whether dealing with small or large numbers, a good researcher needs to keep good records. Each questionnaire therefore should be numbered.

Advantages of Questionnaire

Questionnaires are economical. In terms of materials, money and time it can supply a considerable amount of research data:

- It is easier to arrange
- It supplies standardized answers
- It encourages pre-coded answers
- It permits wide coverage
- It helps in conducting depth study.

Disadvantages

- It is reliable and valid, but slow.
- Pre-coding questions can deter them from answering
- Pre-coded questions can bias the findings towards the researcher
- Postal questionnaire offer little opportunities to check the truthfulness of the answers
- It cannot be used with illiterate and small children.

Irrespective of the limitations general consensus goes in favor of the use of questionnaire. Its quality should be improved and we should be restricted to the situations for which it is suited.

CHECKLIST

A checklist is a type of informational job aid used to reduce failure by compensating for potential limits of human memory and attention. It helps to ensure consisting and completeness in carrying out a task. A basic example is 'to do list'. A more advanced checklist which lays out tasks to be done according to time of a day or other factors.

The checklist consists of a list of items with a place to check, or to mark yes or no.

Purpose

The main purpose of checklist is to call attention to various aspects of an object or situation, to see that nothing of importance is overlooked. For example, if you have to go for outing for a week, you have to list what things you have to take with you. Before leaving home, if you will check your baggage with the least there will be less chance of forgetting to take any important things, like toothbrush, etc. it ensures the completeness of details of the data.

Responses to the checklist items are largely a matter of fact, not of judgment. It is an important tool in gathering facts for educational surveys.

Uses of Checklist

Checklists are used for various purposes. As we have discussed that we can check our requirements for journey, birthday list, proforma for passport, submitting examination form or admission form, etc. in every case, it we will check before doing the work, then there is less chance of overlooking any, important things.

As it is useful in over daily life, it is also useful in educational field in the following way:

- To collect acts for educational surveys.
- To record behavior in observational studies.
- To use in educational appraisal, studies of school buildings, property, plan, textbooks, instructional procedures and outcomes, etc.
- To rate the personality
- To know the interest of the subjects also. Kuder's interest inventory and Strong's Interest Blank are also checklists.

Hints on Constructing Checklist

- Items in the checklist maybe continuous or divided into groups of related items

- Items should be arranged in categories and the categories in a logical or psychological order
- Terms used in the items should be clearly defined
- Checklist should be continuous and comprehensive in nature
- A pilot study should be taken to make it standardized
- Checklist can be constructed in four different ways by arranging items differently.
    I. In one of the arrangement all items found in a situation are to be checked. For example, a subject maybe asked to check ( ) in the blank side of each activity undertaken in a school.
    II. In the second form, the respondent is asked to check with a 'yes' or 'no' or asked to encircle or underline the response to the given item. For example, (1) Does your school have a house system?
    III. Yes/No
    IV. In this form, all the items are positive statements with checks ( ) to be marked in a column of a right. For Example, (1) The school functions as a community center ( ).
    V. The periodical tests are held: fortnightly, monthly, quarterly, and regularly.
    VI. The investigator has to select anyone of the format appropriate to his problem and queries or the combination of many as it requires.

Analysis and Interpretation of Checklist Data

The tabulation and quantification of checklist data is done from the responses. Frequencies are counted, percentages and averages calculated, central tendencies, measures of variability and co-efficient of correlation completed as and when necessary. In long checklists, where related items are grouped together category wise, the checks are added up to give total scores for the category wise total scores can be compared between themselves or with similar scores secured through other studies.

The conclusions from checklist data should be arrived at carefully and judiciously keeping in view the limitations of the tools and respondents.

Advantages

- Students can measure their own behavior with the help of checklist
- Easy and simple to use and frame the tools
- Wanted and unwanted behaviors can be included
- Personal social development can be checked.

Limitations

- Only the presence or absence of the ability can be tested
- Yes or no type judgment can only be given
- How much cannot be tested through checklist.

For example, you want to test the story telling still of a student. You can check only whether the student developed or not developed the skill but you cannot study how much he/she has developed? When the researcher wants to check 'yes' or 'no' of any ability, the checklist can be used.

PSYCHOLOGICAL TESTS

Among the most useful and most frequently employed tools of educational research psychological tests occupy a very significant position. Psychological tests are described to describe and measure a sample of certain aspects of human behavior or inner qualities.

They yield objective descriptions of some psychological aspects of an individual's personality and translate them in quantitative terms.

As we have mentioned earlier there are various kinds of psychological tests. In this unit we will discuss 'Aptitude tests' and 'Inventories'.

Aptitude tests: 'Aptitude tests attempt to predict the capacities or the degree of achievement that maybe expected from individuals in a particular activity'.

Aptitude is a means by which one can find the relative knowledge of a person in terms of his intelligence and also his knowledge in general.

Purpose

The purpose of aptitude test is to test a candidate's profile. Aptitude test helps to check one's knowledge and filters the good candidates. The ability of creativity and intelligence is proved by the aptitude test. It always checks the intelligence and fastness of the person in performance.

Importance of Aptitude Test

Research data show that individually administered aptitude tests have the following qualities:

- They are excellent predictors of future scholastic achievement
- They provide ways for comparison of a child's performance with other in a same situation
- They provide a profile of strength and weaknesses
- They assess difference among individuals.

Uses of Aptitude Test

Aptitude tests are valuable in making program and curricula decisions. In general they have three major uses:

- *Instructional:* Teacher can use aptitude test results to adopt their curricula to match the level of students or to design assignments for students who differ widely.
- *Administrative:* Result of aptitude tests help in determining the programs for college on the basis of aptitude level of high school. It can also be identify students to be accelerated or given extra attention, for exampling and in predicting job training performance.
- *Guidance:* It helps the counsellors to help the parents and students. Parents develop realistic expectations for their Child's performance and students understand their own strength and weaknesses.

Intelligence tests are also a kind of aptitude test as they describe and measure the general ability which enters into the performance of every activity and thus predict the degree of achievement that maybe expected from individuals in various activities.

Aptitude test, however have proved of great value for research in educational and vocational guidance, for research in selection of candidates for particular course of study or professional training and for research of the complex causal relationship type.

CHARACTERISTICS OF DATA COLLECTION

Measurement is the assigning of numbers to observations in order to quantify phenomena. In health care, many of these phenomena, such as quality of life, patient adherence, morbidity, and drug efficacy, are abstract concepts known as theoretical constructs. Measurement involves the operationalization of these constructs in defined variables and the development and application of instruments or tests to quantify these variables. Key indicators of the quality of a measuring instrument are the reliability and validity of the measures. In addition, the responsiveness of the measure to change is of interest in many health care applications where improvement in outcomes as a result of treatment is a primary goal of research.

Validity and reliability are two important characteristics of behavioral measure and are referred to as psychometric properties.

VALIDITY

Validity is often defined as the extent to which an instrument measures what it purports to measure. Validity requires that an instrument is reliable, but an instrument can be reliable without being valid. For example, a scale that is incorrectly calibrated may yield exactly the same, albeit inaccurate, weight values. A multiple choice test intended to evaluate the counselling skills of nursing students may yield reliable scores, but it may actually evaluate drug knowledge rather than the ability to communicate effectively with patients in making a recommendation.

While we speak of the validity of a test or instrument, validity is not a property of the test itself. Instead, validity is the extent to which the interpretations of the results of a test are warranted, which depends on the test's intended use (i.e. measurement of the underlying construct). Much of the research conducted in health care involves quantifying attributes that cannot be measured directly. Instead, hypothetical or abstract concepts (constructs), such as severity of disease, drug efficacy, drug safety, burden of illness, patient satisfaction, health literacy, quality of life, quality of provider patient communication, and adherence to medical regimens, are measured.

Hypothetical constructs cannot be measured directly and can only be inferred from observations of specified behaviors or phenomena that are thought to be indicators of the presence of the construct. Measurement of a construct requires that the conceptual definition be translated into an operational definition. An operational definition of a construct links the conceptual or theoretical definition to more concrete indicators that have numbers applied to signify the 'amount' of the construct.

Validity evidence is built overtime, with validations occurring in a variety of populations. Comprehensive literature reviews on measurement approaches are therefore critical in guiding the selection of measures and measurement instruments.

- *Face validity:* The concern of face validity is to not alienate the test taker. Basically face validity is to what extent, to the naïve, casual test-taker does the test measure what it purports to measure. If an employee is completing a measure of job satisfaction, but realizes that there are items that appear to be geared toward honesty or integrity, the validity of the job satisfaction measure maybe diminished because of the lack of face validity.
- *Construct validity:* This type of validity is a judgment based on the accumulation of evidence from numerous studies using a specific measuring instrument. Evaluation of construct validity requires examining the relationship of the measure being evaluated with variables known to be related or theoretically related to the construct measured by the instrument. For example, a measure of quality of life would be expected to result in lower scores for chronically ill patients than for healthy college students. Correlations that fit the expected pattern contribute evidence of construct validity. All evidence of

validity, including content- and criterion-related validity, contributes to the evidence of construct validity.

- *Content validity:* This type of validity addresses how well the items developed to operationalize a construct provide an adequate and representative sample of all the items that might measure the construct of interest. Because there is no statistical test to determine whether a measure adequately covers a content area or adequately represents a construct, content validity usually depends on the judgment of experts in the field.
- *Criterion-related validity:* This type of validity provides evidence about how well scores on the new measure correlate with other measures of the same construct or very similar underlying constructs that theoretically should be related. It is crucial that these criterion measures are valid themselves. With one type of criterion-related validity—predictive validity—the criterion measurement is obtained at sometime after the administration of the test, and the ability of the test to accurately predict the criterion is evaluated. For example, surrogate outcomes such as blood pressure and cholesterol levels are based on their predictive validity in projecting the risk of cardiovascular disease, even though some of these associations have been recently questioned. Another type of criterion-related validity is concurrent validity. In establishing concurrent validity, scores on an instrument are correlated with scores on another (criterion) measure of the same construct or a highly related construct that is measured concurrently in the same subjects. Ideally, the criterion measure would be considered to be the gold standard measure of the construct. This strategy of determining the validity of a measure might be seen in a situation in which a new instrument has some advantage over the gold standard measure, such as an increased ease of use or reduced time or expense of administration. These advantages would justify the time and effort involved in the development and validation of a new instrument. An example of such a situation is a researcher developing a self-administered version of an instrument that had been validated for person-to-person interviewer administration.

RELIABILITY

According to classical test theory, any score obtained by a measuring instrument (the observed score) is composed of both the 'true' score, which is unknown, and 'error' in the measurement process.

The true score is essentially the score that a person would have received if the measurement were perfectly accurate. The process of developing and validating an instrument is in large part focused on reducing error in the measurement process. There are different means of estimating the reliability of any measure. According to Crocker and Algina, 1 the test developer has a responsibility to "identify the sources of measurement error that would be most detrimental to useful score interpretation and design a reliability study that permits such errors to occur so that their effects can be assessed." Pretesting or pilot testing an instrument allows for the identification of such sources.

Refinement of the instrument then focuses on minimizing measurement error.

Reliability estimates are used to evaluate (1) the stability of measures administered at different times to the same individuals or using the same standard (test-retest reliability) or (2) the equivalence of sets of items from the same test (internal consistency) or of different observers scoring a behavior or event using the same instrument (interrater reliability). Reliability coefficients range from 0.00 to 1.00, with higher coefficients indicating higher levels of reliability.

- *Stability:* Stability of measurement, or test-retest reliability, is determined by administering a test at two different points in time to the same individuals and determining the correlation or strength of association of the two sets of scores.

  The same process maybe used when calibrating a medical measurement device, such as a scale. The timing of the second administration is critical when tests are administered repeatedly.

  Ideally, the interval between administrations should be long enough that values obtained from the second administration will not be affected by the previous measurement (e.g. a subject's memory of responses to the first administration of a knowledge tests, the clinical response to an invasive test procedure) but not so distant that learning or a change in health status could alter the way subjects respond during the second administration.
- *Internal consistency:* Internal consistency gives an estimate of the equivalence of sets of items from the same test (e.g. a set of questions aimed at assessing quality of life or disease severity). The coefficient of internal consistency provides an estimate of the reliability of measurement and is based on the assumption that items measuring the same construct should correlate. Perhaps the most widely used method for estimating internal consistency reliability is Cronbach's alpha. Cronbach's alpha is a function of the average inters correlations of items and the number of items in the scale.

  It is used for summated scales such as quality-of-life instruments, activities of daily living scales, and the Mini Mental State Examination. All things being equal, the greater the number of items in a summated scale, the higher Cronbach's alpha tends to be, with the major gains being in additional items up to approximately 10, when the increase in reliability for each additional item levels off.

This is one reason why the use of a single item to measure a construct is not optimal. Having multiple items to measure a construct aids in the determination of the reliability of measurement and, in general, improves the reliability or precision of the measurement.

- *Split-half reliability:* Requires only one administration, especially appropriate when the test is very long. The most commonly used method to split the test into two is using the odd-even strategy. Since longer tests tend to be more reliable, and since split-half reliability represents the reliability of a test only half as long as the actual test, a correction formula must be applied to the coefficient. Spearman-Brown prophecy formula is used. Split-half reliability is a form of internal consistency reliability.
- *Interrater reliability:* Interrater reliability (also called inter observer agreement) establishes the equivalence of ratings obtained with an instrument when used by different observers. If a measurement process involves judgments or ratings by observers, a reliable measurement will require consistency between different raters. Interrater reliability requires completely independent ratings of the same event by more than one rater. No discussion or collaboration can occur when reliability is being tested. Reliability is determined by the correlation of the scores from two or more independent raters (for ratings on a continuum) or the coefficient of agreement of the judgments of the raters. For categorical variables, Cohen's 5 kappa is commonly used to determine the coefficient of agreement. 2 Kappa is used when two raters or observers classify events or observations into categories based on rating criteria. Rather than a simple percent agreement, kappa takes into account the agreement that could be expected by chance alone. Often, observational instruments or rating scales are developed to evaluate the behaviors of subjects who are being directly observed.

However, any measure that relies on the judgments of raters or reviewers requires evidence that any independent, trained expert would come to the same conclusion. Thus, interrater reliability should be established when data are abstracted from medical charts or when diagnoses or assessments are made for research purposes. Interrater reliability in research such as this depends on developing precise operational definitions of variables being measured as well as having observers well trained to use the instrument. Interrater reliability is optimized when criteria are explicit and raters are trained to apply the criteria. Raters must be trained how to make a decision that an event has occurred or how to determine which point on a scale measuring strength or degree of a phenomenon (e.g. a 3-point scale measuring seriousness of a disease) should be applied. The more that individual judgment is involved in a rating, the more crucial it is that independent observers agree when applying the scoring criteria.

Before data gathering begins, training should include multiple cases in which raters respond to simulated situations they will encounter and rate, interrater reliability is calculated, disagreements are clarified, and a criterion level of agreement is met. Interrater reliability should again be verified throughout the study. Even when established observational instruments are being used or criteria are explicit, research that relies on observations or judgments should check reliability, and the study protocol should include procedures to determine the level of observer agreement.

In most studies, a percentage of observations (e.g. number of charts reviewed) is randomly selected for scoring by two independent raters rather than requiring that two raters judge all observations. In addition, data to establish the consistency with which the primary rater applies the criteria overtime are important for establishing the reliability of the instrument.

Rater drift can occur when an individual rater alters the way he or she applies the scoring criteria (i.e. becoming more lenient or stringent) overtime. Investigators who build in reliability checks throughout the study as data are collected rather than waiting until the end of data collection can identify instances where interrater reliability has begun to deteriorate, perhaps due to rater drift.

TECHNIQUES OF DATA COLLECTION

In dealing with any real life problem it is often found that data at hand are inadequate, and hence, it becomes necessary to collect data that are appropriate. There are several ways of collecting the appropriate data which differ considerably in context of money costs, time and other resources at the disposal of the researcher.

Primary data can be collected either through experiment or through survey. If the researcher conducts an experiment, he observes some quantitative measurements, or the data, with the help of which he examines the truth contained in his hypothesis. But in the case of a survey, data can be collected by anyone or more of the following ways:

Observation

Observational techniques are methods by which an individual or individuals gather firsthand data on programs, processes, or behaviors being studied. They provide evaluators with an opportunity to collect data on a wide range of behaviors, to capture a great variety of interactions, and to openly explore the evaluation topic. By directly observing operations and activities, the evaluator can develop a holistic perspective, i.e. an understanding of the context within which the project operates. This maybe especially important where it is not the event that is of interest, but rather how that event may fit into, or be affected by, a sequence of events. Observational approaches also allow the evaluator to learn about issues the participants or staff maybe unaware of or that they are unwilling or unable to discuss candidly in an interview or focus group.

When to Use Observations

Observations can be useful during both the formative and summative phases of evaluation. For example, during the formative phase, observations can be useful in determining whether or not the project is being delivered and operated as planned. During the summative phase, observations can be used to determine whether or not the project has been successful. The technique would be especially useful in directly examining teaching methods employed by the faculty in their own classes after program participation. Exhibit 16 shows the advantages and disadvantages of observations.

Advantages:

- It provides direct information about behavior of individuals and groups
- It permits evaluator to enter into and understand situation/context
- It provides good opportunities for identifying unanticipated outcomes
- It exists in natural, unstructured, and flexible setting.

Disadvantages

- It is expensive and time consuming
- It needs well-qualified, highly trained observers; may need to be content experts
- It may affect behavior of participants
- Selective perception of observer may distort data
- Behavior or set of behaviors observed maybe atypical.

Survey or Questionnaire

Surveys are a very popular form of data collection, especially when gathering information from large groups, where standardization is important. Surveys can be constructed in many ways, but they always consist of two components: questions and responses. While sometimes evaluators choose to keep responses 'open ended', i.e. allow respondents to answer in a free flowing narrative form; most often the 'close-ended' approach in which respondents are asked to select from a range of predetermined answers is adopted. Open-ended responses maybe difficult to code and require more time and resources to handle than close-ended choices. Responses may take the form of a rating on some scale (e.g. rate a given statement from 1 to 4 on a scale from 'agree' to 'disagree'), may give categories from which to choose (e.g. select from potential categories of partner institutions with which a program could be involved), or may require estimates of numbers or percentages of time in which participants might engage in an activity (e.g. the percentage of time spent on teacher-led instruction or cooperative learning).

Although surveys are popularly referred to as paper-and-pencil instruments, this too is changing. Evaluators are increasingly exploring the utility of survey methods that take advantage of the emerging technologies. Thus, surveys maybe administered via computer-assisted calling, as e-mail attachments, and as web-based online data collection systems. Even the traditional approach of mailing surveys for self-guided response has been supplemented by using facsimile for delivery and return.

Selecting the best method for collecting surveys requires weighing a number of factors. These included the complexity of questions, resources available, the project schedule, etc. For example, web-based surveys are attractive for a number of reasons. First, because the data collected can be put directly into a database, the time and steps between data collection and analysis can be shortened. Second, it is possible to build in checks that keep out-of-range responses from being entered.

However, at this time, unless the survey is fairly simple (no skip patterns, limited use of matrices), the technology needed to develop such surveys can require a significant resource investment. As new tools are developed for commercial use, this problem should diminish.

When to Use Surveys

Surveys are typically selected when information is to be collected from a large number of people or when answers are needed to a clearly defined set of questions. Surveys are good tools for obtaining information on a wide range of topics when in-depth probing of responses is not necessary, and they are useful for both formative and summative purposes.

Frequently, the same survey is used at spaced intervals of time to measure progress along some dimension or change in behavior.

Advantages:

- It is good for gathering descriptive data
- It can cover a wide range of topics
- These are relatively inexpensive to use
- It can be analyzed using a variety of existing software.

Disadvantages:

- Self-report may lead to biased reporting.

- Data may provide a general picture but lack depth.
- May not provide adequate information on context.

Interview

The use of interviews as a data collection method begins with the assumption that the participants' perspectives are meaningful, knowable, and can be made explicit, and that their perspectives affect the success of the project. An in-person or telephone interview, rather than a paper and pencil survey, is selected when interpersonal contact is important and when opportunities for follow-up of interesting comments are desired.

Two types of interviews are used in evaluation research: structured interviews, in which a carefully worded questionnaire is administered, and in-depth interviews, in which the interviewer does not follow a rigid form. In the former, the emphasis is on obtaining answers to carefully phrased questions. Interviewers are trained to deviate only minimally from the question wording to ensure uniformity of interview administration. In the latter, however, the interviewers seek to encourage free and open responses, and there maybe a trade off between comprehensive coverage of topics and in-depth exploration of a more limited set of questions. In-depth interviews also encourage capturing respondents' perceptions in their own words, a very desirable strategy in qualitative data collection. This allows the evaluator to present the meaningfulness of the experience from the respondent's perspective. In-depth interviews are conducted with individuals or a small group of individuals.

When to Use Interviews

Interviews can be used at any stage of the evaluation process. In-depth interviews are especially useful in answering questions such as those suggested by Patton (1990):

- What does the program look and feel like to the participants?
- What do students know about the project?
- What thoughts do students knowledgeable about the program have concerning program operations, processes, and outcomes?
- What are participants' and students' expectations?
- What features of the project are most salient to the participants?
- What changes do participants perceive in themselves as a result of their involvement in the project?

Specific circumstances for which in-depth interviews are particularly appropriate include situations involving complex subject matter, detailed information, high-status respondents, and highly sensitive subject matter.

Advantages:

- It usually yields richest data, details, and new insights
- It permits face-to-face contact with respondents
- It provides opportunity to explore topics in-depth
- It allow interviewer to experience the affective as well as cognitive aspects of responses
- It allow interviewer to explain or help clarify questions, increasing the likelihood of useful responses
- It allow interviewer to be flexible in administering interview to particular individuals or in particular circumstances.

Disadvantages:

- It is expensive and time-consuming
- It requires well-qualified, highly trained interviewers
- Interviewee may distort information through recall error, selective perceptions, desire to please interviewer
- Flexibility can result in inconsistencies across interviews
- Volume of information very large; maybe difficult to transcribe and reduce data.

Tests

As data gathering devices, tests are among the most useful tools of educational research, for they provide the data for most experimental and descriptive studies in education. The instruments have been designed to describe and measure sample of aspects of human behavior. These instruments assess variety of human abilities, potentials achievements and behavior tendencies. They possess different degrees of validity reliability and applicability.

Types of Tests

The following types of tests designed for different purposes are briefly described.

- *Achievement test:* Achievement tests attempt to measure what an individual has learned his present level of performance. Most tests used in schools are achievement tests. They are particularly helpful in determining individual or group status in academic learning. Achievement test scores are used in placing, advancing or retaining students at particular grade revels.
- *Aptitude test:* Aptitude tests seek to assess the level of achievement that an individual can attain in some particular academic or vocational field. In other words, aptitude tests attempt to predict an individual capacity to require improved performance with additional training.

- *Personality test:* It is concerned with the non-intellectual aspect of human behavior. Personality scales are usually self-report instruments. The individual check the responses to certain questions or statements. These instruments yield scores, which are assumed or have been shown to measure certain personality traits or tendencies.

Advantages:

- It provides objective information on what the test taker knows and can do
- It can be constructed to match a given curriculum or set of skills
- It can be score in a straightforward manner
- These are accepted by the public as a credible indicator of learning.

Disadvantages:

- It maybe oversimplified and superficial
- It maybe very time consuming
- It maybe biased against some groups of test takers
- It maybe subject to corruption via coaching or cheating.

Focus Groups

Focus groups combine elements of both interviewing and participant observation. The focus group session is, indeed, an interview—not a discussion group, problem-solving session, or decision-making group. At the same time, focus groups capitalize on group dynamics. The hallmark of focus groups is the explicit use of the group interaction to generate data and insights that would be unlikely to emerge otherwise. The technique inherently allows observation of group dynamics, discussion, and firsthand insights into the respondents' behaviors, attitudes, language, etc.

Focus groups are a gathering of 8 to 12 people who share some characteristics relevant to the evaluation. Originally used as a market research tool to investigate the appeal of various products, the focus group technique has been adopted by other fields, such as education, as a tool for data gathering on a given topic. Initially, focus groups took place in a special facility that included recording apparatus (audio and/or visual) and an attached room with a one-way mirror for observation.

There was an official recorder, who may or may not have been in the room. Participants were paid for attendance and provided with refreshments. As the focus group technique has been adopted by fields outside of marketing, some of these features, such as payment or refreshments, have sometimes been eliminated.

When to use Focus Groups

Focus groups can be useful at both the formative and summative stages of an evaluation. They provide answers to the same types of questions as in-depth interviews, except that they take place in a social context.

Specific applications of the focus group method in evaluations include:

- Identifying and defining problems in project implementation
- Pretesting topics or idea
- Identifying project strengths, weaknesses, and recommendations
- Assisting with interpretation of quantitative findings
- Obtaining perceptions of project outcomes and impacts
- Generating new ideas.

Although focus groups and in-depth interviews share many characteristics, they should not be used interchangeably.

Advantages:

- It is quick and relatively easy to set-up
- Group dynamic can provide useful information that individual data collection does not provide
- It is useful in gaining insight into a topic that maybe more difficult to gather information through other data collection methods.

Disadvantages:

- The discussion can be dominated or side tracked by a few individuals
- Data analysis is time consuming and needs to be well planned in advance
- It does not provide valid information at the individual level
- The information is not representative of other groups.

Schedule Method

In case the informants are largely uneducated and non-responsive data cannot be collected by the mailed questionnaire method. In such cases, schedule method is used to collect data. Here the questionnaires are sent through the enumerators to collect information's. Enumerators are persons appointed by the investigator for the purpose. They directly meet the informants with the questionnaire. They explain the scope and objective of the enquiry to the informants and solicit their cooperation. The enumerators ask the questions to the informants and record their answers in the questionnaire and compile them. The success of this method depends on the sincerity and efficiency of the enumerators. So the enumerator should be sweet-tempered, good-natured, trained and well-behaved.

Schedule method is widely used in extensive studies. It gives fairly correct result as the enumerators directly collect the information. The accuracy of the information depends upon the honesty of the enumerators. They should be unbiased. This method is relatively more costly and time-consuming than the mailed questionnaire method.

Difference between Schedule and Questionnaire

S.No	Questionnaire	Schedule
1.	Questionnaire is generally sent through mail to informants to be answered as specified in a covering letter, but otherwise without further assistance from the sender.	A schedule is generally filled by the research worker or enumerator, who can interpret the questions when necessary.
2.	Data collection is cheap and economical as the money is spent in preparation of questionnaire and in mailing the same to respondents.	Data collection is more expensive as money is spent on enumerators and in imparting trainings to them. Money is also spent in preparing schedules.
3.	Non response is usually high as many people do not respond and many return the questionnaire without answering all questions. Bias due to non response often remains indeterminate.	Non response is very low because this is filled by enumerators who are able to get answers to all questions. But even in this their remains the danger of interviewer bias and cheating.
4.	It is not clear that who replies.	Identity of respondent is not known.
5.	The questionnaire method is likely to be very slow since many respondents do not return the questionnaire.	Information is collected well in time as they are filled by enumerators.
6.	No personal contact is possible in case of questionnaire as the questionna ires are sent to respondents by post who also in turn returns the same by post.	Direct personal contact is established
7.	This method can be used only when respondents are literate and cooperative.	The information can be gathered even when the respondents happen to be illiterate.
8.	Wider and more representative distribution of sample is possible.	There remains the difficulty in sending enumerators over a relatively wider area.

Contd...

Contd...

S.No	Questionnaire	Schedule
9.	Risk of collecting incomplete and wrong information is relatively more under the questionnaire method, when people are unable to understand questions properly.	The information collected is generally complete and accurate as enumerators can remove difficulties if any faced by respondents in correctly understanding the questions. As a result the information collected through schedule is relatively more accurate than that obtained through questionnaires.
10.	The success of questionnaire methods lies more on the quality of the questionnaire itself.	It depends upon the honesty and competence of enumerators
11.	The physical appearance of questionnaire must be quite attractive.	This may not be the case as schedules are to be filled in by enumerators and not by respondents.
12.	This is not possible when collecting data through questionnaire.	Along with schedule observation method can also be used.

SUMMARY

In this unit, we discuss about the sampling and types of sampling are the scientific or probability sampling and the non-scientific or non-probability sampling. The major difference between the two is that while the scientific sampling method allows every member of the population a chance of being selected as a sample, the non-probability method depends more on the decisions of the researcher. The purpose of collecting new relevant data foe a research study, the investigator needs to select proper instruments termed as tools and techniques. Data collection is the step in the research process where the researcher makes contact with the subjects in order to collect the relevant data. Data collection is very important because it is only with the data that the researcher can answer the research questions or test any hypotheses in the research. There are five major methods of data collection and they include observation, interview, questionnaire, mechanical instruments and paper and pencil tests.

Introduction to Analysis of Data

7 unit

INTRODUCTION

Data analysis involves the processing of the coded data into some orderly and summarized pattern in order to recognize relationships and meet the objectives of the study. Analysis can be viewed as the categorization, the aggregation into constituent parts, and the manipulation of data to obtain answers to the research question or questions underlying the research project. A special aspect of analysis is interpretation. The process of interpretation involves taking the results of analysis, making inferences relevant to the research relationships studied, and drawing managerially useful conclusions about these relationships. The analysis of obtained data represents the end of the research process except for the preparation of the report, and everything done prior to this stage has been done so that the proper analysis can be completed and the research questions can be answered.

An Overview of the Analysis Process

The overall process of analyzing and making inferences from sample data can be viewed as a process of refinement that involves a number of separate and sequential steps that maybe identified as part of three broad stages:

- *Tabulation:* Identifying appropriate categories for the information desired, sorting the data into them, making the initial counts of responses, and using summarizing measures to provide economy of description and so facilitate understanding.
- *Formulating additional hypotheses:* Using the inductions derived from the data concerning the relevant variables, their parameters, their differences, and their relationships to suggest working hypotheses not originally considered.

- *Making inferences:* Reaching conclusions about the variables that are important, their parameters, their differences, and the relationships among them. In the tabulation process, appropriate categories are defined for coding the information desired, making the initial counts of responses, and preparing a descriptive summary of the data.

STEPS OF DATA TABULATION

Seven steps are involved in the process of data tabulation:

a. *Categorize:* Define appropriate categories for coding the information collected.
b. *Code:* Assign codes to the respondent's answers.
c. *Create data file:* Enter the data into the computer and create a data file.
d. *Error checking:* Check the data file for errors by performing a simple tabulation analysis to identify errors in coding or data entry. Once errors are identified, data maybe recoded to collapse categories or combine or delete responses.
e. *Generate new variables:* New variables maybe computed by data manipulations that multiply, sum, or otherwise transform variables.
f. *Weight data subclasses:* Weights are often used to adjust the representation of sample subgroups so that they match the proportions found in the population.
g. *Tabulate:* Summarize the responses to each variable included in the analysis.

Defining Categories: Analysis of any sizable array of data often requires that responses be grouped into categories or classes. The identification of response categories early in the study has several advantages. Ideally, it forces the analyst to consider all possible interpretations and responses to the questionnaire. It often leads to improvements in the questionnaire or observation forms. It permits more detailed instruction of interviewers and results in higher consistency in interpreting responses. Editing problems are also reduced.

The definition of categories allows for identification of the database columns assigned to each question or variable and to indicate the values assigned to each response alternative. Depending on the data collection method, data code sheets can be prepared and pre-coded. Data files are often formatted as comma separated (CSV) free format files, meaning that each variable appears in the same relative position for each respondent with some delimiter (comma, tab, space) between variables. The major data analysis software programs read data files and then display them in a spreadsheet-like database. Often the data are entered directly into the spreadsheet-format data file of the statistical program to be used for analysis. Where data is not collected and formatted electronically, precoding of printed questionnaires will eliminate transcription and thereby decreasing both processing errors and costs. Most of today's computer-based software for telephone (CATI) or online (Surveyz.com, Qualtrics.com) surveys automate this entire process. They not only define the question categories in the database but also automatically build the database and record the completed responses as they are submitted. The data may then be analyzed online, exported to Microsoft Excel™ or imported into a dedicated statistical analysis program such as SPSS.

As desirable as the early definition of categories is, it can sometimes only be done after the data have been collected. This is usually the case when open-end text questions, unstructured interviews, and projective techniques are used.

The selection of categories is controlled by both the purposes of the study and the nature of the responses. Useful classifications meet the following conditions:

- *Similarity of response within the category*: Each category should contain responses that, for purposes of the study, are sufficiently similar that they can be considered homogenous.
- *Differences of responses between categories*: Differences in category descriptions should be great enough to disclose any important distinctions in the characteristic being examined.
- *Mutually exclusive categories*: There should be an unambiguous description of categories, defined so that any response can be placed in only one category.
- *Categories should be exhaustive*: The classification schema should provide categories for all responses.

The use of extensive open-end questions often provides rich contextual and anecdotal information, but is a practice often associated with fledgling researchers. Open end questions, of course, have their place in marketing research. However, the researcher should be aware of the inherent difficulties in questionnaire coding and tabulation, not to mention their tendency to be more burdensome to the respondent. All of this is by way of saying that any open-end question should be carefully checked to see if a closed-end question (i.e. check the appropriate box) can be substituted without doing violence to the intent of the question. Obviously, sometimes this substitution should not be made.

Editing and Coding

- *Editing:* Editing is the process of reviewing the data to ensure maximum accuracy and clarity. Editing should be conducted as the data is being collected. This applies to the editing of the collection forms used for pretesting as well as those for the full-scale project. Careful editing early in the collection process will often catch misunderstandings of instructions, errors in recording, and other problems at a stage when it is still possible to eliminate them for the later stages of the study. Early editing has the additional advantage of permitting the questioning of interviewers while the material is still relatively fresh in their minds. Obviously, this has limited application for printed questionnaires, though online or CATI surveys can be edited even when data is being collected.

Editing is normally centralized so as to ensure consistency and uniformity in treatment of the data. If the sample is not large, a single editor usually edits all the data to reduce variation in interpretation. In those cases where the size of the project makes the use of more than one editor mandatory, it is usually best to assign each editor a different portion of the data collection form to edit. In this way the same editor edits the same items on all forms, an arrangement that tends to improve both consistency and productivity.

Typically, interviewer and respondent data are monitored to ensure that data requirements are fulfilled. Each collection form should be edited to ensure that data quality requirements are fulfilled. Regarding data obtained by an interviewer (and to an extent self-report) the following should be specifically evaluated:

- *Legibility of entries*: Obviously the data must be legible in order to be used. Where not legible, although it maybe possible to infer the response from other data collected, where any real doubt exists about the meaning of data it should not be used.
- *Completeness of entries*: On a fully structured collection form, the absence of an entry is ambiguous. It may mean either that the respondent could not or would not provide the answer that the interviewer failed to ask the question or that there was a failure to record collected data.
- *Consistency of entries*: Inconsistencies raise the question of which response is correct. (If a respondent family is indicated as being a non watcher of game shows for example, and a later entry indicates that they watched *Wheel of Fortune* twice during the past week, an obvious question arises as to which is correct). Discrepancies maybe cleared up by questioning the interviewer or call backs to the respondent. When discrepancies cannot be resolved, discarding both entries is usually the wisest course of action.
- *Accuracy of entries*. An editor should keep an eye out for any indication of inaccuracy in the data. Of particular importance is the detection of any repetitive response patterns in the reports of individual interviews. Such patterns may well be indicative of systematic interviewer bias or interviewer/respondent dishonesty.

- *Coding:* Coding is the process of assigning responses to data categories and numbers are assigned to identify them with the categories. *Precoding* refers to the practice of assigning codes to categories and sometimes printing this information on structured questionnaires and observation forms before the data are collected. The interviewer is able to code the responses when interpreting the response and marking the category into which it should be placed.

  Postcoding refers to the assignment of codes to responses after the data are collected. Postcoding is most often required when responses are reported in an unstructured format (open-ended text or numeric input). Careful interpretation and good judgment are required to ensure that the meaning of the response and the meaning of the category are consistently and uniformly matched.

  Once a complete code has been established, after postcoding, a formal coding manual or codebook is often created and made available to those who will be entering or analyzing the data.

  Like good questionnaire construction, good coding requires training and supervision. The editor-coder should be provided with written instructions, including examples. He or she should be exposed to the interviewing of respondents and become acquainted with the process and problems of collecting the data, thus providing aid in its interpretation. The coder also should be aware of the computer routines that are expected to be applied, insofar as they may require certain kinds of data formats.

  Whenever possible (and when cost allows) more than one person should do the coding, specifically the postcoding. By comparing the results of the various coders, a process known as determining *inter coder reliability*, any inconsistencies can be brought out. In addition to the obvious objective of eliminating data coding inconsistencies, the need for recoding sometimes points to the need for additional categories for data classification and may sometimes mean that there is a need to combine some of the categories. Coding is an activity that should not be taken lightly. Improper coding leads to poor analyzes and may even constrain the types of analysis that can be completed.

CLASSIFICATION

'The process of dividing the data into different groups (viz. classes) which are homogeneous within but heterogeneous between them is called a classification'.

It helps in understanding the salient features of the data and also the comparison with similar data. For a final analysis it is the best friend of a statistician.

Methods of Classification

The data is classified in the following ways:

- According to attributes or qualities this is divided into two parts:
  a. Simple classification
  b. Multiple classification
- According to variable or quantity or classification according to class intervals.
  - *Qualitative classification:* When facts are grouped according to the qualities (attributes) like religion, literacy, business, etc. the classification is called as qualitative classification.
  - *Simple classification:* It is also known as classification according to Dichotomy. When data (facts) are divided into groups according to their qualities, the classification is called as 'Simple Classification'. Qualities are denoted by capital letters (A, B, C, D ....) while the absence of these qualities are denoted by lower case letters (a, b, c, d, ..., etc.) For example:

Population (N)
↓
↓ (A) Male   ↓ (a) Female

  - *Manifold or multiple classification:* In this method data is classified using one or more qualities. First, the data is divided into two groups (classes) using one of the qualities. Then using the remaining qualities, the data is divided into different subgroups. For example, the population of a country is classified using three attributes: sex, literacy and business as,

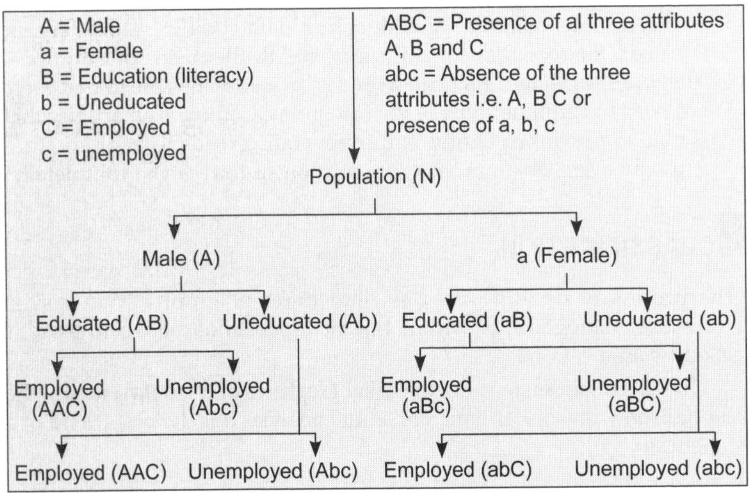

Classification According to Class Intervals or Variables

The data which is expressed in numbers (quantitative data), is classified according to class-intervals. While forming class-intervals one should bear in mind that each and every item must be covered. After finding the least value of an item and the highest value of an item, classify these items into different class-intervals. For example, if in any data the age of 100 persons ranging from 2 years to 47 years, is given, then the classification of this data can be done in this way:

Table 1

Age in years	No. of persons
0 – 10	5
10 – 20	9
20 – 30	32
30 – 40	34
40 – 50	20

In deciding on the grouping of the data into classes, for the purpose of reducing it to a manageable form, we observe that the number of classes should not be too large. If it were so then the object of summarization would be defeated. The number of classes should also not be too small because then we will miss a great deal of detail available and get a distorted picture. As a rule one should have between 10 and 25 classes, the actual number depending on the total frequency. Further, classes should be exhaustive; they should not be overlapping, so that no observed value falls in more than one class. Apart from exceptions, all classes should have the same length.

According to the Class-intervals in Classification the Following Terms are Used

- *Class-limits:* A class is formed within the two values. These values are known as the class-limits of that class. The lower value is called the lower limit and is denoted by l1 while the higher value is called the upper limit of the class and is denoted by l2. In the example given above, the first class-interval has l1 = 0 and l2 = 10.
- *Magnitude of the class-intervals:* The difference between the upper and lower limits of a class is called the magnitude or length or width of a class and is denoted by ' i ' or ' c '. Thus i ° (l2 – l1).
- *Mid-value or class-mark:* The arithmetical average of the two class limits (i.e. the lower limit and the upper limit) is called the mid-value or the class mark of that class-interval. For example, the mid-value of the class-interval (0 – 10) is

  $$\frac{l_1 + l_2}{2\,2} = \frac{0 + 10}{} 5, \text{ of } (10 - 20) \text{ it is } \frac{10 + 20}{2} = 15$$

  and so on.

- *Class frequency:* The units of the data belong to anyone of the groups or classes. The total number of these units is known as the frequency of that class and is denoted by fi or simply f. In the above example, the frequencies of the classes in the given order are 5, 9, 32, 34 and 40 respectively.

Classification According to the Class-intervals

- Exclusive method
- Inclusive method.

- *Exclusive method:* In this method the upper limit of a class becomes the lower limit of the next class. It is called 'Exclusive' as we do not put any item that is equal to the upper limit of a class in the same class; we put it in the next class, i.e. the upper limits of classes are excluded from them. For example, a person of age 20 years will not be included in the class-interval (10–20) but taken in the next class (20–30), since in the class interval (10–20) only units ranging from 10–19 are included. The exclusive-types of class-intervals can also be expressed as: 0 and below 10 or 0–9.9, 10 and below 20 or 10–19.9, 20 and below 30 or 20–29.9 and so on.
- *Inclusive method:* In this method the upper limit of any class interval is kept in the same class-interval. In this method the upper limit of a previous class is less by 1 from the lower limit of the next class interval. In short this method allows a class-interval to include both its lower and upper limits within it. For example:

Table 2

Inclusive method		Inclusive	
Class	**Frequency**	**Class**	**Frequency**
0 – 4	5	0 – 4.9	5
5 – 9	7	5 – 9.9	7
10 – 14	9	10 – 14.9	9
15 – 19	12	15 – 19.9	12
20 – 24	11	20 – 24.9	11
25 – 29	14	25 – 29.9	14

Class boundaries: Weights are recorded to the nearest Kg The class-intervals 60–62 includes all measurements from 59.50000... to 62.50000 ... Kg; the variable being a continuous one. These numbers, indicated briefly by the exact numbers 59.5 and 62.5, are called class-boundaries or true class limits. The smaller number 59.5 is the lower class boundary and the larger one 62.5 is the upper class boundary.

In any problem if the class-intervals are given as the inclusive type, then they should first be converted into the exclusive-type. For this we require a correction factor.

Correction factor = ½ (the upper limit of a class - the lower limit of the next class) which is generally 0.5.

Now you subtract it from the lower limits and add it to the upper limits of the class-intervals given in the inclusive-method. The class-intervals given above can be written after correction as:

Table 3

Class	Frequency
0 – 4.5	5
4.5 – 9.5	7
9.5 – 14.5	9
14.5 – 19.5	12
19.5 – 24.5	11
24.5 – 29.5	14

To obtain class-intervals when their mid-values are given, use the following formulae:

Lower limit (l_1) = m – $i/_2$ and upper limit (l_2) = m + $i/_2$ where m = mid-value and i = class-length.

For example, we are given some mid-values as 72, 77, 82, 87 ... Now; consider the first mid-value 72 and also the differences between successive mid-values.

We have 77 – 72 = 5, 82 – 77 = 5, 87 – 82 = 5....which gives the class-length i = 5.

For the first class-interval, l1 = m – $i/_2$ = 72 – $5/_2$ = 69.5 and l2 = 72 + $5/_2$ = 74.5.

Thus the first class-interval is 69.5 – 74.5 and other class-intervals then are 74.5 – 79.5, 79.5 – 84.5, 84.5 – 89.5.

Open-end class intervals: In any question when the lower limit of the first class-interval or the upper limit of the last class-interval, are not given then subtract the class length of the next immediate class-interval from the upper limit. This will give us the lower limit of the first class-interval. Similarly add the same class length to the lower limit of the last class-interval. But always notice that the lower limit of the first class (i.e. the lowest class) must not be negative or less than 0. For example,

Table 4

With open ends	Completed classes	With open ends	Completed classes
Below 10	0 – 10	Below 10	0 – 10
10 – 20	10 – 20	10 – 25	10 – 25
20 – 30	20 – 30	25 – 40	25 – 40
30 – 40	30 – 40	40 – 70	40 – 70
40 – 50	40 – 50	above 70	70 – 100
above 50	50 – 60		

Relative frequency distribution: The relative frequency of a class is the frequency of the class divided by the total number of frequencies of the class and is generally expresses as a,percentage.

Example: The weights of 100 persons were given as under:

Weigjts (in Kgs)	60 – 62	63 – 63	66 – 68	69 – 71	72 – 74
No. of persons (f_1)	5	18	42	27	8

Solution:

Table 5

Relative Frequency Table		
Weight (in Kg)	No. of persons (f_1)	Relative frequency
60 – 62	5	$\frac{5}{100}$ × 5% or 0.05
63 – 65	18	$\frac{18}{100}$ × 18% or 0.18
66 – 68	42	$\frac{42}{100}$ × 42% or 0.42
69 – 71	27	$\frac{27}{100}$ × 27% or 0.27
72 – 74	8	$\frac{8}{100}$ × 8% or 0.08
Total	$\sum f_1 = 100$	

Note: The word frequency of a class means, the number of times the class is repeated in the data or the total number of items or observations of the data belongs to that class.

Cumulative frequency: Many a times the frequencies of different classes are not given. Only their cumulative frequencies are given. The total frequency of all values less than or equal to the upper class boundary of a given class-interval is called the cumulative frequency up to and including that class interval. In this situation both the limits of a class-interval are not written; either lower or upper limit is written. These cumulative frequencies are called less than or more than cumulative frequencies. For example,

Class-interval	0 – 10	10 – 20	20 – 30	30 – 40	40 – 50
Frequency	4	9	5	12	15

Table 6

Less than cumulative frquency		More than cumulative frequency	
(Upper limits)	(cum. freq.)	(Lower limits)	(cum. freq.)
Less than 10	4	More than 0	45 = 41 + 4
Less than 20	4 + 9 = 13	More than 10	41 = 32 + 9
Less than 30	13 + 5 = 18	More than 20	32 = 27 + 5
Less than 40	18 + 12 = 30	More than 30	27 = 15 + 12
Less than 50	30 + 15 = 45	More than 40	15

Preparation of frequency distribution: We shall now study how to classify the raw data in a tabular form. Consider the data collected by one of the surveyors, interviewing about 50 people. This is as follows:

Size of the shoes: 2, 5, 6, 8, 2, 5, 6, 7, 6, 8, 7, 4, 3,.. This is called the raw data. Here some values repeat themselves. For instance the size 5 is repeated 10 times in 50 people. We say that the value of 5 of the variate has the frequency of 10. Frequency means the number of times a value of the variate or an attribute, as the case maybe, is repeated in the data. A table which shows each value of the characteristic with its corresponding frequency is known as a frequency distribution. The procedure of preparing such a table is explained as below:

Discrete variate: Consider the raw data which gives the size of shoes of 30 persons:

2, 5, 6, 4, 5, 7, 4, 4, 6, 2
3, 5, 5, 4, 5, 6, 5, 4, 3, 2
4, 4, 5, 4, 5, 5, 3, 2, 4, 4

The least value is 2 and the highest is 7. All sizes are integers between 2 and 7 (both inclusive). We can prepare a frequency distribution table as follows:

Table 7

Sizes of shoes	Tally Marks	Frequency
2	IIII	4
3	IIII	3
4	~~IIII~~ ~~IIII~~	10
5	~~IIII~~ ~~IIII~~	9
6	III	3
7	I	1
Total		**30**

In this example the size difference from 2 to 7 is very small. If the range of a variate is very large, it is inconvenient to prepare a frequency distribution for each value of the variate. In such a case we divide the variate into convenient groups and prepare a table showing the groups and their corresponding frequencies. Such a Table is called a *grouped frequency distribution.*

Consider the marks (out of 100) of 50 students as below:

40, 39, 43, 62, 30, 47, 33, 31, 17, 28
36, 29, 40, 32, 39, 24, 57, 42, 15, 30
50, 52, 47, 65, 31, 07, 37, 47, 17, 20
25, 53, 65, 85, 89, 56, 55, 41, 43, 10
44, 40, 69, 22, 40, 65, 39, 36, 71, 12

The range of the variate (marks) is very large. Also we are eager to know the performance of the students. The passing limit is 35 and above. Marks between 35 and 44 form the third class (or grade). Marks ranging between 45 to 59 are considered as second class and 60 to 100 form the first class. Thus we have a grouped frequency distribution as:

Table 8

Marks	Tally Marks	Frequency
0 – 34	𝍸 𝍸 𝍸 I	16
35 – 44	𝍸 𝍸 𝍸 III	18
45 – 59	𝍸 IIII	9
60 – 100	𝍸 II	7
Total		**50**

PRESENTATION AND INTERPRETATION OF DATA USING DESCRIPTIVE STATISTICS

Analysis of data in general way involves a number of closely related operations, which are performed with the purpose of summarizing the collected data, organizing these in such a manner that they answer the research questions. Thus in the process of analysis, hypotheses are subjected to statistical tests of significance to determine with what validity data can be said to indicate any conclusions.

For example, the description of the sample characteristics and analysis and interpretation of data collected from 200 male and female students. The data were analyzed based on the objectives and hypotheses, using descriptive statistics.

Description of Sample Characteristics

The frequency and percentage of the sample in relation to their demographic characteristics are presented in the following Table.

Table 9: Frequency and percentage distribution of sample characteristics n = 200

Sl No.	Variables	Frequency (f)	Percentage (%)
1.	**Age** (a) < 20 years (b) > 20 years	 134 66	 67 33
2.	**Gender** (a) Male (b) Female	 100 100	 50 50
3.	**Religion** (a) Hindu (b) Muslim (c) Christian (d) Any other	 120 8 72 Nil	 60 4 36 Nil
4.	**Source of information on CAD** (a) Magazine & News paper (b) Books & Journals (c) Radio & Television (d) Pamphlets	 99 34 67 Nil	 49.5 17 33.5 Nil

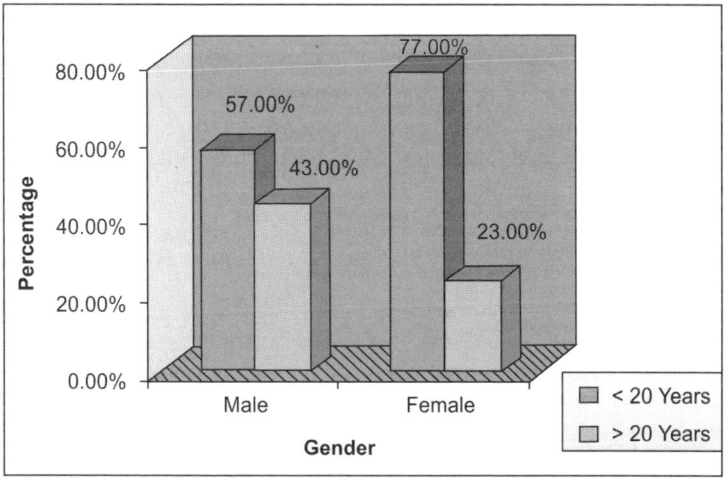

Fig. 7.1: Column diagram depicting percentage distribution of sample characteristics based on age and sex

The data in Figure shows that most of the females (77%) in comparison to males (57%) were within the age group of < 20 years. Only

(43%) of males and (23%) of females were above 20 years but less than 30 years.

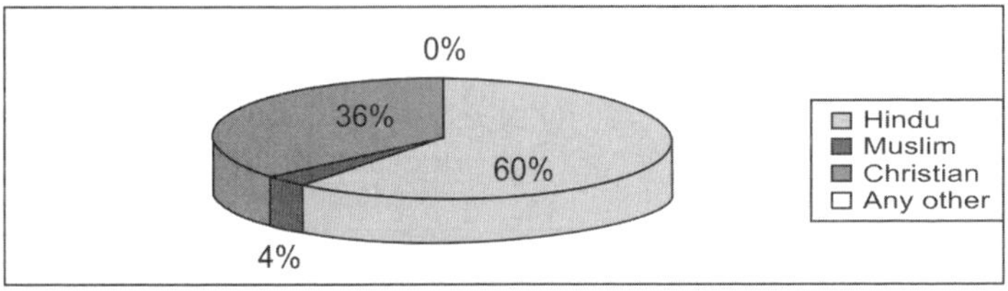

Fig. 7.2: Distribution of sample characteristics based on religion

The data in Figure shows that 120 (60%) of the college students were Hindus, 72 (36%) students were Christians and remaining 8 (4%) students were Muslim.

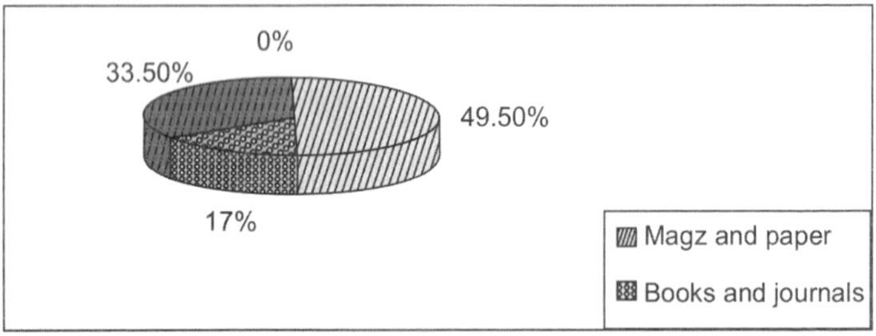

Fig. 7.3: Distribution of sample characteristics based on source of information

The data in figure shows that 99 (49.5%) students got the information of CAD from Magazine and News paper, 67 (33.5%) students had the information through Radio and Television and remaining 34 (17%) students got the information from Books and Journals. None of the students had the information through pamphlets.

SUMMARY

In this unit we discuss about the data analysis is the process of summarizing; presenting and describing the data collected from research in such a way that relationships can be established and inferences draw. The descriptive statistics are those measures that enable the researcher to describe the data or facts as contained in them. The unit on interpretation and discussion of findings counts a lot to the researcher.

Writing of Research Report

8 unit

INTRODUCTION

Research experience is as close to a professional problem-solving activity as anything in the curriculum. It provides exposure to research methodology and an opportunity to work closely with a faculty advisor. It usually requires the use of advanced concepts, a variety of experimental techniques, and state-of-the-art instrumentation. Preparation of a comprehensive written research report is an essential part of a valid research experience, and the student should be aware of this requirement at the outset of the project. It maybe expected that concrete outcomes of any research project would be student presentation of research results at a professional meeting and/or co-authorship on a journal publication.

However, while this is a most desirable outcome, it is not a substitute for a well-written comprehensive report, produced by the student with substantive critique and correction by the faculty mentor, which demonstrates that the student has a full grasp of the scope of the problem, the techniques/instrumental methods used.

Organization of the Research Report

Most scientific research reports, irrespective of the field, parallel the method of scientific reasoning. That is the problem is defined, a hypothesis is created, experiments are devised to test the hypothesis, experiments are conducted, and conclusions are drawn. The exact format of scientific reports is often discipline dependent with variations in order and content. The student is encouraged to adopt the format that is most appropriate to the discipline of the research. Many journals offer a formatting template to aid the author. One example of such a framework is as follows:

- Title
- Abstract

- Introduction
- Experimental details or theoretical analysis
- Results
- Discussion
- Conclusions and summary
- References

Title and Title Page

The title should reflect the content and emphasis of the project described in the report. It should be as short as possible and include essential key words.

The author's name (e.g. Ajay Gauttam) should follow the title on a separate line, followed by the author's affiliation (e.g. Department of Pharmacy, Oxford College of Pharmacy, Bangalore), the date, and possibly the origin of the report (e.g. In partial fulfilment of a Senior Thesis Project under the supervision of Professor Danielle F Green, June, 2009).

All of the above could appear on a single cover page. Acknowledgments and a table of contents can be added as preface pages if desired.

Abstract

The abstract should concisely describe the topic, the scope, the principal findings, and the conclusions. It should be written last to reflect accurately the content of the report. The length of abstracts varies but seldom exceeds 200 words.

A primary objective of an abstract is to communicate to the reader the essence of the paper. The reader will then be the judge of whether to read the full report or not. Were the report to appear in the primary literature, the abstract would serve as a key source of indexing terms and key words to be used in information retrieval. Author abstracts are often published verbatim in Chemical Abstracts.

Introduction

'A good introduction is a clear statement of the problem or project and the reasons for studying it'. The nature of the problem and why it is of interest should be conveyed in the opening paragraphs. This section should describe clearly but briefly the background information on the problem, what has been done before (with proper literature citations), and the objectives of the current project. A clear relationship between the current project and the scope and limitations of earlier work should be made so that the reasons for the project and the approach used will be understood.

Experimental Details, Computation Procedures, or Theoretical Analysis

This section should describe what was actually done. It is a succinct exposition of the laboratory and computational details, describing procedures, techniques, instrumentation, special precautions, and so on. It should be sufficiently detailed that other experienced researchers would be able to repeat the work and obtain comparable results.

In theoretical reports, this section would include sufficient theoretical or mathematical analysis to enable derivations and numerical results to be checked. Computer programs from the public domain should be cited. New computer programs should be described in outline form.

If the experimental section is lengthy and detailed, as in synthetic work, it can be placed at the end of the report so that it does not interrupt the conceptual flow of the report. Its placement will depend on the nature of the project and the discretion of the writer.

Results

In this section, relevant data, observations, and findings are summarized. Tabulation of data, equations, charts, and figures can be used effectively to present results clearly and concisely. Schemes to show reaction sequences maybe used here or elsewhere in the report.

Discussion

The crux of the report is the analysis and interpretation of the results. What do the results mean? How do they relate to the objectives of the project? To what extent have they resolved the problem? Because the 'Results' and 'Discussion' sections are interrelated, they can often be combined as one section.

Conclusions and Summary

A separate section outlining the main conclusions of the project is appropriate if conclusions have not already been stated in the 'Discussion' section. Directions for future work are also suitably expressed here.

A lengthy report, or one in which the findings are complex, usually benefits from a paragraph summarizing the main features of the report: the objectives, the findings, and the conclusions.

The last paragraph of text in manuscripts prepared for publication is customarily dedicated to acknowledgments. However, there is no rule about this, and research reports or senior theses frequently place acknowledgments following the title page.

References

Thoroughness and currency of literature references acknowledge foundational work, direct the reader to published procedures, results, and interpretations, and play a critical role in establishing the overall scholarship of the report according to following criteria:

Books

- Author AA. *Title of Book. Location: Publisher.*
- Author AA, Author BB. *Title of book. Location: Publisher;* 2004.
- Jha AS, Kulshrestha S, Chauhan R. *Research Methodology.* New Delhi: APH Publishing Corporation; 2009.

Chapter in a Book

- Author AA. Title of chapter. In A. Editor, B. Editor, and C. Editor (Eds.), *Title of book* (p./pp. page number/s). Location: Publisher.
- Patel, A. (1997). Adolescence and development. In Kulshrestha, A (Ed.), *Advanced Psychology,* New Delhi: APH Publishing Corporation.; 2004. PP. 258-72.

Journals, Magazines, Newspapers in Print Format

The journal title and the volume number are in italics. Issue numbers are not required if the journal is continuously paged. If paged individually, the issue number is required and it is in regular type in parentheses adjacent to the volume number.

Journals Articles

- Author AA, Author BB, Author CC. Title of article. *Title of Journal, volume* (issue, when appropriate); (2004).
- Author AA, Author B B, Author CC. Title of article. *Title of Journal, xx, xxx-xxx.*

One Author

- Jha AS. Defeating Life: The impact on Life. *Voice of Research;* (2008):*53*(12), PP. 40-45.
- Kulshrestha SS. An Experimental Evaluation of Divorce. *Journal of Psychology;* 2003, *68,* 43-56.

Two to Seven Authors [List all authors]

Jha AS, Kulshrestha SS, Patel RS. Physical Development in Early Adolescence. *Journal of Psychology;* 2009, *PP*. 50, 348-373.

Eight or More Authors [List the first six authors, ... and the last author]

Kulshrestha SS, Patel RS. Wolchik SA, West SG. et al. An Experimental Evaluation of Remarriage. *Journal of Psychology*; 2000, PP. 68, 43-56.

Magazine Articles

- Author AA. Title of article. *Title of Magazine, volume;* 2004.
- Kulshreshtha, A, Kulshrestha S. Cognitive Development. *Science Today;* 2009, *PP 235, 9-17.*

No Author and Bracketed Descriptive Information

The Physical Development [Letter to the editor]. (2000, May 19). *The Indian Times Magazine, 5.*

Newspaper Articles

- Author AA. Title of article. Title of *Newspaper;* 2004.
- Dubey A. Duty and Responsibility of a Teacher. *The Times of India;* 2008, *P* 6.

Newspaper Article with No Author and Discontinuous Pages

- Moral development. *The Indian Express;* 2004, *PP* 1, 4.
- Generic debuts. *The Times of India;* 2000, *PP* 1, 4.

Review Articles

- Author AA. Review title [Review of the medium Title of item reviewed]. *Title of Periodical,* and publication information following format for journal, magazine, or newspaper, as appropriate; 2004.
- Jha S. Regrets [Review of the motion picture The life of unwanted]. *The Era Bros;* 2004, PP 121, 66-7.

Review is Untitled

Raval R M. [Review of the book The History of Medieval India]. *College and Research Libraries;* 2007, PP 58, 487-8.

Others

Reports, Theses:

Jha AS. *A Study of Creativity and its Components in relation to certain Variables.* Ph.D dissertation, Department of Education, Gujarat University; 1992.

Conference Papers:

(a) Published (referenced as a chapter in an edited book):

- Kulshrestha SS, Jha AS. An analysis of linear programming. In: Kulshreshtra A, Patel RS. Linear programming; 2004 PP 182-91.

- APH Publication Corporation. International Seminar conducted at the Annual Convention of the All India Association for Educational Research, Rajkot, Gujarat, India; 2006.

(b) *Unpublished more than six authors:*

- Kulshrestha SS, Kulshreshtra A, Jha AS, Kulshrestha, LS, et al.. Enriching Curriculum through Local Wisdom International Seminar conducted at the Annual; 2004.

Preparing the Manuscript

The personal computer and word processing have made manuscript preparation and revision a great deal easier than it used to be. It is assumed that students will have access to word processing and to additional software that allows numerical data to be graphed, chemical structures to be drawn, and mathematical equations to be represented. These are essential tools of the technical writer. All manuscripts should be carefully proofread before being submitted. Preliminary drafts should be edited by the faculty advisor (and/or a supervising committee) before the report is presented in final form.

Useful Texts

Writing the Laboratory Notebook, Kanare HM, American Chemical Society, Washington, DC, 1985.

This book describes among other things the reasons for note keeping, organizing and writing the notebook with examples, and provides photographs from laboratory notebooks of famous scientists.

ACS Style Guide: Effective Communication of Scientific Information, Coghill, AM, Garson, LR; 3rd Edition, American Chemical Society, Washington, DC, 2006.

This volume is an invaluable writer's handbook in the field of chemistry. It contains a wealth of data on preparing any type of scientific report and is useful for both students and professional chemists. Every research laboratory should have a copy. It gives pointers on the organization of a scientific paper, correct grammar and style, and accepted formats in citing chemical names, chemical symbols, units, and references.

There are useful suggestions on constructing tables, preparing illustrations, using different fonts, and giving oral presentations. In addition, there is a brief overview of the chemical literature, the way in which it is organized and how information is disseminated and retrieved. A selected bibliography of other excellent guides and resources to technical writing is also provided. See also The Basics of Technical Communicating. Cain, B. E.; ACS Professional Reference Book American Chemical Society: Washington, DC, 1988.

Write Like a Chemist, Robinson MS, Stoller FL, Costanza-Robinson MS, Jones JK, Oxford University Press, Oxford, 2008.

This book addresses all aspects of scientific writing. The book provides a structured approach to writing a journal article, conference abstract, scientific poster and research proposal. The approach is designed to turn the complex process of writing into graduated, achievable tasks.

SUMMARY

In this unit we discuss about the communicating research findings is an important step in the research process that reveals what was done to others. Only the researcher can provide meaning to the research and so is in a position to communicate the findings. The reports follow particular guidelines depending on the readers or audience. For academic thesis and dissertations, there are guidelines usually in chapters that the report would comply with. For articles to be published in journals, the guidelines are also provided. For reports that have to be presented at conferences, the guidelines are given and the researcher adheres strictly to those for the work to be accepted. The parts of a research report include, title, abstract, introduction, method, results, discussion conclusions, recommendations, and references/appendix. Research reports should be written in simple and clear language.

Introduction to Research Statistics

9 unit

INTRODUCTION

Statistics is concerned with scientific methods for collecting, organizing, summarising, presenting and analyzing data as well as deriving valid conclusions and making reasonable decisions on the basis of this analysis. Statistics is concerned with the systematic collection of numerical data and its interpretation. The word 'statistic' is used to refer to numerical facts, such as the number of people living in particular area and the study of ways of collecting, analyzing and interpreting the facts.

Statistics is defined differently by different authors over a period of time. In the olden days statistics was confined to only state affairs but in modern days it embraces almost every sphere of human activity. Therefore a number of old definitions, which was confined to narrow field of enquiry, were replaced by more definitions, which are much more comprehensive and exhaustive.

Secondly, statistics has been defined in two different ways—Statistical data and statistical methods. The following are some of the definitions of statistics as numerical data.

- Statistics are the classified facts representing the conditions of people in a state. In particular they are the facts, which can be stated in numbers or in tables of numbers or in any tabular or classified arrangement.
- Statistics are measurements, enumerations or estimates of natural phenomenon usually systematically arranged, analyzed and presented as to exhibit important interrelationships among them.

Definitions

- According to *AL Bowley* 'Statistics are numerical statement of facts in any department of enquiry placed in relation to each other'.

- According to *Bowley gives* another definition for statistics, which states 'statistics maybe rightly called the scheme of averages'. This definition is also incomplete, as averages play an important role in understanding and comparing data and statistics provide more measures.
- According to *Croxton and Cowden* 'Statistics maybe defined as the science of collection, presentation analysis and interpretation of numerical data from the logical analysis.'

Inferential and Descriptive Statistics

There are four main stages in doing research: designing a study, collecting the data, obtaining descriptive statistics, and perhaps performing some inferential statistics. Statistics are a set of tools for obtaining insight into a psychological phenomenon.

- Descriptive statistics summarize the data, making clear any trends, patterns, etc. which maybe lurking within them; they consist of visual displays such as graphs, and summary statistics such as means.
- Inferential statistics attempt to make inferences about the parent population on the basis of the limited samples actually obtained. The term inferential statistics is usually reserved for the various statistical tests used for comparing two or more groups of subjects within an experiment, etc. (Although in effect, most of statistics in psychology involves a process of trying to make inferences about humanity on the basis of a few undergraduate subjects!).

Samples and Populations

In statistics, the terms sample and population have special meanings. A sample is a limited subset from a population, and a population is the entire set of things under consideration. What constitutes a population will vary according to what it is you are trying to make extrapolations to: usually the population to which we are trying to generalize from our sample consists of the entire human race.

However, if you are interested only in making claims about the behavior of three-toed.

Amazonian sloths, then you might be able to get access to the entire population of sloths if there were not very many of them in existence. Normally, we have to obtain data from a limited sample of subjects because it is impossible to obtain data from the entire population to which they belong.

Types of Data used in Statistics

It is important to know what kind of data you are dealing with, as certain statistics can only be used validly with certain kinds of data:

- *Nominal (Categorical) data:* Numbers are used only as names for categories. Therefore they are not really acting as numbers, but just serving as labels. If the numbers can be replaced by letters or names, then you are dealing with nominal data. So, if you had four groups, you could label them '1', '2', '3' and '4', but it would mean just the same as if they were entitled 'A', 'B', 'C', and 'D'. You cannot do any statistics or arithmetic on nominal data, in just the same way as you cannot add together A and B. The numbers on footballers' jerseys are the classic example of nominal data: adding together players at positions 1 and 2 does not give you the player at position 3.
- *Ordinal (Rank) data:* Things can be ordered in terms of some property such as size, length, speed, time, etc. However, successive points on the scale are not necessarily spaced equally apart. To rank Grand Prix racers in terms of whether they finish first, second, third, and so on, is to measure them on an ordinal scale: all that you know for certain is the order of finishing—the difference between first and second placed finishers maybe quite different from the difference between those placed second and third. In psychology, most attitude scales (e.g. seven-point scales which run from '1' for 'completely disagree' through to '7' for 'completely agree') are making measurements on an ordinal scale.
- *Interval data:* These are measured on a scale on which measurements are spaced at equal intervals, but on which there is no true zero point (although there maybe a point on the scale which is arbitrarily named 'zero'). The classic examples are the Fahrenheit and Centigrade temperature scales. On the Centigrade scale, a rise of 'one degree' represents an increase in heat by the same amount, whether one is talking about the shift from 5 degrees to 6 degrees, or from 90 degrees to 91 degrees. However, because the zero point on the scale is arbitrary, one cannot make any statements about ratios of quantities on the scale: thus it is not permissible to say that 26 degrees is twice 13 degrees or half of 52 degrees.
- *Ratio data:* This scale is the same as the interval scale, except that there is a true zero on the scale, representing a complete absence of the thing in question which is being measured. Measurements of height, weight, length, time are all measurements on ratio scales. With this kind of scale, the intervals are equally spaced and we can make meaningful statements about the ratios of quantities measured. Thus, an increase in length between 9 inches and 10 inches is the same as an increase in length between 90 inches and 91 inches; and additionally, we can say that 6 inches is twice 3 inches, and half of 12 inches. The concept of levels of measurement may seem rather abstract and confusing now,

but it will prove important in helping us to decide which statistics are appropriate for our data. For example, some statistical tests can only be used with nominal data, and others can only be used with interval or ratio data.

Measures of Central Tendency

These are single numbers which attempt to convey some impression of what constitutes 'typical' performance. The three most commonly encountered are the mean, median and mode. Each has advantages and disadvantages as a summary description of our data.

Mean

Mean is what most people commonly refer to as an average? The mean refers to the number you obtain when you sum-up a given set of numbers and then divide this sum by the total number in the set. Mean is also referred to more correctly as arithmetic mean.

$$\text{Mean} = \frac{\text{Sum of elements in set}}{\text{Number of elements in set}}$$

Given a set of ***n*** elements from a_1 to a_n

$$a_1, a_2, a_3, a_4, \text{..........} a_{n-1}, a_n$$

The mean is found by adding up all the a's and then dividing by the total number, ***n***

$$\text{Mean} = \frac{a_1 + a_2 + a_3 + a_4 + \text{........} + a_{n-1}, a_n}{\text{Number of elements in set}}$$

This can be generalized by the formula below:

$$\text{Mean} = \frac{1}{n} \sum_{i=0}^{n} a_i$$

Mean example problems

Example 1

Find the mean of the set of numbers below

3, 4, – 1, 22, 14, 0, 9, 18, 7, 0, 1

Solution

The first step is to count how many numbers there are in the set, which we shall call n

$$n = 10$$

The next step is to add up all the numbers in the set

$$\text{Sum} = 3 + 4 + -1 + 22 + 14 + 0 + 9 + 18 + 7 + 0 + 1$$

$$\text{Sum} = 77$$

The last step is to find the actual mean by dividing the sum by n

$$\text{Mean} = \frac{\text{sum}}{n}$$

$$\text{Mean} = \frac{77}{10}$$

$$\text{Mean} = 7.7$$

Mean can also be found for grouped data, but before we see an example on that, let us first define frequency.

Frequency in statistics means the same as in everyday use of the word. The frequency an element in a set refers to how many of that element there are in the set. The frequency can be from 0 to as many as possible. If you are told that the frequency an element a is 3, that means that there are 3 as in the set.

Example 2

Find the mean of the set of ages in the table below:

Age (years)	Frequency
10	0
11	8
12	3
13	2
14	7

Solution

The first step is to find the total number of ages, which we shall call n. Since it will be tedious to count all the ages, we can find n by adding up the frequencies:

$n = 0 + 8 + 3 + 2 + 7$

$n = 20$

Next we need to find the sum of all the ages. We can do this in two ways: we can add up each individual age, which will be a long and tedious process; or we can use the frequency to make things faster.

Since we know that the frequency represents how many of that particular age there are, we can just multiply each age by its frequency, and then add up all these products.

$\text{Sum} = (10 \times 0) + (11 \times 8) + (12 \times 3) + (13 \times 2) + (14 \times 7)$

$\text{Sum} = 0 + 88 + 36 + 26 + 98$

$\text{Sum} = 248$

The last step is to find the mean by dividing the sum by n

$$\text{Mean} = \frac{248}{20}$$

Population Mean vs Sample Mean

In the introduction to statistics section, we defined a population and a sample whereby a sample is a part of a population.

In statistics there are two kinds of means: Population mean and sample mean. A population mean is the true mean of the entire population of the data set while a sample mean is the mean of a small sample of the population. These different means appear frequently in both statistics and probability and should not be confused with each other.

Population mean is represented by the Greek letter μ (pronounced mu) while sample mean is represented by x (pronounced *x bar*). The total number of elements in a population is represented by N while the number of elements in a sample is represented by n. This leads to an adjustment in the formula we gave above for calculating the mean.

$$\text{Population means } \mu = \frac{1}{n}\sum_{i=1}^{N} a_i$$

$$\text{Population means } \mu = \frac{1}{n}\sum_{i=1}^{N} a_i$$

The sample mean is commonly used to estimate the population mean when the population mean is unknown. This is because they have the same expected value.

Median

The median is defined as the number in the middle of a given set of numbers arranged in order of increasing magnitude. When given a set of numbers, the median is the number positioned in the exact middle of the list when you arrange the numbers from the lowest to the highest. The median is also a measure of average. In higher level statistics, median is used as a measure of dispersion. The median is important because it describes the behavior of the entire set of numbers.

Example 3

Find the median in the set of numbers given below

15, 16, 15, 15, 16, 18, 19, 20, 11

Solution

From the definition of median, we should be able to tell that the first step is to rearrange the given set of numbers in order of increasing magnitude, i.e. from the lowest to the highest

7, 11, 15, 15, 16, 18, 19, 20, 21

Then we inspect the set to find that number which lies in the exact middle.

~~7~~, ~~11~~, ~~15~~, ~~15~~, 16, ~~18~~, ~~19~~, ~~20~~, ~~21~~

Lets try another example to emphasize something interesting that often occurs when solving for the median.

Example 4

Find the median of the given data

13, 0, 5, 8, – 8, –5, 10, 7, 1, 0, 0, 4, 6, 16

Solution

As in the previous example, we start off by rearranging the data in order from the smallest to the largest.

– 8, – 5, 0, 0, 0, 1, 4, 5, 6, 7, 8, 10, 13, 16

Next we inspect the data to find the number that lies in the exact middle.

~~–8~~, ~~–5~~, ~~0~~, ~~0~~, ~~0~~, ~~1~~, 4, 5, ~~6~~, ~~7~~, ~~8~~, ~~10~~, ~~13~~, ~~16~~

We can see from the above that we end up with two numbers (4 and 5) in the middle. We can solve for the median by finding the mean of these two numbers as follows:

$$\text{Median} = \frac{4+5}{2}$$

$$\text{Median} = \frac{9}{2}$$

$$\text{Median} = 4.5$$

Mode

The mode is defined as the element that appears most frequently in a given set of elements. Using the definition of frequency given above, mode can also be defined as the element with the largest frequency in a given data set.

For a given data set, there can be more than one mode. As long as those elements all have the same frequency and that frequency is the highest, they are all the modal elements of the data set.

Example 5

Find the mode of the following data set.

3, 12, 15, 3, 15, 8, 20, 19, 3, 15, 12, 19, 9

Solution

Mode = 3 and 15

Mode for Grouped Data

As we saw in the section on data, grouped data is divided into classes. We have defined mode as the element which has the highest frequency in a given data set. In grouped data, we can find two kinds of mode: the Modal Class, or class with the highest frequency and the mode itself, which we calculate from the modal class using the formula below.

$$\text{Mode} = L + \left(\frac{f_1 - f_0}{2f_1 - f_0 - f_2}\right) \times h$$

Where:

- L is the lower class limit of the modal class
- f_1 is the frequency of the modal class
- f_0 is the frequency of the class before the modal class in the frequency table
- f_2 is the frequency of the class after the modal class in the frequency table
- h is the class interval of the modal class

Example 6

Find the modal class and the actual mode of the data set below

Number	Frequency
1 – 3	7
4 – 6	6
7 – 9	4
10 – 12	2
13 – 15	2
16 – 18	8
19 – 21	1
22 – 24	2
25 – 27	3
28 – 30	2

Solution

$$\text{Modal class} = 10 - 12$$

$$\text{Mode} = L + \left(\frac{f_1 - f_0}{2f_1 - f_0 - f_2}\right) \times h$$

Where:

- $L = 10$
- $f_1 = 9$
- $f_0 = 4$
- $f_2 = 2$
- $h = 3$

Therefore,

$$\text{Mode} = 10 + \left(\frac{9 - 4}{(2 \times 9) - 2 - 4}\right) \times 3$$

Solving the above using the order of operations:

$$\text{Mode} = 10 + \left(\frac{5}{12}\right) \times 3$$

$$\text{Mode} = 10 + 1.25$$
$$\text{Mode} = 11.25$$

Range

The range is defined as the difference between the highest and lowest number in a given data set.

Range = Highest Value – Lowest Value

Example 7

Find the range of the data set below

3, 12, 15, 3, 15, 8, 20, 19, 3, 15, 12, 19, 0

Solution

Range = 20 – 3 = 17

- *Assumed mean:* In the section on averages, we learned how to calculate the mean for a given set of data. The data we looked at was ungrouped data and the total number of elements in the data set was not that large. That method is not always a realistic approach especially if you are dealing with grouped data. That is where the assumed mean comes into play.

  Assumed mean, like the name suggests, is a guess or an assumption of the mean. Assumed mean is most commonly denoted by the letter *a*. It does not need to be correct or even close to the actual mean and choice of the assumed mean is at your discretion except for where the question explicitly asks you to use a certain assumed mean value. Assumed mean is used to calculate the actual mean as well as the variance and standard deviation as we shall see later.

  Assumed mean can be calculated from the following formula:

$$x = a + \left(\frac{\Sigma f_i u_i}{\Sigma f_i}\right) \times h$$

  It is very important to remember that the above formula only applies to grouped data with equal class intervals.

Now let us define each term used in the formula:

- x is the mean which we are trying to find.
- a is the assumed mean.
- h is the class interval which we looked at in the section on data.
- fi is the frequency of each class, we find the total frequency of all the classes in the data set ($\sum f_i$) by adding up all the f_i's

- Each u_i is found from the following formula:

$$u_i = \frac{d_i}{h}$$

Where h is the class interval and each d_i is the difference between the mid element in a class and the assumed mean.

d is calculated from the following formula:

$$d_i = x_i - a$$

Where x is the midpoint of a given class.

x is obtained from the following:

$$x = \frac{\text{Upperclass boundary + Lowerclass boundary}}{2}$$

x_i is the number in the middle of a given class.

Therefore u_i becomes

$$\underline{x}_i = \frac{x_i - a}{h}$$

Let's try an example to see how to apply the assumed mean method for finding mean.

Example 1

The student body of a certain school were polled to find out what their hobbies were. The number of hobbies each student had was then recorded and the data obtained was grouped into classes shown in the table below. Using an assumed mean of 17 and find the mean for the number of hobbies of the students in the school.

Number of hobbies	Frequency
0 – 4	45
5 – 9	58
10 – 14	27
15 – 19	30
20 – 24	19
25 – 29	11
30 – 34	8
35 – 40	2

Solution: We have been given the assumed mean a as 17 and we know the formula for finding mean from the assumed mean as

We can find the class interval by using the class limits as follows:

We now have one component we need and we are one step closer to finding the mean.

So we can solve the rest of this problem using a table whereby we find each remaining component of the formula and then substitute at the end:

Hobbies	Frequency f_i	x_i	$d_i = x_i - a$	$u_i = d_i/h$	f_iu_i
0 – 4	45	2	–15	–3	–135
5 – 9	58	7	–10	–2	–116
10 – 14	27	12	–5	–1	–27
15 – 19	30	17	0	0	0
20 – 24	19	22	5	1	19
25 – 29	11	27	10	2	22
30 – 34	8	32	15	3	24
35 – 40	2	37	20	4	8
	$\sum f_i = 200$				$\sum f_iu_i = -202$

$$\bar{x} = a + \frac{\Sigma f_i u_i}{\Sigma f_i} \times h$$

Substituting

$$\bar{x} = 17 + \frac{-202}{200} \times \underline{5}$$

$$\bar{x} = 17 - 5.05$$

$$\bar{x} = 11.95$$

The mean number of hobbies is **11.95.**

Cumulative frequency: It is defined as a running total of frequencies. The frequency of an element in a set refers to how many of that element there are in the set. Cumulative frequency can also defined as the sum of all previous frequencies up to the current point.

The cumulative frequency is important when analyzing data, where the value of the cumulative frequency indicates the number of elements in the data set that lie below the current value. The cumulative frequency is also useful when representing data using diagrams like histograms.

Cumulative Frequency Table

The cumulative frequency is usually observed by constructing a cumulative frequency table. The cumulative frequency table takes the form as in the example below.

Example 1

The set of data below shows the ages of participants in a certain summer camp. Draw a cumulative frequency table for the data.

Age (years)	Frequency
10	3
11	18
12	13
13	12
14	7
15	27

Solution: The cumulative frequency at a certain point is found by adding the frequency at the present point to the cumulative frequency of the previous point.

The cumulative frequency for the first data point is the same as its frequency since there is no cumulative frequency before it.

Age (years)	Frequency	Cumulative Frequency
10	3	3
11	18	3 + 18 = 21
12	13	21 + 13 = 34
13	12	34 + 12 = 46
14	7	46 + 7 = 53
15	27	53 + 27 = 80

- *Cumulative Frequency Graph:* It also known as an Ogive, is a curve showing the cumulative frequency for a given set of data. The cumulative frequency is plotted on the y-axis against the data which is on the x-axis for un-grouped data. When dealing with grouped data, the Ogive is formed by plotting the cumulative frequency against the upper boundary of the class. An Ogive is used to study the growth rate of data as it shows the accumulation of frequency and hence its growth rate.

Example 2

Plot the cumulative frequency curve for the data set below:

Age (years)	Frequency
10	5
11	10
12	27
13	18
14	6
15	16
16	38
17	9

Solution:

Age (years)	Frequency	Cumulative Frequency
10	5	5
11	10	5 + 10 = 15
12	27	15 + 27 = 42
13	18	42 + 18 = 60
14	6	60 + 6 = 66
15	16	66 + 16 = 82
16	38	82 + 38 = 120
17	9	120 + 9 = 129

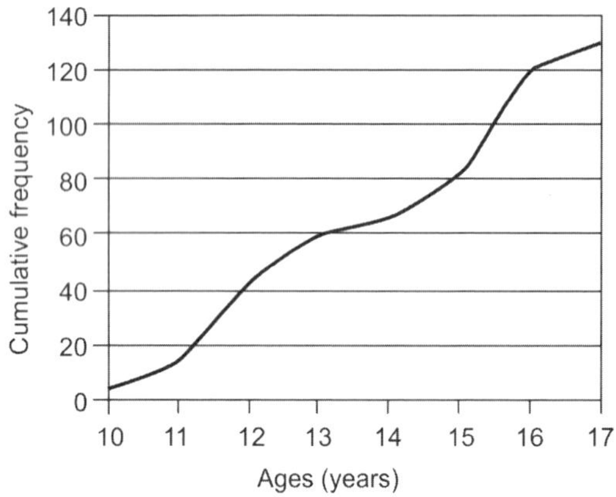

Fig. 9.1: Cumulative frequency graph (ogive)

- *Percentile:* It is a certain percentage of a set of data. Percentiles are used to observe how many of a given set of data fall within a certain percentage range; for example; a thirtieth percentile indicates data that lies the 13% mark of the entire data set.
- *Calculating percentiles:* Let designate a percentile as P_m where m represents the percentile we are finding, for example for the tenth percentile, $m\}$ would be 10. Given that the total number of elements in the data set is N
- *Quartiles:* The term quartile is derived from the word quarter which means one fourth of something. Thus a quartile is a certain fourth of a data set. When you arrange a date set increasing order from the lowest to the highest, then you divide this data into groups of four, you end up with quartiles. There are three quartiles that are studied in statistics.
  (a) *First quartile (Q_1):* When you arrange a data set in increasing order from the lowest to the highest, then you proceed to divide this

data into four groups, the data at the lower fourth (1⁄4) mark of the data is referred to as the *first uartile.*

The First Quartile is equal to the data at the 25th percentile of the data. The first quartile can also be obtained using the Ogive whereby you section off the curve into four parts and then the data that lies on the last quadrant is referred to as the first quartile.

(b) *Second quartile (Q_2):* When you arrange a given data set in increasing order from the lowest to the highest and then divide this data into four groups , the data value at the second fourth (2⁄4) mark of the data is referred to as the *second quartile.*

This is the equivalent to the data value at the half way point of all the data and is also equal to the data value at the 50th percentile.

The second quartile can similarly be obtained from an Ogive by sectioning off the curve into four and the data that lies at the second quadrant mark is then referred to as the second data. In other words, all the data at the half way line on the cumulative frequency curve is the second quartile. The second quartile is also equal to the median.

(c) *Third quartile (Q_3):* When you arrange a given data set in increasing order from the lowest to the highest and then divide this data into four groups, the data value at the third fourth (3⁄4) mark of the data is referred to as the *third quartile.*

This is the equivalent of the the data at the 75th percentile. The third quartile can be obtained from an Ogive by dividing the curve into four and then considering all the data value that lies at the 3⁄4 mark.

Calculating quartiles from cumulative frequency: As mentioned above, we can obtain the different quartiles from the Ogive, which means that we use the cumulative frequency to calculate the quartile.

Given that the cumulative frequency for the last element in the data set is given as *fc*, the quartiles can be calculated as follows:

$$Q_1 \text{ position} = \frac{(f_c + 1)}{4}$$

$$Q_2 \text{ position} = \frac{2(f_c + 1)}{4}$$

$$Q_3 \text{ position} = \frac{3(f_c + 1)}{4}$$

The quartile is then located by matching up which element has the cumulative frequency corresponding to the position obtained above.

Example 3

Find the first, second and third quartiles of the data set below using the cumulative frequency curve.

Age (years)	Frequency
10	5
11	10
12	27
13	18
14	6
15	16
16	38
17	9

Solution:

Age (years)	Frequency	Cumulative Frequency
10	5	5
11	10	15
12	27	42
13	18	60
14	6	66
15	16	82
16	38	120
17	9	129

$$f_c = 129$$

$$Q_1 \text{ position} = \frac{(129 + 1)}{4} = 32.5$$

$$Q_2 \text{ position} = \frac{2(129 + 1)}{4} = 65$$

$$Q_3 \text{ position} = \frac{3(129 + 1)}{4} = 97.5$$

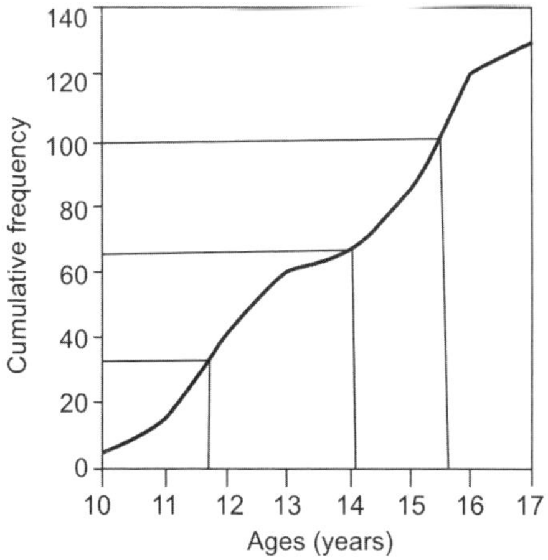

Fig. 9.2: Cumulative frequency graph

From the Ogive, we can see the positions where the quartiles lie and thus can approximate them as follows:

$$Q_1 = 11.5$$
$$Q_2 = 14.5$$
$$Q_3 = 15.5$$

- *Interquartile range:* The interquartile range is the difference between the third quartile and the first quartile.

$$\text{Interquartile range} = Q_3 - Q_1$$

Dispersion - Deviation and Variance

Dispersion

It measures how the various elements behave with regards to some sort of central tendency, usually the mean. Measures of dispersion include range, interquartile range, variance, standard deviation and absolute deviation. We have already looked at the first two in the averages section, so let us move on to the other measures.

Deviation

Absolute deviation for a given data set is defined as the average of the absolute difference between the elements of the set and the mean (average deviation) or the median element (median absolute deviation).

The average deviation is calculated as follows:

$$\text{Average deviations} = \frac{1}{n}\sum_{i=1}^{n}(x_1 - \bar{x})$$

Which means that the average deviation is the average of the differences between each element of the data set and the mean.

The median absolute deviation is calculated as follows:

$$\text{Median absolute deviations} = \frac{1}{n}\sum_{i=1}^{n}(x_1 - median)$$

Example 1

The heights of a group of 10 students randomly selected from a given school are as follows (in *ft*):

5.5, 3.5, 4.6, 6.1, 5.7, 5.11, 4.9, 5.0, 5.0, 5.5

- Find the absolute deviation from the mean
- Find the absolute deviation from the median.

Solution:

- To find the absolute deviation from the mean, we need to first find the mean of the heights.

  We know that the mean $\bar{x}$ is given by:

$$\bar{x} = \frac{1}{n}\sum_{i=1}^{n} x_i$$

  Using the above, we calculate the mean as:

$$\bar{x} = \frac{5.5 + 3.5 + 4.6 + 6.1 + 5.7 + 5.11 + 4.9 + 5.0 + 5.0 + 5.5}{10}$$

$$\bar{x} = \frac{50.91}{10}$$

$$\bar{x} = 5.091$$

  The mean height is 5.091 *ft*.

  The deviation from the mean for each of the elements in the data set is obtained by subtracting the mean from that element, as follows:

  For 5.5:

$$5.5 - \bar{x}$$
$$= 5.5 - 5.091 = 0.409$$

  We find all the deviations and then take their average (remember that we only consider their absolute values):

  Sum of deviations from the mean =

  $|5.5 - 5.091| + |3.5 - 5.091| + |4.6 - 5.091|$
  $+ |6.1 - 5.091| + |5.7 - 5.091| + |5.11 - 5.091|$
  $+ |4.9 - 5.091| + |5.0 - 5.091| + |5.0 - 5.091| + |5.5 - 5.091|$
  $= 0.409 + 1.591 + 0.491 + 1.009 + 0.609 + 0.019 + 0.191 + 0.091 + 0.091 + 0.409$
  $= 4.91$

Absolute deviations from the mean = $\frac{4.91}{10} = 0.491$

- To find the absolute deviation from the median, we need to first find the median height for the data set.

  We know that to find the median value, we arrange the elements in the data set in ascending or descending order and the find that element that lies in the middle.

  5.5, 3.5, 4.6, 6.1, 5.7, 5.11, 4.9, 4.9, 5.0, 5.0, 5.5

  Arranged in ascending order from the smallest to the largest:

  3.5, 4.6, 4.9, 5.0, 5.0, 5.5, 5.5, 5.7, 5.11, 6.1

  Finding the median:

  3.5, ~~4.6~~, ~~4.9~~, ~~5.0~~, 5.0, 5.5, 5.5, ~~5.7~~, ~~5.11~~, ~~6.1~~

  Since we had an even number of elements in the data set, it comes as no surprise that we are unable to obtain a median by canceling out corresponding elements. We are left with two elements and so we find their mean which then becomes our median.

  $$\text{Median} = \frac{5.0 + 5.5}{2} = 5.25$$

  Having obtained our median as 5.25, we can proceed to find the average deviation from the median using the same steps as in the previous question.

  sum of deviations from the mean =

  $|5.5 - 5.25| + |3.5 - 5.25| + |4.6 - 5.25| + |6.1 - 5.25|$

  $+ |5.7 - 5.25| + |5.11 - 5.2| + |4.9 - 5.25| + |5.0 - 5.25|$

  $+ |5.0 - 5.25| + |5.5 - 5.25|$

  $= 0.25 + 1.75 + 0.65 + 0.85 + 0.45 + 0.14 + 0.35 + 0.25 + 0.25 + 0.25 = 5.19$

  $= 4.91$

  Absolute deviations from the mean = $\frac{5.19}{10} = 0.519$

Variance

- Variance, as the name suggests, is a measure of how different the elements in a given population are. Variance is used to indicate how spread out these elements are from the mean of the population. There are two kinds of variance: popuiation variance and sample variance.

  Population variance is the variance of the entire population and is denoted by σ^2 while sample variance is the variance of a sample space of the population; and is denoted by S^2.

Standard deviation

- It is the square root of variance. Standard deviation is a measure of how precise the mean of a population or sample is. It is used to indicate trends in the elements in a given data set with respect to the mean, i.e. the spread of these elements from the mean.

Just as we have a population and sample variance, we also have a population and sample standard deviation. Population standard deviation is denoted by σ while the sample standard deviation is denoted by S.

Although absolute deviation is also a measure of dispersion, variance and standard deviation are better measures because of the way they are calculated. Calculating variance involves squaring the differences (deviations) between the element and the mean and this makes the differences larger and thus more manageable. Making the differences larger adds a weighting factor to them making trends easier to spot.

The population variance can be calculated from the following:

$$\sigma^2 = \frac{1}{n}\sum_{i=1}^{n}(x_i - \mu)^2$$

Where μ is the population mean.

The sample variance is given by

$$S^2 = \frac{1}{n-1}\sum_{i=1}^{n}(x_i - \bar{x})^2$$

Where $\bar{x}$ is the sample mean.

Standard deviation is simply the square root of variance, so we can calculate it by taking the square root of the above variance formulae:

Population standard deviation

$$\sigma = \sqrt{\frac{1}{n}\sum_{i=1}^{n}(x_i - \mu)^2}$$

Where μ is the population mean.

Sample standard deviation

$$S = \sqrt{\frac{1}{n-1}\sum_{i=1}^{n}(x_i - \bar{x})^2}$$

Where $\bar{x}$ is the sample mean.

The difference in calculating σ^2 and S^2 is the average if found using the number of elements in the set for σ^2. By contrast, we use one less than the sample space size for S^2. The reason for this is that by using $n-1$ we ensure that S^2 is an unbiased estimator of σ^2.

Inferential Statistical Method

Inferential statistics are the statistics that enables inferences or conclusions to be made in a study about a population or given data from a sample. Inferential statistics are based on the laws of probability.

Statistical inferences consist mainly of estimating parameters and testing hypothesis. Examples of inferential statistics include – *t* test, Analysis of Variance (ANOVA), Chi square test, Analysis of Covariance (ANCOVA); to mention but a few.

The correlation coefficient mentioned under measurement in the earlier unit is often called a bi-variate statistics because it can be used as an inferential and descriptive statistics.

The *t* test is the statistic most commonly used for the testing of hypotheses that applies to differences between two groups, while the Analysis of Variance procedure can handle three or more groups as well as more than one independent variable.

The Chi square is most frequently used in connection with hypothesis relating to differences in proportions. Details of the computation of these can be obtained from any standard statistics textbook. You will be provided with some of them in the reading references at the end of this unit.

Hypothesis Testing and Levels of Significance

The null hypothesis is a statement that no relationship exists between the variables under study, and that any observed relationships are due to chance or sampling fluctuations. It is the null hypothesis that is often used in hypothesis testing.

The level of significance is always specified for statistical tests once testing of hypothesis is involved. The level of significance attaches a probability error to the rejection of the null hypothesis. The level often adopted in most studies is 0.05 or 5% level. Rejecting the null hypothesis of no difference means that there is less than 5% chance of observing the data if null hypothesis is true.

Two types of errors are possible with the rejection and/or acceptance of the null hypothesis.

Type 1 error: This error refers to rejection of the null hypothesis when it is true. The researcher in this situation concludes falsely that a difference is there when in fact, there is no difference.

Type 2 error: It is to accept the null hypothesis when it is false; to conclude wrongly that a difference does not exist when in reality, there is a difference.

One strategy to avoid both errors is to ensure that the sample size is increased in the study.

SUMMARY

In this unit we discuss the descriptive statistics are those measures that enable the researcher to describe the data or facts as contained in them.

Examples include the simple arithmetic mean or average. The inferential statistics are those that enable the researcher to make inferences or draw conclusions. Measures of central tendency and measures of dispersion are descriptive statistics and provide means of expressing how close and how wide apart the observations in a distribution are respectively. The mean and the standard deviation are the most useful of the measures respectively. Inferential statistics are used for hypothesis testing, and the level of significance used is usually 0.05 or 5%. Type 1 and Type 2 errors could occur when the null hypothesis is rejected wrongly and when it is accepted where it should be rejected respectively.

Application and Utilization of Research in Nursing Practices

10 unit

INTRODUCTION

Utilization of research findings is a major aspect of research in any field. It is the proceeds of research that give rise to new information, new methods, procedures and the basis for progression of any profession. Research is the only way to provide evidence or proof of what works and what does not. Many organizations spend lots of funds on research in order to improve their work situations and make a difference in people's lives. Utilization of findings is often not easy, because many are not enthusiastic to try new methods. They would rather continue as they are, but part of the responsibility of the researcher is to share the information about the research and its contribution in such a way that interests will enable other people to adopt or replicate the studies in order to make use of the findings.

Research Utilization vs Evidence Based Practice

The terms *research utilization* and *evidence-based practice (EBP)* are sometimes used synonymously. Although there is overlap between the two concepts, they are, in fact, distinct. Research utilization (RU), the narrower of the two terms, is the use of the findings from a disciplined study or set of studies in a practical application that is unrelated to the original research. In projects that have had research utilization as a goal, the emphasis is on translating empirically derived knowledge into real-world applications.

EBP involves making clinical decisions on the basis of the best possible evidence. Usually, the best evidence comes from rigorous research, but EBP also uses other sources of credible information.

The Utilization of Nursing Research

During the 1980s and early 1990s, *research utilization* became an important buzz word, and several changes in nursing education and nursing research were prompted by the desire to develop a knowledge base for nursing practice. In education, nursing schools increasingly began to include courses on research methods so that students would become intelligent research consumers. In the research arena, there was a shift in focus toward clinical nursing problems. These changes, coupled with the completion of several large research utilization projects, played a role in sensitizing the nursing community to the desirability of using research as a basis for practice; they were not enough, however, to lead to widespread integration of research findings into the delivery of nursing care. Research utilization, as the nursing community has come to recognize, is a complex and nonlinear phenomenon that poses professional challenges.

The Research Utilization Process: Rogers' Diffusion of Innovations Theory

Several theorists have developed models of how knowledge gets disseminated and used. The most noteworthy is one that has influenced several research utilization projects in the nursing community, Rogers' (1995) Diffusion of Innovations Theory.

Rogers postulates that knowledge diffusion is an evolutionary process by which an innovation is communicated overtime to members of a social system. The key elements in this process, all of which influence the rate and extent of innovation adoption, include the following:

- *The innovation* is the new idea, practice, or procedure that, if adopted, will result in changes; the nature of the innovation strongly affects decisions about adoption.
- *Communication channels* are the media through which information about the innovation is transmitted, and can include both mass media (e.g. journal articles, the Internet), or individual, face-to-face communication. Communication is most effective when there are shared beliefs, values, and expectations on the part of the sender and receiver of information.
- *Time* is a component of the theory in that the process of knowledge diffusion occurs overtime; there are varying amounts of time that elapse between the creation of the knowledge and its dissemination, and between knowledge awareness and the decision to use or reject the innovation.
- *The social system* is the set of interrelated units that solve problems and seek to accomplish a common goal; diffusion occurs within social systems that vary in their norms and receptivity to innovations.

Rogers characterized the innovation adoption process as having five stages: knowledge, persuasion, decision, implementation, and confirmation.

During the *knowledge stage,* individuals or groups become aware of the innovation, and during the *persuasion stage,* they form a positive attitude toward it. In the *decision stage,* a choice is made about whether to adopt or reject the innovation.

The innovation is actually put into use during the *implementation stage.* Finally, the effectiveness of the innovation is evaluated during the *confirmation stage,* and decisions get made about continuation or discontinuation of the innovation.

Recent research on utilization has challenged the linear nature of the process, and Rogers himself acknowledges that stages can sometimes be skipped, but the general model has been a useful way to think about the research utilization process in nursing.

Evidence-Based Practice

The research utilization/innovation diffusion process begins with an empirically based innovation or new idea that gets scrutinized for possible adoption in practice settings. EBP, by contrast, begins with a search for information about how best to solve specific practice problems.

Types of Evidence and Evidence Hierarchies

There is no consensus about what constitutes usable evidence for EBP, but there is general agreement that findings from rigorous studies are paramount.

There is, however, some controversy about what constitutes 'rigorous' research. In the initial phases of the EBP movement, there was a definite bias toward reliance on information from randomized clinical trials (RCTs), a bias stemming in part from the fact that the initial focus (e.g. at the Cochrane Collaboration) was on evidence about interventions rather than about other aspects of health care practice. This bias, in turn, led to some resistance to EBP by nurses who felt that evidence from qualitative and non-RCT studies would be ignored.

As Closs and Cheater (1999) have noted, "Some antagonism towards EBN (evidence-based nursing) seems to derive from viewing it as an unwelcome extension of the positivist tradition". Positions about what constitutes useful evidence have loosened, but there have nevertheless been efforts to develop *evidence hierarchies* that rank studies according to the strength of evidence they provide. Several such hierarchies have been developed, many based on the one proposed by Archie Cochrane. Most hierarchies put meta-analyzes of RCT studies at the pinnacle and other types of nonresearch evidence (e.g. clinical expertise) at the base.

As one example, Stetler, Brunell, Giuliano, Morse, Prince, and Newell-Stokes (1998) developed a six-level evidence hierarchy that also assigns grades on study quality (from A to D) within each of the six levels. The levels (from strongest to weakest) are as follows:

- Meta-analyzes of controlled studies
- Individual experimental studies
- Quasi-experimental studies (e.g. time series, non-equivalent control group) or matched case-control studies
- Non-experimental studies (e.g. correlational, descriptive, qualitative studies)
- Program evaluations, research utilization studies, quality improvement projects, case reports
- Opinions of respected authorities and of expert committees.

To date, there have been relatively few published studies of RCTs (level ii) in nursing, and even fewer published meta-analyzes of RCT nursing studies (see for example, Cullum, 1997). Therefore, evidence from other types of research will play an important role in evidence-based nursing practice.

Moreover, the evidence hierarchies are sensibly applied only to certain types of questions, such as questions about the effectiveness of interventions.

Many other clinical questions of importance to nurses can best be answered with rich descriptive and qualitative data from level iv and v studies.

Another issue is that there continue to be clinical practice questions for which there are relatively few research data. In such situations, an EBP will have to draw on other sources. Goode (2000) described an EBP model developed at the University of Colorado Hospital that has been includes nine non research sources of evidence that can be used to supplement the core (i.e. findings from disciplined research). These nine alternative sources include the following: benchmarking data (e.g. national rates for caesarean deliveries); cost-effectiveness analyzes; pathophysiologic data; retrospective or concurrent chart review; quality improvement and risk data; international, national, and local standards; institutional data collected for infection control purposes; patient preferences; and clinical expertise.

Thus, although EBP encompasses research utilization, both research and non-research sources of information play a role in EBP. Nurses and other health care professionals must be able to locate evidence, evaluate it, and integrate it with clinical judgment and patient preferences to determine the most clinically effective solutions to health problems.

Barriers to using Research in Nursing Practice

The next section of this chapter describes approaches to undertaking a research utilization or EBP project. First, however, we review some of the barriers to research utilization and research-based EBP in nursing because it is useful to take these barriers into account in the planning and implementation of efforts to integrate research into practice.

Several studies that have explored nurses' perceptions of barriers to research utilization have yielded remarkably similar results about constraints clinical nurses face (Funk, Tornquist, & Champagne, 1995).

Research-Related Barriers

For many nursing problems, the state-of-the-art of research knowledge is fairly primitive. Results reported in the literature may not merit translation into practice if methodologic flaws are extensive. Thus, one impediment to using research in practice is that, for many nursing problems, a solid base of valid and trustworthy study results has not been developed.

As we have repeatedly stressed, most studies have flaws, and so if nurses were to wait for 'perfect' studies before basing clinical decisions on research findings, they would have a very long wait indeed. It is precisely because of the limits of research methods that replication is essential. When repeated efforts to address a research question in different settings yield similar results, then there can be greater confidence in the findings. Single studies rarely provide an adequate basis for making changes in nursing practice. Therefore, another constraint to using research evidence is the dearth of published replications.

Nurse-Related Barriers

Studies have found that many clinical nurses have characteristics that constrain the use of research evidence in practice. One issue concerns nurses' educational preparation and their research skills. Many have not received any formal instruction in research, and may lack the skills to judge the merits of a study. Courses on research methodology are now typically offered in baccalaureate nursing programs, but the ability to critique a research report is not necessarily sufficient for effectively incorporating research results into daily decision-making.

Nurses' attitudes toward research and their motivation to engage in EBP have repeatedly been identified as potential barriers. Studies have found that the more positive the attitude, the more likely is the nurse to use research in practice.

Some nurses see research utilization as little more than a 'necessary evil' (Thompson, 2001), but there has been a trend toward more positive attitudes.

Another characteristic is one that is common to most humans: People are often resistant to change. Change requires effort, retraining, and restructuring of work habits. Change may also be perceived as threatening (e.g. changes maybe perceived as affecting job security). Thus, there is likely to be some opposition to introducing innovations in the practice setting. However, there is evidence from a survey of more than 1200 nurses that nurses value nursing research and want to be involved in research-related activities (Rizzuto, Bostrom, Suter, and Chenitz, 1994).

Organizational Barriers

Many of the major impediments to using research in practice stem from the organizations that train and employ nurses. Organizations, perhaps to an even greater degree than individuals, resist change, unless there is a strong organizational perception that there is something fundamentally wrong with the status quo. To challenge tradition and accepted practices, a spirit of intellectual curiosity and openness must prevail.

In many practice settings, administrators have established procedures to reward competence in nursing practice; however, few practice settings have established a system to reward nurses for critiquing nursing studies, for using research in practice, or for discussing research findings with clients. Thus, organizations have failed to motivate or reward nurses to seek ways to implement appropriate findings in their practice. Research review and use are often considered appropriate activities only when time is available, but available time is usually limited. In several studies of barriers to RU, one of the greatest reported barriers was 'insufficient time on the job to implement new ideas.'

Organizations also maybe reluctant to expend resources for RU/EBP activities or for changing organizational policy. Resources maybe required for the use of outside consultants, staff release time, library materials and Internet access, evaluating the effects of an innovation, and so on. With the push toward cost containment in health care settings, resource constraints may therefore pose a barrier to change—unless the project has cost containment as an explicit goal.

EBP will become part of organizational norms only if there is a commitment on the part of managers and administrators. Strong leadership in health care organizations is essential to making EBP happen.

Models for Evidence-Based Nursing Practice

During the 1980s and 1990s, a number of different models of research utilization were developed. These models offered guidelines for designing and implementing a utilization project in a practice setting.

The most prominent of these models were the previously mentioned Diffusion of Innovations Theory, the Stetler model, and the Iowa model. The latter two models have been updated to incorporate EBP processes, rather than research utilization processes alone.

The *Stetler Model* of Research Utilization (Stetler, 1994) was designed with the assumption that research utilization could be undertaken not only by organizations, but by individual clinicians and managers. It was a model designed to promote and facilitate critical thinking about the application of research findings in practice. The updated and refined model is based on many of the same assumptions and strategies as the original, but provides "an enhanced approach to the overall application of research in the service setting". The current model, presented graphically in involves five sequential phases:

- *Preparation:* In this phase, nurses define the underlying purpose and outcomes of the project; search, sort, and select sources of research evidence; consider external factors that can influence potential application and internal factors that can diminish objectivity; and affirm the priority of the perceived problem.
- *Validation.* This phase involves a utilization focused critique of each source of evidence, focusing in particular on whether it is sufficiently sound for *potential* application in practice. (The process stops at this point if the evidence sources are rejected.)
- *Comparative evaluation and decision-making:* This phase involves a synthesis of findings and the application of four criteria that, taken together, are used to determine the desirability and feasibility of applying findings from validated sources to nursing practice.
- *Translation/Application:* This phase involves activities to:
  - Confirm how the findings will be used (e.g. formally or informally).
  - Spell out the operational details of the application, and implement them. The latter might involve the development of a guideline, detailed procedure, or plan of action, possibly including plans for formal organizational change.
- *Evaluation:* In the final phase, the application is evaluated. Informal use of the innovation versus formal use would lead to different evaluative strategies.

Although the Stetler model originally was designed as a tool for individual practitioners, it has also been the basis of formal research utilization and EBP projects by groups of nurses.

SUMMARY

In this unit we discuss about the utilization of research findings is important to update practice in all aspects of nursing: Education, clinical practice, home care, community, etc. Utilization of research findings depends on the relevance of the findings to the needs and problems of the practitioners. The participation of the research personnel would be seen as facilitator for utilization of findings. There is need for support from managers and employers to give time for training and costs for the application of research findings in practice to ensure evidence based practice. Barriers to research utilization include lack of knowledge of research by nurses, lack of facilities needed to implement findings, lack of time to read research, poor access to research information/reports, and lack of competency to read and interpret research findings. A major strength to ensure utilization would be continued professional development and in service education programs for practitioners and involvement of research personnel in the utilization of findings.

PROFORMA FOR THE SYNOPSIS

Name of College/University

1. Name of the candidate and address
2. Name of the institution
3. Course of study and subject
4. Date of admission to the course
5. Title of the topic
6. Brief resume of the intended work:
    - 6.1 Introduction
    - 6.2 Need for the study
    - 6.3 Review of literature
    - 6.4 Statement of the problem
    - 6.5 Objectives of the study
    - 6.6 Hypotheses of the study
    - 6.7 Variables under study
      Independent variables
      Dependent variables
    - 6.8 Operational definitions
    - 6.9 Assumptions
7. Material and methods:
    - 7.1 Source of data
    - 7.2 Method of collection of data:
        - 7.2.1 Research approach

7.2.2 Research design
7.2.3 Setting of the study
7.2.4 Population
7.2.5 Sample size
7.2.6 Sampling technique
7.2.7 Sampling criteria
Inclusion criteria
Exclusion criteria
7.2.8 Tool for data collection
7.2.9 Data analysis method
Descriptive statistics
Inferential statistics
7.3 Does the study require any interventions to be conducted on patients or other humans or animals
7.4 Has the ethical clearance been obtained from your institution?

8. List of references
9. Signature of the student
10. Remarks of the guide
11. Name and designation of the guide:
    11.1 Guide name and address
    11.2 Signature of the guide
    11.3 Head of the department
    Name and address
    11.4 Signature of the hod
12. Remarks of principal
13. Signature of the principal

3

Section

Professional Trends and Adjustment

COURSE DESCRIPTION

Hrs. 45

Course description

This course is designed to help students develop an understanding of the career opportunities available, limitations of nursing profession professional development.

General Objectives

Upon completion of this course the students will able to:

- Describe nursing as a profession and the criteria of a profession
- Identify various professional responsibilities of a nurse
- Describe various professional organizations related to nursing and health identify the need for in-service and continuing education in nursing
- Demonstrate skills in application of knowledge of professional etiquettes in the practice of nursing in any health care setting.

Course content

Unit 11: Introduction to Nursing as a Profession

- Definition and criteria of nursing profession
- Evolution of nursing profession in India
- Educational preparation of a professional nurse
- Qualities/characteristics and role of a professional nurse.

Unit 12: Professional Ethics

- Meaning and relationship of professional ethics and etiquettes
- Code of ethics for nurses, INC, ICN code of ethics and Nightingale pledge
- Procedure for employment: locating a position, applying and accepting a position, resignation from a position.

Unit 13: Personal and Professional Growth/Development

- Continuing Education:
  - Meaning and importance of continuing education
  - Scope of continuing education
  - Planning and financing for continuing education
  - In-service education: definition, need participation.

- Career in Nursing:
  - Opportunities available in hospital, community, teaching and other related special organizations
  - International influence and aid
  - Nursing in the future.

Unit 14: Legislation in Nursing

- Purpose and importance of laws in nursing, legal terms.
- Common legal hazards in nursing
- Health laws and regulations affecting nurses in India at different levels; center and state. Consumer protection bill and its impact in nursing practice
- Fundamental conduct and service rule and instructional rules
- Regulation and reciprocities.

Unit: 14: Professional and Related Organizations

- *Professional organization:* Trained nurses association of India (TNAI), Student Nurse Association, International council of Nurses (ICN), Indian Nursing Council (INC), State Nursing councils, Commonwealth Nurses Federation (CNF), Nurses league of Christian Medical Association.
- *Related organizations and their contribution to nursing:* World Health Organization (WHO), Red Cross, St. John's ambulance, UNICEF, World Bank, etc.

Introduction to Nursing as a Profession

11 unit

INTRODUCTION

Nursing profession is that assumes responsibility for the continuous care of the sick, injured, disabled, and the dying persons. Nursing is also responsible for encouraging the health of individuals, families, and communities in medical and community settings. Nurses are actively involved in health care research, management, policy deliberations, and patient advocacy. Nurses with post baccalaureate preparation assume independent responsibility for providing primary health care and speciality services to individuals, families, and communities.

Professional nurses work both independently and in collaboration with other health care professionals such as physicians. Professional nurses supervise the work of nurses who have limited licenses, such as licensed practical nurses (LPNs). Professional nurses also oversee the work of nursing assistants in various settings.

Nursing is the largest, the most diverse, and one of the most respected of all the health care professions. The demand for nursing remains high, and projections suggest that such demand will substantively increase. Advances in health care technology, rising expectations of people seeking care, and reorganization of health care systems require a greater number of highly educated professionals. Demographic changes, such as large aging populations in many countries of the world, also fuel this demand.

DEFINITION OF NURSING

Although nursing practice varies both through its various specialities and countries, these nursing organizations offer the following definitions:

- According to *International Council of Nurses* 'Nursing encompasses autonomous and collaborative care of individuals of all ages, families, groups and communities, sick or well and in all settings. Nursing includes the promotion of health, prevention of illness, and the care of ill, disabled and dying people. Advocacy, promotion of a safe environment, research, participation in shaping health policy and in patient and health systems management, and education are also key nursing roles'.

- According to *American Nurses Association* 'Nursing is the protection, promotion, and optimization of health and abilities; prevention of illness and injury, alleviation of suffering through the diagnosis and treatment of human responses; and advocacy in health care for individuals, families, communities, and populations'.
- According to *Virginia Avenel Henderson* 'The unique function of the nurse is to assist the individual, sick or well, in the performance of those activities contributing to health or its recovery (or to peaceful death) that he would perform unaided if he had the necessary strength, will or knowledge'.
- According to *Florence Nightingale,* the founder of modern nursing 'Nursing is the care which puts a person in the best possible condition for nature to restore or preserve health, to prevent or to care disease or injury'.
- Nursing is provision of optimal conditions to enhance the person's reparative processes and prevent the reparative process from being interrupted.
- The practice of nursing is defined as diagnosing and treating human response to actual or potential health problems through such services as case finding, health teaching, health counselling and provision of support to or restoration of life and well-being and executing medical regimes prescribed by licensed or otherwise legally authorized physician or dentist.
- Nursing is directed toward meeting both the health and illness need and man who is viewed holistically as having physical, emotional, psychological intellectual, social and spiritual.
- Nursing is a humanistic science dedicated to compassionate concern with maintaining and promoting health, preventing illness and caring for and rehabilitating the sick and disabled.
- Nursing is a deliberate action, a function of the practical intelligence of nurses and action to bring about humanely desirable conditions in persons and their environments.
- As a practice discipline nursing's scientific body of knowledge is used to provide an essential service to people, that is to promote ability to affect health positively.

CRITERIA OF NURSING PROFESSION

Nursing is gaining recognition as a profession. Profession has been defined as an occupation that requires extensive education or a calling that requires special knowledge, skill, and preparation. A profession is generally distinguished from other kinds of occupations by:

- *Its requirement of prolonged, specialized training to acquire a body of knowledge pertinent to the role to be performed:* Specialized education is an important aspect of professional status. In modern times, the trend in education for the professions has shifted toward programs in colleges and universities. Many nursing educators believe that the undergraduate nursing curriculum should include liberal arts education in addition to the biologic and social sciences and the nursing discipline.
- *An orientation of the individual toward service, either to a community or to an organization:* A service orientation differentiates nursing from an occupation pursued primarily for profit. Many consider altruism (selfless concern for others) the hallmark of a profession. Nursing has a tradition of service to others. This service, however, must be guided by certain rules, policies, or codes of ethics. Today, nursing is also an important component of the health care delivery system.
- *Ongoing research:* Increasing research in nursing is contributing to nursing practice. Nursing research has focused on practice-related issues, studies were often related to the nature if the knowledge base underlying nursing practice.
- *Code of ethics:* Nurses have traditionally placed a high value on the worth and dignity of others. The nursing profession requires integrity if its members; that is, a member is expected to do what is considered right regardless of the personal cost. Ethical codes change as the needs and values of society change. Nursing has developed its own codes of ethics.

EVOLUTION OF NURSING PROFESSION IN INDIA

Nursing in Ancient Times

Ancient history shows records of nursing. What we know about the care of the sick in ancient times has been discovered through songs and findings of archaeologists. People were interested in the mysteries of life, birth, disease and death. Men lived very close to nature and life was very simple also people made few changes except when men were compelled to do so. Men attributed spiritual value to all natural objects, believing that objects in nature such as trees or rivers had spirit or soul. Objects in nature became friends such as water and trees, while storms and poisonous plants became enemies. Attitudes changed according to man's ability to control nature. They thanked friendly harmless objects for their help and tried to cooperate with the unfriendly, threatening situations.

Disease was believed to be caused by evil spirits within the body. The body had to undergo unpleasant experiences to get rid of these evil spirits. Men thought disease was caused by their failure to satisfy the gods, or was punishment for their sins. These ideas are still prevalent today even among highly civilized and intelligent people.

People were ignorant of the laws of nature. People were beaten to get rid of evil spirits, sudden fright, loud noises and magic ceremonies were also used to get rid of evil spirit. Holes on the bodies were made for the evil spirits to escape. Sacrifices were offered as a treatment. Care was given by the man who knew the signs and symptoms of evil spirits and knew what to do in certain conditions. He wore a strange dress and used magic words. He took his role as a priest. He attempted to understand and control the forces of health and disease. The skill of primitive men in fighting disease has given us many medical and surgical treatments. Massage, fomentation, bone setting, amputations, hot and cold baths, abdominal sections and heat to control hemorrhage are some of the skills gained from primitive men.

Nursing in Greek and Roman Medicine

People in Greece believed that medicine was of divine origin and was represented by many gods. Apollo, the sun god, represented health and medicine, his son Aesculapius, was the god of healing and his daughter, Hygeia, was the goddess of health. Temples were built for gods. A priest physician was incharge of it. People came to the temple and believed that during their sleep god would appear and prescribe them treatment. They used special diets and massage bath.

Hippocrates gave scientific views to medicine. He was known as the father of medicine. He taught doctors signs and symptoms of diseases. The treatment was based on diagnosis. He developed ways of doing physical examination and taking histories. Stress was given on good health by giving good diet, fresh air and maintaining cleanliness. He gave instructions in hot applications, poultices, cold sponge for fever, fluid for kidney diseases and mouth washes. Rome learnt a lot from Greece about medicine. Rome built good sanitation, good roads and bridges. There were pubic baths for men and women; drinking water was brought by channel or large pipes. Drainage system and sewage were made. They built market places and hospitals. Old women and men of good character did nursing in those days.

Nursing in Modern Times

The modern form of nursing was started by Florence Nightingale. Before that, it was influenced by religious groups. In the 15th and 16th centuries, nursing was dominated in Europe by religious bodies including Benedictine and Augustinian sisters, Franciscan brothers and sisters of charity. Original motivation for caring for the sick was in order to ensure one's salvation by engaging in self-sacrificing work. That is why nursing was considered as a noble work. Today, the salvation has been replaced by a desire to serve people, nation and the world with the help of scientific technology.

Actually, Florence Nightingale (1820–1910) revived nursing during her life time. She said, "Nursing is to help the patient to live."

She was one of the most influential reformers of her time. Even today, her writings remain as relevant as they were 120 years ago. Her own practical experiences combined with her own aims for the nursing profession gave her a greater insight into problems of hospital administration than her contemporaries. Her social position enabled her to give ideas to the committees, which controlled the voluntary hospitals in those days. But above all, she had the determination to use every weapon she possessed including charm and social pressure to achieve the objective she had in mind, thus becoming the greatest publicist the profession has ever had. After the Crimean War of 1854, nursing could never be the same again. Florence Nightingale's adventure in Crimea drew public attention on an enormous scale to the problems of nursing role in transforming the recruitment, training and practice of the new profession.

Nursing in India

The earliest Indian medicine was Ayur Veda Medicine found in Veda 5000 BC About 1400 BC Charaka, the father of medicine, wrote a book on internal medicine. From these books we learn the hospitals were large and well equipped. Surgery had advanced to a high level. Doctors and attendants or nurses had to be people of high moral character. King Ashoka BC 226–250, built monasteries and houses for travellers, hospitals for men and animals were founded. Hygienic practice was adapted; cleanliness of body was a religious duty. First importance was given to prevention of diseases. Doctors and nurses were expected to be skilful and trustworthy. They had to keep their nails short. Nurses were usually men or old women.

In 1857 the India Mutiny turned Miss Nightingale's interest to the health of the Army in India. It was for this purpose the Royal Commission was appointed in 1859. In 1868, a sanitary department was established.

In March 1888, ten qualified British nurses arrived in India to look after the British Army in India. In 1905, during the British rule in India, missionary nurses arrived as members of Missionary Medical Association. This was the very start of formalized nursing service in India.

Gradually, the increasing need of adequately trained nurses led to creation of South India Examining Board in 1911 and the North India Examining Board in 1912. It was the mission hospital nursing leaders who laid the foundation of systematic Nursing education in India. However, the mid India Board of Examination was started in 1934. But this was not regulated for registration. State-wise councils started developing from 1935 onwards. Indian Nursing Council (INC) Act was passed by the Parliament in 1947. The Nursing Council upgraded the educational requirements which permitted only matriculated candidates to seek admission to the schools. Now, India has State-wise registration councils in 19 states. (TNAI yearbook 2000–2001).

The Central Government granted an approval to the Bhore Committee's (1946) recommendations by starting two colleges of Nursing in Delhi (1946) and Vellore (1947). This provided university degree level courses. With the efforts of Professor S. Radhakrishnan (the then Chairman of University Education Commission), Nursing education in the country was integrated into the system of higher education.

Over decades, there has been an improvement in the availability of nursing education in India.

EDUCATIONAL PREPARATION OF A PROFESSIONAL NURSE

- *Practical nurse education:* Practical nursing has been in existence for many years. In the past the practical nurse was the family, friends or community members who was called to the home during emergencies. These were lay people who gained the experience through self taught. The first formal education in practical nursing was started in 1892. The duration of training was 3 months and students were called attendants. The curricula of practical nursing includes child and elderly care, cooking and care of the sick at home.
- *Licensed practical nursing:* This program provided by high school, community colleges, vocational schools, hospitals, and a variety of health agents. These programs usually last one year and provide both classroom and clinical experiences. At the end, the graduate takes national council licensing examination to obtain a license as a practical or vocational nurse. In Ethiopia the international licensed examination was given up to 1977. Later on national was given and stopped 1997.

- *Registered nursing:* In the United States, most basic education for registered nurses is provided in three types of programs, diploma, associate degree, and baccalaureate programs in Canada, the 2-years, 3-years or more diploma and baccalaureate programs prepare registered nurses.
- *Diploma:* Today's diploma nursing program have changed markedly from the original nightingale model, becoming hospital-based education programs that provide a rich clinical experience for nursing students these programs programs may last two or more years and are often associated with colleges or universities. In Ethiopia the diploma program required 8th grade and stayed for 4 years, then the requirement was changed to 10th to 12th grade and staying 2 to 3 years.
- *Associate degree:* In 1980 as a solution to the acute shortage of nurses that came about because of World War II. Associated degree programs are offered in united state in junior colleges as well as in college and universities.
- *Baccalaureate degree:* Although baccalaureate nursing education programs were established in universities in both united state and Canada in the early 1900s. In 1960s the number of the students enrolled in these programs increased markedly. In Ethiopia this programme was started in Jimma university in 1993. Later on the program continued in Della, Alemaya and Gonedr.
- *Master's programs:* Master's programs generally take from 11/2 to 2 years to complete. In 1995 the numbers of nurses obtaining master's degree increased. The mastered program has been proposed in September, 2005 in Ethiopia.
- *Doctoral programs:* Doctoral programs in nursing, which award the degree of doctor of nursing science (DNS). The program, began in the 1960s in united state.
- *Continuing education:* To formalize experiences designed to enlarge the knowledge or skills of practitioners.
- *In-service education:* Program is administered by an employer; it is designed to update the knowledge or skills of employees.

QUALITIES OF A PROFESSIONALLY NURSE

The professional nurse is outstanding in his/her area of care, this he/she is able to achieve by employing certain qualities at his/her disposal. These special qualities differentiate him/her from all other members of the health team.

- *Honest:* One of the qualities that make the nurse outstanding is honesty. He/she is taught to be truthful at all times when dealing with the patient and his family, and when dealing with colleagues and other members of the health team. By so doing, he is able to earn everyone's confidence/trust.

- *Caring:* The nurse is able to give the client proper attention. He/she is compassionate in taking care of the clients; the comfort of the patient is of utmost importance to him/her.
- *Empathetic:* He/she is able to understand the feelings of the patient and treat him the way he/she would love to be treated.
- *Observant:* The nurse is an observant person; she is able to monitor/observe the client closely to know when there is improvement in his condition or when there is deterioration. He/she is also able to observe his environment whether it is safe or not.
- *Skilful:* He is skilful in handling the problems of the patient. These skills which are enhanced by his training enable him to properly deal with his client's problems.
- *Decisive:* He/she is able to analyze situations and take prompt decisions.
- *Confidential:* The nurse is able to hold in confidence whatever information he has concerning his clients. He does not divulge the client's personal information to any other person.
- *Physically fit:* The nurse is physically fit because the job is demanding—it involves lifting, hours of standing, long periods of procedures, etc.
- *Emotionally stable:* He is also emotionally stable; he should be in his right state of mind. It takes emotional stability for a person to take right decisions and also be accountable for his actions.
- *Good interpersonal skills:* He should possess good interpersonal skills to be able to interact with other members of the health team. He should be able to interact with doctors, pharmacists, physiotherapists, dentists, nutritionists, etc.
- *Teachable:* The nurse should be someone who is willing to learn what would add value to his/her life.
- *Respect:* He must have respect for the rights of the patient and other members of the medical team. He should particularly be willing to respect the cultural differences, religious rights, etc. of the clients.
- *Good communicator:* He should also possess good communication skills in order to effectively act as a link between the medical team and the client. He should be able to communicate also with his colleagues.
- *Flexible:* The nurse should also be fairly flexible in his approach to work. He should be able to adapt when there is a change in work schedule/situations.
- *Hospitable:* He should be friendly to the patient and family, as well as to professional colleagues. He should be able to give the clients a smile when dealing with them.

- *Obedient:* Nursing is a disciplined profession; therefore the nurse must be willing to obey hierarchy and also obey laid down rules of the profession.
- *Neat:* The professional nurse is always neat. He is conscious of his environment and makes sure he is not a vehicle for the spread of microorganisms.
- *Cautious:* The nurse is careful while dealing with the patient, his colleagues and members of the health team. He tries to avoid all forms of errors while compiling his records and other documents.
- *Intelligent:* The nurse must be an intelligent person who is able to take initiative on his/her own; and must be able to interpret prescriptions and the nursing care plan. He mustn't be someone who would not kill the patient or make irreparable errors as a result of his unintelligent decisions.
- *Agile:* The nurse is supposed to be an agile person and must be able to respond swiftly to all situations. Time is of the essence while dealing with human lives; he/she must be able to act fast to save situations before they deteriorate.

CHARACTERISTICS OF A PROFESSIONALLY NURSE

Although the physician treats the disease, the nurse is the healthcare provider that treats the patient. First and foremost, nurses assess and care for the patients' needs, emotional responses and define the barriers to care. As patient advocates, the nurse is the coordinator of the patient's medical care, family interactions, other healthcare providers and the physician's orders. Although nurses practice in hospitals, skilled nursing centers, medical centers and outpatient clinics, those who have committed themselves to the service of the community continue to demonstrate similar attributes that are indicative of successful careers in nursing.

- *Empathy:* The most important quality for a nurse is to embody empathy. According to the study Empathy and the Quality of Care, empathy is a multidimensional concept that enables the caregiver to identify, share emotions and provide care for the patient in distress. The basic definition of nursing is caring and empathy is at the core of nursing.
- *Detail oriented:* Nurses perform patient assessments, manage medical equipment and administer medication. The nurse's role has a zero tolerance for error where the smallest mistake may result in a life-threatening event. Nurses provide detailed documentation and pay close attention to the transcription of physician orders. Those who are oriented to the finest details in patient care are superior in the nursing field.

- *Communication:* Nurses provide care for and interact with people of various ages, multicultural backgrounds and specific needs and requirements. According to the study Magnet Environments for Professional Nursing Practice, nurses of excellence take the time to listen, understand and protect the patient's cultural beliefs.
- *Intuition:* The best nurses use experience, scientific knowledge, and instinct when assessing patients. Intuition in nursing is defined as the immediate understanding of a problem without the necessity of conscious thought. Nurses pick-up on the smallest cues, nuances and seemingly unrelated patient statements that may render further investigation. Through intuition, superior nurses save lives and prevent further illness.
- *Physical endurance:* Maintaining physical health is a vital part of enduring the stressful and high-energy demands of the nursing profession. Nurses lift heavy patients, move weighty medical equipment, and may spend 12 hours or more on their feet during a shift. Accomplished nurses observe a healthy diet and perform regular exercise.
- *Emotional stability:* During the course of a work day, nurses need to be ready to handle difficult emergencies, be witness to human suffering, and experience stressful situations. Gifted nurses should be able to cope with these events well by using the power of their own spirituality or by accepting that life is a cycle of inevitable events.
- *Critical thinking:* Nurses must be able to obtain autonomy through critical thinking skills that arm them with the ability to respond to the constant changes and needs of a patient in their charge. As nurses build on practical knowledge, gain experience and continue educational endeavors, the intellectually disciplined process allows the nurse to recognize possible patient problems. According to the Bureau of Labor Statistics, critical thinking is an important quality that allows nurses to take action and make referrals.
- *Coordinator of services:* Nurses lead the allied healthcare team and coordinates care with other providers. The top nurses effectively convey the patient's requests and condition to other members of the medical team for optimal care, time management and efficiency.
- *Patience:* For nurses in any career field or speciality, patience is an integral part of success. Great nurses understand that patience can overcome anxiety, misunderstandings and help patients and colleagues feel empowered by good decisions.
- *Dedication:* Successful nurses focus on the needs of their patients and provide the best possible care under any circumstances. These dedicated nurses continue to enhance their education, become leaders in their field, and teach novice nurses in their speciality.

ROLE OF A PROFESSIONAL NURSE

- *Care provider:* Caring/comforting involve knowledge and sensitivity to what matter and what is important to the client.
- *Communicator/helper:* Effective communication is an essential element of all helping profession, including nursing. It helps the client to explain the internal feeling.
- *Teacher/educator:* Teacher refers to activities by which the teacher helps the student to learn. The client also need education based on the case.
- *Counselor:* Counseling is a process of helping a client to recognized and copes with stressful psychological or social problem, to develop improved interpersonal relationships and promote personal growth.
- *Client advocate:* An advocate pleads the cause of others or argues or pleads for a cause or proposal.
- *Change agent:* A change agent is a person or group who initiates changes or who assists others in making modification in them or in the system.
- *Leader:* Leadership is defined as mutual process of interpersonal influence through which the nurse helps a client make decision in establishing and achieving goals to improve the client well being.
- *Manager:* Management defines manager as who plans, gives direction, developing staff, monitoring operations, giving rewards fairly and representing both staff member and administration as needed.
- *Researcher:* Majority of researchers in nursing are prepared at doctoral and post doctoral level. Although an increasing number of clinicians and nurses with masters degree are beginning to practice it.

SUMMARY

In this unit we discuss about nursing is a humanistic science dedicated to compassionate concern with maintaining and promoting health, preventing illness and caring for and rehabilitating the sick and disabled. In ancient India, male nurses staffed early Hospitals and women served as midwives and nursed ill family members. A profession is a calling that requires special knowledge and skilled preparation. A profession is generally distinguished from other kinds of occupation by: Its requirement of prolonged specialized training acquiring a body of knowledge pertinent to the role to be performed and an orientation of the individual to ward service, ether to community or organization.

12 unit

Professional Ethics

INTRODUCTION

The *Code of Ethics for Registered Nurses* serves as a foundation for nurses' ethical practice. It provides guidance for ethical relationships, responsibilities, behaviors and decision-making, and it is to be used in conjunction with the professional standards, laws and regulations that guide practice. The code serves as a means of self-evaluation and self-reflection for ethical nursing practice and provides a basis for feedback and peer review. It also serves as an ethical basis from which nurses can advocate for quality work environments that support the delivery of safe, compassionate, competent and ethical care.

Nurses recognize the privilege of being part of a self-regulating profession and have a responsibility to merit this privilege. The code informs other health-care professionals as well as members of the public about the ethical commitments of nurses and the responsibilities nurses accept as being part of a self-regulating profession.

MEANING OF PROFESSIONAL ETHICS

Ethics is concerned with 'right and wrong', although agreeing what is 'right' can be challenging. An understanding of ethics is essential to the delivery of skilled professional care. It is vital that nurses appreciate the value of ethics in their work. Ethics is relevant to clinical, practice-based issues and affects all areas of the professional nursing role. To apply ethics effectively, nurses must develop reasoning skills and understand the concepts and principles that assist ethical analysis. The terms 'ethical' and 'moral' are used interchangeably.

RELATIONSHIP BETWEEN PROFESSIONAL ETHICS AND ETIQUETTES

Professional ethics introduces students to the fundamentals of nursing ethics. Nursing students learn about the decision-making process to solve ethical dilemmas, understanding barriers and consequences when making ethical decisions, and the process for blowing the whistle when unethical situations arise. The fundamental responsibility of the nurse is to promote health, prevent illness, restore health and to alleviate suffering. The need for nursing is universal; inherent in nursing is respect for life, dignity and rights of man. It embraces nationality, race, creed, color, age, and gender, politic or social status. Ethic is based on moral issues as inter-alia and relate to the society or group you serve.

Etiquette is another name for good manner; it tells us how to behave in everyday situation. This includes respect to the senior, clients and relations, staff and community. These are some ethics/etiquette which when respected have implication on the leadership role and the image of the Nurse.

- Nurse should report to duty punctually.
- The nurse should be courteous when spoken to.
- Correct and prescribe uniform must be worn, kept neat and tidy.
- All activities should be directed towards patients care.
- Dangling ear rings should not be worn.
- Address patients and clients by their names respectfully.
- Avoid absenteeism and always seek permission from your superior when you want to leave your department or unit.
- The nurse should not loiter around after the day's work unless she has very important thing to do or visiting hours.
- The nurse should behave politely in public and protect the image of the profession.
- Should serve the community to the best of his ability.
- The nurse should apply and practice hospital economy effectively.
- Finger nails should kept short, neat and should not be painted.
- The nurse should not smoke or chew gum while in uniform.
- The nurse should not come to duty drunk nor drink while on duty.
- Hairstyle should be neat and avoid hair ornaments and flowers should not be worn as self beautification.
- Report and refer any illness to the appropriate quarters
- Attend to patients promptly and listen to their complaints and needs.
- Should avoid shouting and calling colleagues across the ward as this could be embarrassing and disturbing.

- All communication with patients should be based on her care.
- Patients' information should be kept confidential.
- Nurses should not use noisy shoes as this will disturb the patients.
- All instructions and messages regarding to patients as maybe directed by the sister or ward charge should be reported and action taken immediately.
- The nurse should give comprehensive nursing care to all manners of patients in respect of tribe, age religion and race.

The Activities of the Nurses are Reflected on the Following

- *Nurse and people:* To provide care, promote an environment in which the values, customs and spiritual beliefs of individuals are respected.
- *Nurse and practice:* The nurse personal responsibility for nursing practice and maintaining competence by continuous learning.
- *Nurse and society:* The nurse share with other citizens the responsibility for initiating and supporting actions to meet the health and social needs of the public.
- *Nurse and co-workers:* The nurse sustains cooperative relationship with coworkers in nursing and other members of health team.
- *Nurse and the profession:* The nurse play the major role in determining and implementing desirable standards of nursing practice and nursing education.

The public perception of nurses are enormous ranging from cruelty to patients, using vulgar language, bickering, backbiting and apportioning blame on the release of patients' confidential, lack of decorum, non sympathetic and I do not care attitude towards patients care.

CODE OF PROFESSIONAL CONDUCT FOR NURSES

Each nurse (registered or enrolled) is accountable for his/her practice. In the exercise of his/her professional responsibilities, each nurse has an obligation to uphold and adhere to the code of professional conduct for nurses. The code aims to make explicit the standards for professional conduct that nurses shall act at all times in their course of duty. It may also serve to provide the public with a basis for decisions regarding standards of professional conduct.

The code of professional conduct for nurses highlights eight aspects of professional conduct that nurses are to comply within discharging their professional duties.

a. *Respect the dignity, uniqueness, values, culture and beliefs of patients/ clients and their families in the provision of nursing care:*
   - The nurse recognizes and respects the uniqueness and dignity of each patient/client and responds to his/her need for care.

- The nurse seeks assistance and advice from appropriate personnel in care situations where he/she finds difficulties in providing due care for the patients/clients due to conflict of personal belief.
- The nurse treats with consideration and respect the wishes and decisions of patients/clients and their families when planning and delivering care.

b. *Hold in confidence personal information obtained in a professional capacity:*
   - The nurse ensures that the information given by the patients/clients in confidence will only be used for the purposes for which it was given.
   - The nurse protects the information obtained in the course of professional practice and discloses only with the patient's/client's consent, or in exceptional circumstances, such as where a court order is made for disclosure.
   - When personal information is required for teaching, research or quality assurance procedures, the nurse takes care to protect the patients/client's anonymity and privacy.

c. *Safeguard informed decision-making and the well-being of patients/clients in the provision of care:*
   - The nurse provides patients/clients and their families with accurate and relevant information to the best of the nurse's knowledge to facilitate them to make informed judgments and decisions.
   - In situations where patients are mentally incapacitated or unable to decide or speak for they regarding choices of care/treatment, the nurse should endeavor to ensure that the perspective of the patient/client is represented by an appropriate representative.

d. *Provide safe and competent nursing care:*
   - The nurse promotes a safe and therapeutic environment in the provision of nursing care.
   - The nurse is responsible and accountable for individual nursing judgments and actions.
   - The nurse ensures that there is no action or omission of responsibility that is detrimental to the interests and safety of patients/clients.
   - The nurse uses judgment in relation to individual knowledge, qualifications and competence when accepting or delegating duties or responsibilities.
   - The nurse collaborates with nursing colleagues and other members of healthcare team to advocate health care environments conducive to safe and competent care.
   - The nurse practices and maintains the best possible standard of care within the reality of her/his working conditions.

- The nurse does not condone or connive at any action that may jeopardize the safety of patients/clients.
- The nurse raises objection to practices that compromise safe and appropriate care to patients/clients.
- The nurse reports to an appropriate person or authority any circumstances in which safe and appropriate care cannot be provided.
- The nurse plays his/her rightful role in the healthcare establishments.

e. *Maintain the agreed standard of practice:*
- The nurse is responsible for ensuring that the standard of nursing practice is congruent with the agreed standards of the profession.
- The nurse participates in identifying, implementing and evaluating evidence-based practices.
- The nurse recognizes the need for lifelong learning and participates in continuing nursing education.
- The nurse is active in updating her knowledge and skills at regular intervals to enhance professional competence.
- The nurse observes occupational health and safety at work, and observes the health and safety rules for fostering self and other colleagues well-being and safety in practice situations.

f. *Foster the trust that is inherent in the privileged relationship between nurses and their patients/clients:*
- The nurse fosters a therapeutic relationship with patients/clients and their families and is vigilant that such a relationship is not abused.
- The nurse promotes and preserves the trust from their patients/clients and does not cause his/her patients/clients any physical or psychological harm.
- The nurse does not abuse his/her patients'/clients' property.

g. *Uphold the image of nurses and the profession by refusing advantages:*
- The nurse declines any gift, favor or hospitality offered for the purpose of obtaining preferential treatment.
- The nurse ensures that his/her professional status is not misused in the promotion of commercial products or services.
- The nurse ensures that his/her professional judgment is not influenced by any commercial considerations.
- The nurse declares to the appropriate authority any financial or other interests in accordance with prevailing laws and regulations.

h. *Practice in accordance with laws of Indian/International relevant to the area of nursing practice:*
- The nurse observes the laws of Indian relevant to nursing and health care practices.

- There are many ordinances which have a direct or indirect application to nursing. The following is a selected list of ordinances related to nursing practice. It is not intended to be exhaustive examples:
  - Antibiotics Ordinance
  - Births and Deaths Registration Ordinance
  - Dangerous Drugs Ordinance
  - Human Organ Transplant Ordinance
  - Mental Health Ordinance
  - Midwives Registration Ordinance.

CODE OF ETHICS FOR NURSES (INDIAN NURSING COUNCIL)

The code of ethics for nurses aims to make explicit the fundamental moral commitments of the profession; provide nurses with a basis for ethical practice and to indicate to the community the values that nurse's hold.

The code of ethics for nurses is organized around four broad value statements and seventeen provisions that represent the morals and ideals of the profession and are regarded as central to ethical nursing practice. The four broad value statements are:

a. Respect life, and improve quality of life
b. Respect individual rights and dignity
c. Be responsive to society's needs, and work towards a healthy community through partnership
d. Strive for excellence, and assure quality of care.

The provisions articulated in each value statement are ethical responsibilities that nurses should act upon in order to enact the broad values in practice situations. For each of these statements, the scope of responsibilities identified extends beyond individuals to include families, communities and society. By upholding these values in practice, it is envisaged that nurses can improve their personal quality, provide quality nursing care and earn the trust of those under their care.

These value statements are based on the following general principles

- People's needs are universal. Nursing service is provided for people throughout their life span.
- Inherent in nursing is the respect for life, dignity and rights of individuals, and improvement in the quality of life.
- Nurses should serve all people irrespective of race, nationality, creed, color, age, gender, politics or social status.

- The fundamental responsibilities of nurses are to promote health, prevent illness, restore health, and alleviate suffering caused by ill health.
- *Respect life, and improve quality of life:*
  - Nurses should encourage the individual, the family and the community to improve the quality of life.
  - Nurses should ensure patient/client safety when delivering nursing services.
  - Nurses should provide information and consultation in accordance with and adjustable to patients'/clients' and their families' capacity and needs.
  - Nurses should respect the wishes of the dying patients/clients, and ensure that they have peace and dignity at the time of death.
- *Respect individual rights and dignity:*
  - Nurses should respect the individual's spiritual beliefs, values and customs.
  - Nurses should hold in confidence patients'/clients' information and be prudent in their use of the information.
  - Nurses should respect patients'/clients' and their families' wishes, encouraging them to participate in planning and implementing nursing care.
  - Nurses should take appropriate action to safeguard the individual's rights and dignity.
  - Nurses should value truthfulness and integrity and put oneself in the place of another.
- *Be responsive to society's needs, and work towards a healthy community through partnership:*
  - Nurses should share the responsibility in raising the health consciousness of the community.
  - Nurses should collaborate with others in initiating and supporting actions that work towards the goal of 'health for all'.
  - Nurses should use health care resources efficiently and effectively through partnerships with the community.
  - Nurses should coordinate their services with those of medical and social groups in rendering health services to individuals, families and the community, as appropriate.
- *Strive for excellence, and assure quality of care:*
  - Nurses should seek truth from facts, and use scientific evidence in finding the best possible ways to provide nursing services for the well-being of patients/clients.
  - Nurses should maintain the highest standards of nursing care possible, actually seeking improvement on the existing service.

- Nurses should exercise professional judgment in accepting responsibilities and delegating nursing activities to others.
- Nurses should value research and development for the promotion of nursing knowledge and skills.

ICN CODE OF ETHICS

An international code of ethics for nurses was first adopted by the International Council of Nurses (ICN) in 1953. It has been revised and reaffirmed at various times since, most recently with this review and revision completed in 2012.

Nurses have four fundamental responsibilities: to promote health, to prevent illness, to restore health and to alleviate suffering. The need for nursing is universal. Inherent in nursing is a respect for human rights, including cultural rights, the right to life and choice, to dignity and to be treated with respect. Nursing care is respectful of and unrestricted by considerations of age, color, creed, culture, disability or illness, gender, sexual orientation, nationality, politics, race or social status. Nurses render health services to the individual, the family and the community and coordinate their services with those of related groups.

The ICN code of ethics for nurses has four principal elements that outline the standards of ethical conduct.

ELEMENTS OF THE CODE

Nurses and People

- The nurse's primary professional responsibility is to people requiring nursing care.
- In providing care, the nurse promotes an environment in which the human rights, values, customs and spiritual beliefs of the individual, family and community are respected.
- The nurse ensures that the individual receives accurate, sufficient and timely information in a culturally appropriate manner on which to base consent for care and related treatment.
- The nurse holds in confidence personal information and uses judgment in sharing this information.
- The nurse shares with society the responsibility for initiating and supporting action to meet the health and social needs of the public, in particular those of vulnerable populations.
- The nurse advocates for equity and social justice in resource allocation, access to health care and other social and economic services.

- The nurse demonstrates professional values such as respectfulness, responsiveness, compassion, trustworthiness and integrity.

Nurses and Practice

- The nurse carries personal responsibility and accountability for nursing practice, and for maintaining competence by continual learning.
- The nurse maintains a standard of personal health such that the ability to provide care is not compromised.
- The nurse uses judgment regarding individual competence when accepting and delegating responsibility.
- The nurse at all times maintains standards of personal conduct which reflect well on the profession and enhance its image and public confidence.
- The nurse, in providing care, ensures that use of technology and scientific advances are compatible with the safety, dignity and rights of people.
- The nurse strives to foster and maintain a practice culture promoting ethical behavior and open dialogue.

Nurses and the Profession

- The nurse assumes the major role in determining and implementing acceptable standards of clinical nursing practice, management, research and education.
- The nurse is active in developing a core of research-based professional knowledge that supports evidence-based practice.
- The nurse is active in developing and sustaining a core of professional values.
- The nurse, acting through the professional organization, participates in creating a positive practice environment and maintaining safe, equitable social and economic working conditions in nursing.
- The nurse practices to sustain and protect the natural environment and is aware of its consequences on health.
- The nurse contributes to an ethical organizational environment and challenges unethical practices and settings.

Nurses and Co-workers

- The nurse sustains a collaborative and respectful relationship with co-workers in nursing and other fields.
- The nurse takes appropriate action to safeguard individuals, families and communities when their health is endangered by a co-worker or any other person.

- The nurse takes appropriate action to support and guide co-workers to advance ethical conduct.

NIGHTINGALE PLEDGE

This modified 'Hippocratic Oath' was composed in 1893 by Mrs Lystra E Gretter and a Committee for the Farrand Training School for Nurses, Detroit, Michigan. It was called the *Florence Nightingale Pledge* as a token of esteem for the founder of modern nursing.

'I solemnly pledge myself before God and in the presence of this assembly, to pass my life in purity and to practice my profession faithfully. I will abstain from whatever is deleterious and mischievous, and will not take or knowingly administer any harmful drug. I will do all in my power to maintain and elevate the standard of my profession, and will hold in confidence all personal matters committed to my keeping and all family affairs coming to my knowledge in the practice of my calling. With loyalty will I endeavor to aid the physician in his work, and devote myself to the welfare of those committed to my care'.

PROCEDURE FOR EMPLOYMENT

Registered nurses (RNs), regardless of speciality or work setting, perform basic duties that include treating patients, educating patients and the public about various medical conditions, and providing advice and emotional support to patients' family members. RNs record patients' medical histories and symptoms help to perform diagnostic tests and analyze results, operate medical machinery, administer treatment and medications, and help with patient follow-up and rehabilitation.

Employment is expected to grow more slowly in hospitals-health care's largest industry: than in most other health care industries. While the intensity of nursing care is likely to increase, requiring more nurses per patient, the number of inpatients (those who remain in the hospital for more than 24 hours) is not likely to grow by much. Patients are being discharged earlier, and more procedures are being done on an outpatient basis, both inside and outside hospitals. Rapid growth is expected in hospital outpatient facilities, such as those providing same-day surgery, rehabilitation, and chemotherapy.

LOCATING A POSITION

Overall job opportunities are expected to be excellent for registered nurses. Employers in some parts of the country and in certain employment settings report difficulty in attracting and retaining an adequate number of RNs, primarily because of an aging RN workforce and a lack of younger workers to fill positions. Enrolments in nursing programs at all levels have increased more rapidly in the past few years as students seek jobs with stable employment. However, many qualified applicants are being turned away because of a shortage of nursing faculty. The need for nursing faculty will only increase as many instructors near retirement. Many employers also are relying on foreign-educated nurses to fill vacant positions.

Even though overall employment opportunities for all nursing specialities are expected to be excellent, they can vary by employment setting. Despite the slower employment growth in hospitals, job opportunities should still be excellent because of the relatively high turnover of hospital nurses. RNs working in hospitals frequently work overtime and night and weekend shifts and also treat seriously ill and injured patients, all of which can contribute to frequently: critical care units, emergency departments, and operating rooms generally will have more job openings than other departments. To attract and retain qualified nurses, hospitals may offer signing bonuses, family-friendly work schedules, or subsidized training. A growing number of hospitals also are experimenting with online bidding to fill open shifts, in which nurses can volunteer to fill open shifts at premium wages. This can decrease the amount of mandatory overtime that nurses are required to work.

Although faster employment growth is projected in physicians' offices and outpatient care centers, RNs may face greater competition for these positions because they generally offer regular working hours and more comfortable working environments. There also maybe some competition for jobs in employment services, despite a high rate of employment growth, because a large number of workers are attracted by the industry's relatively high wages and the flexibility of the work in this industry.

Generally, RNs with at least a bachelor's degree will have better job prospects than those without a bachelor's. In addition, all four advanced practice specialities-clinical nurse specialists, nurse practitioners, nurse-midwives, and nurse anesthetists will be in high demand, particularly in medically underserved areas such as inner cities and rural areas.

APPLYING FOR THE JOB

When you reply to a job advertisement, you should receive an application pack containing some or all of the following:

- An application form
- A job description/person specification
- Information about the school or local authority.

Read through everything, highlighting key words and phrases.

The person specification outlines the qualifications, experience, knowledge and skills required. Your application will need to evidence how you meet each of these requirements. Ensure your application is targeted directly at the specific school and job: do not use a generic teaching job application.

Applications usually ask the applicant at the minimum for your name, phone number, and address. In addition to this applications also ask for previous employment information, educational background, emergency contacts, references, as well as any special skills the applicant might have.

The three categories application fields are very useful for discovering are; physical characteristics, experience, and socio-environmental factors.

The Interview

When you receive an offer of an interview, confirm as promptly as possible that you will attend. Try and arrange to visit the school prior to the interview day. Interviews will focus on your application, your teacher training and school experience, previous work experience, interests, suitability for the particular school, and what you can contribute. Be prepared with specific examples to evidence your skills.

Interviewers Look For

- Excellent communication skills.
- Positive social skills with pupils and co-workers, with the ability to motivate.
- Classroom management skills.
- Professional knowledge and understanding of your subject.
- A personal philosophy about, and a commitment to, the teaching of your subjects the ability to reflect on what you have gained from your course and placements and awareness of your own development needs and a positive choice for that school and/or local authority (LA).

Types of Interview

The format and style of the interview varies depending on where it is held and who it is conducted by. Be aware of your body language–smile and try to look relaxed. A firm handshake and eye contact when you meet the panel and answer questions can make a good initial impression.

Pool Interviews

- These are usually held in the offices of the local authority and the panel maybe made-up of a head teacher, an inspector/adviser and perhaps a school governor.

- The result of the interview is usually given a few days later.
- Even if you are successful, you can expect to be interviewed again by any schools interested in you.

Interviews for Specific Posts

- These usually take place at the school concerned and may include a number of other activities.
- Interviews may last up to an hour and panels are likely to be made-up of a combination of teaching staff at different levels of seniority. Governors may also be included. Increasingly pupils are being involved at this stage of the selection process.

Interview Activities

The interview maybe in a typical question and answer format or it could consist of different exercises or activities. These may include:

- *Informal discussions:* These maybe with a senior teacher/head of department or other staff and may take place during a school tour. If so, ensure you show an interest by talking to pupils. This is an opportunity to ask questions, but remember you are still being assessed.
- *Teaching a lesson or part-lesson:* You are likely to be asked to teach a class on a given topic. If this is the case, you will be given prior warning. Check available resources at the school before the day. At your interview, you maybe asked about your lesson focus and learning outcomes and your evaluation of how the lesson went.
- *Group discussion:* These are more common in interviews for secondary posts and topics include:
  - Class management and control.
  - Recent developments in the teaching of your subject.
  - You will be assessed on your knowledge of the topic and ability to work in a group. Be sensitive to others in the group and ensure you take an active part without dominating the discussion.
- *Interview by pupils:* You may have an interview with pupils. This is becoming more common, even at primary level.
- *Presentation:* For more senior roles, you maybe asked to give a short presentation to staff or the interviewing panel. You should be given prior warning of this.

Interview Tips Preparation

If you did your research for your supporting statement and related your skills and experience to the vacancy, you have done much of the groundwork in preparing for the interview. The following points all need to be considered:

- Re-read the job advertisement, and application pack plus your application form/CV (in particular, your supporting statement and any notes you made# when preparing it).
- Ensure you have specific examples from your school experience to demonstrate how you meet the selection criteria, you can take evidence such as photographs, lesson plans, as further evidence.
- Research the teaching profession as a whole, and your own subject in particular. You should be up to date on latest developments and be able to discuss current trends and educational issues, see the Hot topics section in the AGCAS Routes into teaching publication within this series. Reading the educational press regularly is essential.
- Try to anticipate the questions you maybe asked at interview and prepare a rough outline of the answers you will give. Look at some example questions.
- Think about questions to ask the panel: Make sure you have not already been given the answer to your question during the interview.
- Ensure you can demonstrate your commitment to the particular school as well as to the teaching profession as a whole.
- Plan your journey and allow plenty of time to get there.
- Dress smartly; consider this in relation to teaching a sample lesson.

Responding to Questions

- Listen carefully to the questions so you do not misunderstand what is being asked. Ask for clarification if necessary.
- Do no talk too much: you can always pause and ask if they require further details.
- Do not simply answer yes or no.
- Nonverbal communication is very important. How you answer is important to convey motivation and make you stand out.
- Give yourself time to think before responding: you do not need to jump straight into an answer.
- Provide greater depth to support information you put in your application.
- Do not assume that the entire panel has read it thoroughly.
- Try to expand your answers with interesting information about yourself and give examples to evidence your points and highlight your skills.
- Talk rationally about yourself and others: a perceptive, balanced critique of your training course is far more impressive than either excessive praise or blanket criticism.

The way you communicate in the interview will be taken as a reflection of how you communicate in the classroom. Your body language and the clarity of your speech are very important and you should always try to sound positive and enthusiastic.

ACCEPTING A POSITION

Think carefully before you accept or decline the position and if you have other interviews lined up that you wish to attend, ask if you can have more time to make your decision. Bear in mind, however, that the school may give a time limit on getting your answer so that they do not lose their second choice candidate should you decline.

After you have accepted an offer you should receive a written confirmation of appointment, which should also confirm your starting salary point. You should then reply in writing to accept the offer. You may also wish to ask if you can visit the school again before you take-up your post so that you can make some advance preparations.

RESIGNATION FROM A POSITION

A resignation letter can help you maintain a positive relationship with your old employer, while paving the way for you to move on. You never know when you might need that previous employer to give you a reference, so it makes sense to take the time to write polished and professional resignation letters. Your resignation letter also provides official notice that you are terminating your employment with the company. Review these employee resignation letters examples to get ideas for your own letter to use to resign from employment.

When you are resigning from employment, it is proper protocol to provide your employer with a formal resignation letter for your employee file.

A resignation letter should be simple, brief, focused, and to the point. There is no need to elaborate on your reason for leaving. Simply provide information on when you are leaving and let the employer know you appreciate your time with the company.

Sample Resignation Letter

Your Name: ....

Your Address:...

....

Your City, State, Zip Code: ....

Your Phone Number: ....Your Email: ....

Date......................Name:...

Title: ....

Organization: ....
Address: ....
City, State, Zip Code: ....

Dear Mr/Ms Last Name:

I would like to inform you that I am resigning from my position as Staff Nurse/Tutor for the Hospital/Institution, effective August 1.

Thank you for the opportunities for professional and personal development that you have provided me during the last five years. I have enjoyed working for the hospital/Institute and appreciate the support provided me during my tenure with the hospital.

If I can be of any help during this transition, please let me know.

Sincerely,

Your Signature (hard copy letter)

Your Typed Name

SUMMARY

In this unit we have discuss about the nursing code of ethics, values, rights and obligations of patients and nurses. Accountability and responsibility of nurses have to fulfilling their tasks, the harmonious relationship between nurses with patients, partners, and other professions. Nurses recognize the privilege of being part of a self-regulating profession and have a responsibility to merit this privilege. The code informs other health-care professionals as well as members of the public about the ethical commitments of nurses and the responsibilities nurses accept as being part of a self-regulating profession.

Personal and Professional Growth/ Development

13 unit

INTRODUCTION

Individual professional development becomes increasingly important in times of rapid change. The increasing complexity of society will require that extension employees engage in lifelong learning in order to maintain professional expertise. Professional development refers to skills and knowledge attained for both personal development and career advancement. Professional development encompasses all types of facilitated learning opportunities, ranging from college degrees to formal coursework, conferences and informal learning opportunities situated in practice. Professional development is an important part of nursing. It provides growth in areas not always taught in clinical practice. Professional development has been described as intensive and collaborative, ideally incorporating an evaluative stage. There are a variety of approaches to professional development, including workshop attendance, consultation, coaching, and communities of practice, lesson study, mentoring, reflective supervision, and technical assistance.

CONTINUING EDUCATION

A professional nurse engages in lifelong learning that will influence practice and ultimately impact the quality of care that a patient receives. The technical skills and critical thinking acumen demonstrated by the critical care nurse at the bedside are not enough to sustain an evidence-based practice environment. Nurses need to cultivate and internalize a passion for learning throughout their careers. They need to adopt a healthy work environment that gives merit to continuing education (CE). In order to provide the best patient care health professionals should invest in educational opportunities that give them up to date knowledge and skills.

Meaning of Continuing Education

Continuing Nursing Education (CNE) consists of various educational activities that maintain and develop the knowledge, skills and professional practice of nurses/midwives. Nurses/midwives need to maintain their competencies through continuing nursing education in order to provide safe patient care and to keep pace with advances and innovations in healthcare.

- According to *Cooper* 'It is all the learning activities that occurs after an individual has completed his/her basic education'.
- According to *Ofosu* 'It consists of planned learning experiences beyond a basic nursing educational program. These experiences are designed to promote the development of knowledge, skills, and attitudes for the enhancement of nursing practice, thus improving health care to the public'.
- The *Commission defines 'continuing nursing education' as* systematic professional learning experiences obtained after initial licensure designed to augment the knowledge, skills, and judgment of nurses and enrich nurses' contributions to quality health care.

Importance of Continuing Education

Continuing education is necessary for nurses to perform competently, and respond positively to advanced medical, and technological changes in this age of rapid change, and to prevent obsolescence. It is needed to meet the expressed needs or interests of nurses to enable them to provide current and ultimately safe and effective patient care.

- *Earn more knowledge:* This maybe one of the most useful tools a nurse can possess to improve the lives of their patients on a day-to-day basis. Medical advancements and new infectious illnesses are constantly being discovered, as well as updated techniques for treatment and new medications. Therefore, it is important to stay abreast of current research to make sure patients are given the most up-to-date treatment.
- *Broader nursing career opportunities:* For example, a nurse that has obtained a MSN degree can easily move from a hospital job into a research job. Gaining a degree can also mean opportunities to move into a specialty career such as oncology, pediatrics, or becoming a nurse practitioner with a family practice.
- *Future licensing laws may require bachelor's degrees:* Some states require that Registered Nurses (RNs) renew their nursing licenses to stay certified. Renewal of certification may mean completing continuing education classes. Some nurses will even work toward a degree while earning their recertification at the same time.

- *Transitioning from an RN license to a BSN or MSN degree is becoming easier:* There are many online nursing schools that are accredited. They offer courses structured for those who are holding down a full time job and looking to complete a degree that fits into their already busy lifestyle.
- *Employers and hospitals are increasingly looking to hire a nurse who has a BSN:* Nurses with degrees often have an in-depth knowledge of the profession. Nurses with degrees are very often promoted to supervisory positions and awarded higher pay. While earning a BSN, nurses gain decision-making and critical care skills. This makes them eligible for positions such as head or staff nurse, department chief, or administrative manager.

Scope of Continuing Education

A registered nurse shall, with or without compensation or personal profit, practice nursing that incorporates caring for all clients in all settings, is guided by nursing standards consistent with standards established by the National Council of State Boards of Nursing and approved by the board, and shall be limited to:

- Providing comprehensive nursing assessment of the health status of clients, families, groups, and communities.
- Collaborating with a health care team to develop an integrated client-centered plan of health care.
- Developing a plan of nursing strategies to be integrated within the client-centered health care plan that establishes nursing diagnoses, setting goals to meet identified health care needs, prescribing nursing interventions, and implementing nursing care through the execution of independent nursing strategies and prescribed medical regimen.
- Delegating and assigning nursing interventions to implement the plan of care.
- Providing for the maintenance of safe and effective nursing care rendered directly or indirectly.
- Promoting a safe and therapeutic environment.
- Providing health teaching and counseling to promote, attain, and maintain the optimum health level of clients, families, groups, and communities.
- Advocating for clients, families, groups, and communities by attaining and maintaining what is in the best interest of the client or group.
- Evaluating responses to interventions and the effectiveness of the plan of care.
- Communicating and collaborating with other health care professionals in the management of health care and the implementation of the total health care regimen within and across care settings.

- Acquiring and applying critical new knowledge and technologies to the practice of nursing.
- Managing, supervising, and evaluating the practice of nursing.
- Teaching the theory and practice of nursing.
- Participating in the development of policies, procedures, and systems to support the client.
- Other nursing services that require education and training prescribed by the board and in conformance with national nursing standards.

Planning for Continuing Education

- Continuing education offerings are designed by a planning committee comprised of nurses and other health professionals with expertise in the content area. A designed nurse with minimal master's preparation will be appointed to chair the planning, implementation and evaluation of the offering.
- All offering promotion/publicity will include date, location, program title, purpose and objectives, target audience, credentials of major faculty, program schedule, costs and items covered by cost, refund policy for completion of said program, and any other information required by the Board of Nursing.
- For those programs requiring preregistration, telephone registration is possible; however, enrolee registration is assured only following receipt of the designated fee.
- Attendance monitoring procedures are the responsibility of conference coordinator and/or professional staff or designated nurse planner.
- Continuing education offerings reserve the right to cancel a scheduled offering for lack of enrolment needed to support it. Cancellation will be determined one week prior to scheduled date. Offerings cancelled because of inadequate enrolment other non-controllable factors influencing conduct of activity will include notification of faculty and notification of preregistered enrolees with full refund of paid registration fees.
- Syllabi and other handout materials prepared for continuing education offerings adhere to the current copyright laws. Materials from conferences are considered part of the registration fee for the offering and are not for resale.
- Programs developed for continuing education credit will meet with one or more of the Board of Nursing criteria for continuing education:
  - Nursing practice related to health care of patients/clients/families in any setting.
  - Professional growth and development related to nursing practice roles and designed to enhance the delivery of patient care and health service.

  - Sciences upon which nursing practice, nursing education or nursing research is based, i.e. nursing theories and biological, physical, behavioral, computer, social or basic sciences.
  - Social, economic, legal and ethical aspects of health care.
  - Management or administration of health care, health care personnel, or health care facilities.
  - Education of patients or their significant others, students, or personnel in the health care field.
- Complete conference records will be on file in a secure location for each offering including planning, records, purpose, objectives, schedule, faculty with qualifications designated, and list of enrolees, budget, evaluation report, bibliography and other requirements as mandated by the Board of Nursing.
- Admission to offerings with limited enrolment (and so published) will be granted registration on a first come, first served basis.
- Enrolee attendance records will not be released without written request of the individual in question. Such requests are directed to the attention of the Operations Coordinator in a secure location at the College of Nursing.
- Continuing Education Unit (CEU) records are on permanent storage in a secure location in the College of Nursing.
- Cosponsoring programs must meet the criteria required of all accrediting bodies as well as the policies and procedures of the University.
- Enrolee comments regarding continuing education offerings are invited on evaluation forms with any additional comments accepted by sponsoring department of by writing directly to the Board of Nursing. The address of the Board of Nursing shall be listed on the evaluation form, or in the syllabus information for every program.
- Continuing education offerings are designed for registered nurses. Offerings maybe attended by LPNs with the understanding that the offering has been designed specifically for registered nurses.
- Units of measurement used for continuing education courses shall be as follows: 1 contact hour = 50 minutes of didactic instruction, work on learner designed self-study, and clinical or laboratory practicum in an informal offering. 1 CEU = 10 contact hours of instruction.
- The College of Nursing Continuing Nursing Education policies are reviewed annual by the administrative authority.
- Co-sponsored programs require that a College of Nursing designated nurse planner by directly involved in the planning and that the College of Nursing grant its approval to the following:
  - Selection of program content and objectives as determined by a needs assessment of potential participants

- Selection of faculty
- Development of evaluation materials
- Any promotional advance materials distributed to potential registrants
- Contact hours/record keeping.

Regulating Individual Health Professionals

Since the early 1970s, CE for health professionals has been linked directly to licensure, certification, and credentialing. The various regulatory authorities—states for licensure, specialty societies for certification, and health care organizations for credentialing—attempt to ensure that a given health professional's background meets some minimal standard of quality.

Learning tools such as self-assessment, peer evaluation, and learning portfolios should all have a role in supporting the acquisition of knowledge and skills, reinforcing competence, and reassuring the public's trust. However, current licensing and certification systems principally assess learning only by measuring health professionals' participation in CE. Despite some professions' efforts to recognize achievement in knowledge, competence, and performance.

Licensure

In many health professions, professionals are mandated by law to receive a license to practice from a state licensing board and health professionals may hold a license in more than one state. This requirement is arguably the strongest regulatory tool available to assess individual health professionals. However, licensure has been linked only tangentially to performance improvement moreover, while initial licensure establishes the minimum competence required for admission to a profession, it does not guarantee that a health professional will maintain competency or provide a high level of care.

The various professional state boards are represented by national organizations, such as the Federation of State Medical Boards and the National Council of State Boards of Nursing. CE licensure requirements are generally organized around learning activities that often are conducted in groups, such as at conferences and lectures, and the content and processes of learning are under the control of the CE provider. Licensure has been linked only tangentially to performance improvement.

Certification

Certification is the process by which professional specialty societies or credentialing bodies—not regulatory bodies—certify individual health professionals as qualified experts to practice in a particular area of a profession. In professions that require certification, such as medicine (under specialty boards), professionals must regularly repeat the certification processes, which differ by profession and by specialty. The American Board of Medical Specialties has recently adopted new standards for a four-component mandatory maintenance-of-certification program: the components focus on professional standing, lifelong learning and self-assessment, cognitive expertise, and evaluation of performance in practice. Instead of recertification being required once every 10 years, this shift toward a new type of maintenance of certification requires continual engagement in professional development (ABMS, 2009).

Credentialing

Credentialing occurs at the level of health care organizations, such as hospitals and group practices, which employ health professionals. Organizations use credentialing in an attempt to ensure that health professionals are qualified to practice and maintain a minimum level of competence and performance. Many organizations use credentialing as the basis for granting staff privileges, and some organizations also credential health professionals for particular procedures, based on their experience and clinical outcomes. Many organizations develop their own credentialing guidelines. The process can be likened to an audit. Credentialing often includes, at a minimum, review and verification of a health professional's licensure, education, and certification, if applicable.

IN-SERVICE EDUCATION

In-service education is the vehicle by which goals and the multiple articulated means available to achieve them can be explored. It can be used to consider and solve problems, institutes and advance learning elicit and analyze and systematize individual ideas for group; develop the idea of the hospital as another community agency, and struggle to understand ourselves, others and inherent relationships.

Definitions

- In-service education is a planned learning experience provided by the employing agency for its employees.
- According to American Nurse Association, the term in-service to mean those "learning experiences provided in the work setting for the purpose of assisting staff in performing their assigned functions in that particular agency."
- It is the educational opportunities provided by the employer for the employee to attain or to improve his skill on the job efficiency, potential and capabilities.

Needs of In-Service Education

- The rapid scientific and technological advances have greatly altered practice of nursing
- The gap between scientific knowledge and its application grows wider each year
- Elimination of certain illnesses, mainly the communicable diseases
- Most of the successful surgeries performed
- Availability of newer drugs
- Complex machinery.

Objectives of In-Service Education

- To discover potentialities, to alert personnel in working conditions
- To assist nurses in identifying and meeting current bearing needs and those needs generated by changing professional practice
- To disseminate new information from body of nursing knowledge and health sciences through a variety of channels
- To state that an agency recognizes that education of personnel is an important agency function
- To assist the personnel in increasing their personal and professional growth
- To give a belief that every employee will benefit from continuing education service within or outside the agency
- To provide orientation, skill training, management and continuing education
- To achieve the objectives of the hospital, i.e. to develop good atmosphere and effective care
- To retain experienced personnel to foster their continuing development.

Methods of In-service Education

- There are two important methods of in-service education.
  1. Self-directed individual study
  2. Institutional method

Self-directed Individual Study

- It is a method of in-service education where the interest of the person is required for the study. The various methods of individual study are:
  - By developing good reading and writing habits. For this she should approach a good library, refer good books and keep the bibliography records.

- Attending conferences, clinics, seminars, workshops, etc. will broaden the interests.
- Visits to other schools and colleges of nursing and other healthcare institutions will help to exchange and review ideas.
- Attending postgraduate studies, examination for renewal of licence.
- By the use of TV, radio, video, etc.
- By attending social and religious activities.
- Be a member of one or more of allied health organizations to increase the perspective and widen the professional horizons.

Institutional Method

- *Within the institution:*
  - Organization of in-service education program which is based on the need of the public and the patient
  - Meetings and conferences on professional issues
  - Organization of a good hospital library with periodicals and books
  - Publishing bulletins and journals by the institution
  - Bulletin board.
- *Beyond the institution:* Deputation of staff for continuing education, post-certificate courses, MSc nursing courses and sending the staff for professional conferences and encouraging to do correspondence courses and computer technology, so that they maybe able to update their knowledge and skill.

Institutional Methods Include

- *General program:* A common procedure is to arrange for staff nurses a series of doctor's lectures on new developments in medical sciences. Sometimes nursing demonstrations can be included in the plan. The aim is to improve nursing care through an upgrading of the staff by giving more information. They will have greater understanding of their responsibilities and will improve the quality of their nursing practice.

  The highest type of staff education, more acceptably called staff development, results when groups of staff members work together to achieve a common goal. In the process of working together in a democratic manner, the individuals grow both personally and professionally. By working together, morale is improved, interest in the institution increases and greater loyalty to the administration results. The staff develops a sense of belonging when she realizes that her ideas are important and valuable to others. This results in improvement of the quality of her work.

Another one in which staff nurses maybe interested is the organization of the nursing team. If the hospital is considering the establishment of team method of assignment graduate staff nurses might like to study on the requisites for nursing team leadership.

- *Ward program:* Even if the hospital has no in-service program for staff development, the head nurse still has an obligation to her staff to help them grow professionally, if the head nurse were to adopt the methods of general program. This will result in staff development.
  - Planning a program for development of patient care
  - Developing ward routines
  - Delegating specific responsibilities to staff members
  - Studying patient problems and developing patient care plans
  - Planning for institution of nursing team
  - Orientation to the ward and to special experiences.
- *Bedside clinic and nursing care conference:* Bedside clinic and nursing care conference portray the nursing problems typically associated with particular disease or disorder and to give a vivid picture of the related nursing care by associating it with a specific individual.
- *Bedside clinic:* Bedside clinic always entails the presence of the patient. Either the group visits the bedside or the patient is brought to the conference room. The patient is not present for the entire discussion. Before the arrival of the patient, the nurse points out to the group the observations that should be made while he is present. When the patient is no longer needed, he is returned to his room. The discussion follows, questions answered, the material summarized and the most important points are summarized. The clinic usually lasts about 30 minutes.
- *Nursing care conference:* In the nursing care conference the patient is usually not present for any part of the class. This maybe the method of choice when the entire group is well acquainted with the patient and would have nothing new to learn from going to see him.
- *Teaching rounds:* The aim of teaching rounds is to acquaint nurses with all patients on the ward in order that better understanding and more purposeful care must be achieved for each patient. Usually all patients are visited on rounds and the visit is accompanied by a discussion pertaining to each patient's care. Weekly rounds are usually enough, sometimes a group, perhaps only the new patients or those whose condition has markedly changed in the past week.

Approaches to In-service Education Program

There are mainly three approaches:

a. *Centralized approach:* The centralized approach has its origin from the belief that the in-service curriculum ought to emanate from and be conducted by nursing personnel in the control administration of the agency. In this approach, there is a department within the nursing service that is responsible for the educational program. The staff nurses working in this department devote full time to in-service education. The head of the program will be assistant director of nursing service. The staff of the department works with nursing personnel, but is not directly responsible for patient care.

Advantages

- Staff members in this department are responsible for both major parts of the program, i.e. orientation and continuing education
- It is planned for all nursing groups head nurses, staff nurses, aides, etc.
- Budget control and evaluation are facilitated
- It is advantageous when the resources, people, place and things are preplanned
- It is advantageous when committees are directed to work; the specific problems are identified by the administration.

Disadvantages

- Lectures and group discussion do not necessarily meet the needs of staff members in actual work situation on the patient care division. The staff may not be sufficient to work with nurses on each division
- The in-service staff cannot plan program to meet the needs and various interests of nurses employed in the hospital with specialized services
- If the central administration makes most of the decisions that count, the outcome of the issue may not be accepted at times.

b. *Decentralized Approach:* Decentralized approach is based on the conviction that the in-service curriculum for all nursing personnel should be the responsibility of the practicing nurse with whom the personnel work. This is planned by and conducted for the employees for one or more units. Learners themselves should develop and direct the learning experience. The entire in-service education program orientation and continuing education is carried out on each patient care division for the nursing personnel assigned to them.

Advantages

- It is planned for staff members who work together, care for the same patients and share the common nursing goals

- It is planned around the special relevant interest of the employees, e.g. cardiac monitoring classes held in CCU
- Classes are related to clinical problems that are existing
- The qualities like self direction, initiative and participation will be fostered
- The opportunities for face to face communication among the group members are more
- Formal and informal planning, learning and evaluation can be done in the same geographic area or unit
- Learning on the unit from role models in the immediate work situation and from in-service education for unit personnel is possible
- Patient participation-helps to develop mutual trust and respect.

Disadvantages

- Budgeting is difficult when each nursing division has a program:
  - Duplication of efforts occurs when similar material in classes is taught at the same time.
  - If the head nurse does not see this as a priority, employees working with her will have little opportunity for planned learning experience
  - A purely decentralized approach is theoretically possible but practically not probable to prolonged effort. The pressure of getting the work done, time, willingness for involvement, turnover and lack of persisting leadership are factors which initiate against it.

c. *Combined or coordinated approach:* The coordinated approach is compromise between the centralized and decentralized pattern. In this a practicing nurse carries out a large measure of responsibility for the in-service curriculum. The central administration nursing personnel of the agency is responsible for a broad program which is to be imparted to all nursing personnel.

   In this approach, there is a central nursing in-service education department and nurse on each division or on each service—who holds leadership responsibility for staff development activities. When coordination is improved, duplication can be avoided and unity of effort maintained. An added advantage of the coordinated approach is that realistically people will tend to lend support to an effort in which they personally participate or contribute. This approach involves both nursing administration and practitioners in a complementary way.

Factors Affecting In-service Education

The economic, social, medical and technological sciences which affect that society will affect nursing in-service education. The related factors affecting the in-service education programs are:

- *Cost of healthcare:* In-service education may increase the efficiency of nursing services, but it adds additional expenditure on healthcare delivery system
- *Manpower:* In-service education requires qualified human resources, leading to increased human resources
- *Changes:* In nursing practice leads to frequent changes in the programs and in-service education
- Standards and organization for the nursing practices.

CAREER IN NURSING

Nursing, as a career, has always been in demand. Now with more and more private hospitals and nursing homes coming up, the demand for trained nurses has increased manifold. Playing a significant role in the healthcare profession, nurses shoulder a wide variety of responsibilities. Right from taking bedside care of patients to administrating medicines to maintaining day-to-day records of patients to arranging medical equipment—a host of duties are performed by nurses. Now when it comes to courses, wide varieties of options are available for nursing aspirants.

Different Types of Nursing Courses

In India, various Universities and medical colleges provide diploma, graduate and postgraduate nursing courses. Besides, many institutes offer various midwifery courses.

Here are some popular courses that nursing aspirants in India generally pursue:

- *Diploma in nursing:* The duration of the diploma course is of 3 years followed by an internship of 6 months.
- *BSc in nursing:* Students who have Biology, Physics and Chemistry in 10 + 2 can go for graduate program. The course guide of the program covers the basic nitty-gritty about nursing. The duration of the course is 4 years along with an internship of 6 months.
- *MSc in nursing:* Students who have successfully completed their BSc in Nursing can pursue this course. The duration of the course is of 2 years.
- Apart from that, some other midwifery and specialized courses are offered. These include Master of Public Health (MPH), General

Nursing and Midwifery, Multipurpose Health Workers Training, Auxiliary Nurse Midwife/Health Worker (ANM) and so on.

CAREER OPPORTUNITIES IN NURSING

Nurses have extensive career paths, both in hospitals, large or small, public or private, and in the community. Once they choose a certain path, there are still many options open to them. They can also decide to follow a different path at some point in their nursing career, to seek exciting, new challenges.

This level of flexibility and choice provides constant stimulation and job satisfaction for nurses and midwives.

Hospital offers a diverse range of career choices for nurses and provides the opportunity to live and work in different settings, with hospitals in every city across India, as well as in many other countries. Nurses are also always needed overseas.

In hospitals, nurses have the opportunity to rotate through wards or areas which interest them, or they can choose to specialize in one area. In clinical areas, nurses and midwives work as members of a diverse team of health professionals, all dedicated to improving the health status and outcomes of their clients or patients.

Hospitals also present a number of nursing opportunities within areas outside the wards, such as radiology, pathology, operation theaters, management education, research and clinics.

The community offers a wide variety of options for nurse looking for an alternative to work in hospitals. Community roles include working in community health services, district nursing, primary care or working in industry, schools or teaching in higher education.

In fact, many of the roles that nurses perform are required in both hospital and community settings, e.g. mental health and aged care.

Almost all of us have some idea of the roles that nurse perform in general areas within a hospital, such as medical and surgical wards, and in the community, such as residential and aged care services, but the reality is that all these roles are extensive and challenging, contributing lasting positive effects on individual patients, clients and the community as a whole.

- *Aged care or geriatric nurse:* These nurses work in a range of settings, which include the community, hospitals, rehabilitation units and residential care facilities. Aged care nurse perform many different role at various levels. They possess well-developed knowledge and skills specific to older people, in assessment, diagnosis, treatment and evaluation.

  These nurses working in a hospital environment require a thorough understanding of a wide range of age-specific problems and their management. Successful rehabilitation and effective discharge planning requires the ability to liaise closely with community nurses and other health care providers to develop an effective plan of care at home.

These nurse who work in the home or community setting have the opportunity to work independently, in partnership with families and local health care providers, or in small multidisciplinary teams. They are excellent communicators; so they can advocate for residents and other in their care, coordinate multidisciplinary team members and support family members, all of which are integral components of providing aged care.

- *Critical care nurses:* These nurses also work in highly technology areas, such as intensive care and coronary care, where they care for acutely and critically ill patients of all aged and diagnoses, often on a one to one basis. Critical care nursing requiring complex assessment skill and a high level of care, involving the use of technology such as monitors and ventilators. These nurse work closely with all members of the critical care team and also provide emotional support to patients, family and friends.
- *Emergency nurses:* For a different career path, the emergency department in any hospital is a dynamic, changeable place to work. It is a highly technological area that treats the broadest range of injuries, illness and trauma. Emergency nurses require a high level of expertise. They adapt quickly to changing situations, relish unpredictability and work very well as members of an extended team of health professionals.
- *Maternal and child health nurses:* These nurses work in the community to support young children (newborns through to school age) and their families. The main focus of this role is the early detection, intervention and prevention of issues affecting young children and their families, including emotional, social and physical problems.
- *Mental health nurses:* These nurses work with individuals, families and communities to assess mental health needs, develop diagnoses and plan, implement and evaluate appropriate nursing care. They assess levels of dysfunction in their coping abilities and prevent further disability. It also includes implementing treatment, health education, crisis intervention and counseling and case management. These nurse work in wide array of setting, such as hospitals, community based or home care programs, prisons, schools and local, state and federal mental health agencies.
- *Neonatal intensive care nurses:* Neonatal Intensive care, a much specialized intensive care unit, is a relatively new area of practice compared with adult health, or other areas of nursing. It provides the opportunity for neonatal intensive care nurses to devote their expertise to

newborns who need this concentrated level of attention at the beginning of their lives. Babies admitted to a neonatal intensive care unit (NICU) maybe small for their age, premature or sick newborns that require technology care, such as ventilators.

- *Occupational health nurses:* These nurses work in a variety of business and industrial sites. They combine public health concepts with their knowledge of emergency care and the law, and they also provide education to minimize workplace accidents and improve risk management in the workplace.
- *Oncology nurses:* These nurses provide care, support and education, not only to people with cancer, but also to their families and friends. They guide patients experiencing or at risk of developing cancer, through counseling for cancer prevention and the screening process. As part of a dedicated team, they provide acute care right through rehabilitation or palliative care as necessary.
- *Pediatric nurses:* These nurses provide comprehensive care to children of all ages, from newborn to adolescents, and their families, in various settings. They care for the physical, emotional and social aspects of health and illness in their patients, as well as providing education and health promotion for disease prevention. They manage physical and mental disabilities, and acute and chronic illness, such as respiratory infections, asthma, ear, nose and throat infections, cancer, growth and development problems.
- *Palliative care nurses:* These nurses work closely with other healthcare providers, including physicians, social workers and other health workers, to attend to the needs of patients and their families, who face terminal illness and bereavement. They are different from other nursing disciplines in their dedication and commitment to almost exclusively caring for dying patients. Of all rolls within the profession palliative care nursing is one of the most emotionally demanding, often involving round the clock availability, expert management of pain and other symptoms and intensive family support.
- *Remote area nurses:* This nursing area is a challenging and expanded clinical role, with remote area nurses often working without immediate access to doctors. They provide a 24-hour on call emergency service to their client groups, which mainly consist of Aboriginal people, pastoralists and small town, mining and tourist populations.
- *Research nurses:* These nurses are involved within nursing, medical and paramedical research programs. They work for many different organizations, such as teaching and university hospitals, pharmaceutical companies, universities, educational facilities and research institutes. Their roles can include monitoring clients on client trials, such as new medicines, and studies to improve the outcomes of nursing practice or new treatments. The work can be permanent, temporary or

part-time and may depend upon grants or availability of funds from other sources.

INTERNATIONAL INFLUENCE THE CAREER IN NURSING

Changes in professional roles and the movement of people across national and international boundaries make it important to understand healthcare and nursing issues in a global context. Communicating with patients from diverse cultural backgrounds is only one challenge facing nurses today. Nurses need to think and act in ways that are culturally sensitive as they provide care.

Study abroad programs broaden students' perspectives. As students learn about different cultures and the values that drive them, they begin to understand and accept cultural differences in patients and co-workers. While study abroad gives students an opportunity to understand nursing practice and education in different cultures, international students bring cultural diversity and experiences to our doorstep, challenging us to adopt a global perspective.

International collaboration brings together nurses with similar research interests who share their talents and resources to address common areas of concern. Faculty at the School of Nursing are collaborating with international researchers in the areas of chronic disease, technology and genetics. Our international programs and collaborations help advance nursing and healthcare knowledge, and enhance the quality of care given to all patients.

About Nurses Migration

Global nurse migration has been a topic of conversation for several years, particularly as the recognition of nurse shortages has increased. Moreover, while one typically thinks of migration as something that occurs when nurses move from one country to another, the impact of migration can be just as significant when nurses move from one region of the country to another or from one setting to another (rural to urban, for instance).

Reasons why nurses migrate are well known. Push factors, that is, attributes of the source country, include but are not limited to poor working conditions, poor or dangerous environment and limited scope of practice. Pull factors, which are attributes of the destination country, include factors such as better pay, career opportunities, the power of the profession, and health care system needs.

Moreover, what has become increasingly evident is that destination countries have benefited from this migration, while source countries have suffered. Recently, the World Health Organization (WHO) established a code of ethical recruitment in recognition of inequities that exist consequent to migration. While there are concerns, the code is a major step in recognizing the needs of source and destination countries. For example, there are recommendations about the responsibilities that destination countries have regarding the training and retraining of health care providers in source countries. Governments are provided with provisions to help them monitor the alignment of their policies with the code. Thus, expectations for appropriate recruitment of nurses are available to country officials, and to employers within countries.

THE FUTURE OF NURSING

In many ways this is a time of chaos within health care systems around the world. The economic downturn in the global society has impacted on health care. In many places services have been cut and access to services reduced. In addition, new diseases such as AIDS, SARS and the threat of bio-terrorism have entered our lives. New technologies and treatments occur rapidly, but are often expensive, and financing these advances can be difficult. Patients are moved out of hospital rapidly, and those that remain are more acutely ill than they have been in the past.

Those discharged patients often need more assistance at home and in the community than in previous years, and those services can also be expensive. Nurses are a vital part of the health care scene, but nursing shortages have appeared in many areas, shortages that are predicted to worsen overtime.

Chaos theory talks about dissolution of old patterns and development of new. The nursing profession needs to begin to recognize new trends and patterns that are emerging in health care. Change theory tells us that unsettled a time, a form of unfreezing of old patterns, is also an era of opportunity. Changes are inevitable, and both nursing and especially nursing education are in an excellent position to lead rather than follow. But that is not easy. It takes energy, ideas and commitment.

This is our time of opportunity! It is crucial that nurses become involved in the political process and that we teach our students and future leaders how to do that. It is crucial that nurses learn to collect data to document health care needs and our impact on the health of our societies. Nurses must learn how to identify those health care needs of patients, families, communities and societies; to communicate those needs to policy and decision makers and not allow those needs to be lost in the frenzy of cost cutting options. It is crucial that nurses learn to generate new ideas for care, utilizing the new medical and communication technologies that are blossoming daily, but also keeping our high touch together with the high tech. It is crucial that nurses learn the terminology of finance and business concepts that are driving health care systems today and generate those new ideas for care with fiscal responsibility, and seeking new ways to lower costs. It is crucial that nurses learn about implementation strategies for those ideas. That we learn to deal with opposition, and that we can present our arguments well; that we learn to develop coalitions and a supportive constituency; that we learn to compromise in ways that develop win-win situations and that we learn what we can give up and what we cannot. These are major challenges for nurses and nurse educators today and in the future.

Factors Influencing the Future of Nursing

There are a number of external factors that are directly influencing the nursing profession. These need to be taken into account as the profession plans its future:

Changing Community

- There are significant demographic shifts, particularly with the aging population. These and other trends are changing the composition of the workforce.
- In general, community expectations are increasing, including those around work-life balance
- Infrastructure is failing to meet the demands of an increasing number of geographically isolated communities.

Policy and Funding

- Complex and inadequate funding of health and education coupled with the demands of meeting regulatory requirements is placing pressure on both systems. This is exacerbated by the lack of collaboration between key stakeholders
- Health and education are undergoing major reforms at the national and state levels
- National and political influences are driving government policy.

Service Delivery

- Complexity of health care is increasing in response to the diversity of population needs
- Advances in technology, new knowledge and an emphasis on quality and safety are contributing to new models of care
- There is increasing pressure to change the scope/boundaries of clinical practice
- There is a shortage of health professionals to meet demand.

Role and Responsibilities of Nurses in Future

Nursing educators have a major responsibility in this arena and need to be aware of and responsive to new trends and changes in the health care milieu. They and the students they prepare should be a portal through which this information is communicated to nurses in the field, who often do not have sufficient resources or time to keep abreast of new developments. Although strategic planning can be used to develop nursing practice and educational programs of the future, in today's world change is coming rapidly, and those strategic plans cannot be static. Practicing nurses, nurse administrators and nurse educators must respond to changes quickly, as well as being proactive, based on recognition of trends and external environmental dynamics. The following trends are particularly important to monitor and develop methods to favorably impact their course overtime to ensure quality health care:

- *Rapid changes in health care technology and therapies:* It is likely mean continued lowered acute care stays. Driving forces include increasingly sophisticated surgical technologies that are less invasive and promote quicker healing. New therapies may reduce sick time, hopefully even in areas such as cancer, HIV/AIDS and genetic disorders.

  Communication technology has also changed dramatically. However, as those technologies have prolonged the life span, reduced mortality has changed fatal illness into more chronic illness, which may still require care and control. The growth of telemedicine, telenursing, and telehealth will also change the way we function, and have great potential and challenges for the development of new nursing roles. Restraining forces however could include the reduction of research funding, as we deal with the current fiscal crisis, and which may slow potential advances. With lowered acute care stays, many more people will require care in their own communities.

  Nurses need to be better prepared to work within this area; financial issues of care provision need to be addressed and nurses need to be better prepared to work with chronic care needs.
- *Demographic trends, epidemiological trends, and health care statistics:* It helps us recognize health care needs for society and give information for future planning of cost effective services. Increasing life span is a driving force for the development of improved services for the elderly. End of life care has received more attention over the last few years, but nursing research into this area needs to be further developed and findings disseminated. In many societies immigrant issues have created the need for better cultural understanding of health care needs and require resources for care.

- *Flow of resources:* Where is the money going and where is it likely to go? Money flowing into health care in the community will be a driving force for changes in that area, but a blocked flow will be a restraining force to preventive health care services. Nursing input and political power can impact that flow to provide effective health care programs and services.
- *Supply of manpower and competition:* Manpower shortages or surpluses in health care professions impact the utilization of nurses and advanced practice nurses. Who are our competitors for delivery of services and resources? This is a particularly important area in a time of nursing shortage to be sure that less qualified health care workers is not used to substitute for the sake of expedience and reduced costs. How can we develop competitive and marketing strategies? How can we form coalitions to reduce competition? At the same time we need to explore whether more collaborative programs of care can be developed effectively, so that we are not holding onto outmoded ideas of the profession but can develop newer modes, such as advanced practice nursing, to work in interdisciplinary collaboration. Collaborative rather than competitive strategies can strengthen quality of care by better utilizing the expertise of each participant.
- *Role delineation, role confusion:* These are the jobs keeping-up with the expectations of nurses and with advanced practice nursing? How are support worker jobs defined? How do professional standards interact with reality? How many people are required to do the job? Can one person realistically do the job? How can job satisfaction be increased in this era of high stress in the workplace?
- *Public opinion:* Nurses need to be aware of the public perception of their role. Development of coalitions and supporters within communities and media can be a driving force for advanced nursing practice. Consumer or professional opposition can provide barriers to practice, and be a restraining force.
- *Global trends:* We are a global economy and health care services face similar problems internationally. We can learn and benefit from contacts in other countries, and we can offer our services when appropriate to improve overall healthcare in both developing and industrial countries. Global terrorism needs to be addressed, and nurses need to be well prepared to deal with the aftermath and to document its effects on those we care for nurse educators need to incorporate disaster training and stress counseling into the curriculum and to provide workshops in this area for nurses already in practice. It is essential that nurses participate in the political process to reduce this threat.
- *Nursing practice and theory:* Nursing research and theory development need to be supported and findings disseminated to continue to build

our nursing science and incorporate the results into practice. We need to increase our core of nurses who have met high academic standards for carrying out research and provide resources for their activities.

Nursing research and theory also have the potential to contribute to the body of knowledge of other disciplines in the same way that we have borrowed from other theorists to use in our practice. The role of advanced practice nursing has been growing and has demonstrated effectiveness in the health care system. These nurses are now able to provide medical expertise in diagnosing and treating specific conditions, but are not mini-doctors. The medical portion of their practice is only one tool within their whole tool box of nursing competencies for use in providing holistic nursing care and health education. That combination has the potential to strengthen the provision of health care around the world.

SUMMARY

In this unit we discuss about the nursing, a profession that recalls the name of Florence Nightingale is indeed one of the noblest professions in the world. It is the art of caring for sick people with the science of health care. It is a vital component of any form of medical care. Continuing Education (CE) is the process by which health professionals keep up to date with the latest knowledge and advances in health care. The process of preparing Continuing Nursing Education (CNE) activities is assisted by the use of a program planning model. Usually, program planning is viewed as a linear process in which an audience is targeted, needs assessed, purpose identified, etc. There are many benefits to choosing a nurse career. The nurse helps people on a daily basis, and almost always finds the work to be very fulfilling on a personal level. Nurses are able to choose their own specialty, working in the field of nursing or medicine that suits them best. Nursing provides many opportunities for advancement into management, as well as providing job security. To ensure nursing and nurse education remain relevant, the Department of Human Services, Nurse Policy Branch initiated a project to discuss the future role of nursing and inform the future education and preparation of nurses.

Legislation in Nursing

14 unit

INTRODUCTION

As a nurse it has become an important necessity to be aware of the legal aspects associated with caring and helping people in the health industry today. Unfortunately, the more and more negligence cases there are the less and less people want to get into the health care field fearing legal aspects and the inevitable law suites. The first nursing law created was that of nursing registration in 1903.

The Tort Law is the legal aspects of the law that most nurses are more familiar with. This is the law that involved malpractice and negligence cases which many nurses take the time to learn inside and out as this is one of the biggest fears in the produces harm, whether it is unintentional or intentional. Malpractice is a specific type of Tort where the standards of care are no met. This is one of the most common and familiar laws to nurses and something that nurses and doctors alike must be familiar within order to continue their care effectively.

Nurses must take as many precautions as they can during their daily shifts. Recording, documenting and reporting daily routines and decisions is one of the most common ways to make sure on track with patience and in the right. Nurses learn in school/college that proper care of a patient is not only making the right decision but maintaining and organizing their medical/nursing records and reports effectively. The legal aspects of nursing are thought and expected to be kept-up on throughout every nurse's career.

PURPOSES OF LAW IN NURSING

The law serves a number of purposes in nursing:

- To provide a framework for establishing which nursing actions in the care of client are legal?

- To differentiate the nurses responsibility from those of other health professional.
- To establish the boundaries of independent nursing action.
- To assist in maintain a standard of nursing practice by making nurses accountable under the law.

IMPORTANCE OF LAW IN NURSING

- Nurses have more responsibility
- Increased the number of advance practice nurses
- Law is there to assist in the decision-making process involved in nursing practice
- Law is there for the protection of nursing practices
- Law is there for the identification of the risk of liability
- Increase in professional authority, accountability and autonomy in nursing practice.

TYPES OF LAW

Law governs the relationship of private individuals with government and with each other.

Public Law

It is one type of law which deals with an individual's relationship to the state:

- *Constitutional law:* It set of basic laws that defines and limits the powers of government. The nurses maintain rights as an individual. For example, constitutional rights, civil rights, state constitution, etc.
- *Administrative law:* It develops by group who are appointed to governmental administrative agencies like food, drug, cosmetics, social security, nurses practice Act, etc.
- *Criminal law:* These acts or offences against the welfare or safety of the public. For example, controlled substance act, criminal codes, etc.

Civil Law

This type of law which deals with crimes against a person or persons in such legal matters:

- *Contract law:* It is enforcement of agreements among private individuals like promise, mutual understanding and compensation.
- *Tort law:* It is the enforcement of duties and rights among independent of contractual agreements. It is a civil wrong committed on a person

or property stemming from either a direct invasion of some legal right of the person, infraction of some public duty, or the violation of some private obligation by which damages accrue to the person. For example, negligence and malpractice, assault and battery, false imprisonment, invasion of privacy, fraud, defamation, etc.

Classification of Torts

Intentional Torts

Intentional torts are willful acts that violate another's right, e.g. assault, battering, false imprisonment, etc. This is the category of civil law, with which nurses are generally concerned.

- *Assault:* Assault is any intentional threat to bring about harmful or offensive contact. No actual contact is necessary. The law protects clients who afraid of harmful contact. It is an assault for a nurse to threaten to give a client for an X-ray procedure when the client has refused consent. The key issue is the client consent. In an assault lawsuit, if the clients give consent, the nurse is not responsible.
- *Battery:* Battery is un-consented or unlawful touching of a person. For battery to occur, the touching must occur without consent. Remember that consent maybe implied rather than specifically stated. Therefore, if the patient extends an arm for injection, he cannot later charge battery, saying that he was not asked. But if the patient agreed because of a thread (assault), the touching would still be considered battery because the consent was not freely given.
- *False imprisonment:* The tort of false imprisonment occurs with unjustified restraining of a person without legal warrant. For example, this occurs when nurses restrain a client in a bounded area to keep the person from freedom but when it occurs in health care it is most often the basis of a civil suit rather than a criminal case. Anytime a patient needs to be confined for his or her own safety or well-being, it is best to help the understand and agree to that course of action. If the patient is not responsible, the guardian or legal representative may give permission. The third alternative is to objectively document the need in the patients record and obtain a physicians order as soon as possible. Be sure to follow the policies of the facility.

Quasi-intentional Torts

- *Invasion of Privacy:* Invasion of privacy means the intrusion into the personal life of another, without just cause, which can give the person whose privacy, has been invaded a right to bring a lawsuit for damages against the person or entity that intruded. However, public personages are not protected in most situations, since they have placed themselves already within the public eye, and their activities (even personal and sometimes intimate) are considered newsworthy, i.e. of legitimate public interest. However, an otherwise non-public individual has a right to privacy.

- *Defamation:* It is an intentional tort makes derogatory remarks about another.
- *Slander:* Oral defamation of character. It implies defamation in the form of spoken words. If a nurse tells a client that his physician is incompetent, the nurse could be liable for slander.
- *Libel:* Written defamation. It is defamation in the form of written words. If a nurse writes such defamation as mentioned above it is a case of liable.

Unintentional Torts

- *Negligence:* Negligence refers to a failure of an individual to do something that reasonably medical professional person would do under similar situation. It is characterized by inadvertence, thoughtfulness or inattention. It goes without saying that every situation is different, and that is where the law becomes somewhat cloudy. However, when reviewing a nursing negligence case, assumptions and circumstantial evidence are taken into account to determine if there was negligence.

  Examples of Nursing Negligence

  - Failure to use aseptic technique where required.
  - Leaving a foreign object in a patient's body during surgery.
  - Failing to respond promptly to patient symptoms impending disaster.
  - Failing to protect an infirm patient from falling resulting in injuries to patients.
  - Administering wrong medicine to a patient.
  - Administering a care in such a manner that a patient suffers injury, e.g. improper handling of hot water bag: bums to client, etc.
  - Any nurse who does not meet accepted standard of practice or care or who performs duties in a careless fashion, runs a risk of being found negligent.
- *Proof:* There are five main elements in a nursing negligence case, and all elements must be proven in order for a case to be valid. If one or more of the elements is not present, the case maybe difficult to pursue: (1) the nurse had a duty to perform, (2) the appropriate care was apparent in the situation, (3) there was a breach or violation of care, (4) there was an injury proven to result from the nurse's negligence,

and (5) there is proof that damages occurred as a direct result of the situation.

- *Malpractice:* Malpractice is professional misconduct by professional person and concerns, professional actions an in the failure of a person with professional education and skills to act in a reasonable and prudent manner. Medical malpractice is defined as a wrongful act by a physician, nurse, or other medical professional in the administration of treatment or at times, the omission of medical treatment, to a patient under his or her care.

Types of Nursing Malpractice

Nursing malpractice takes many forms, including:

- Medication errors: giving a patient the wrong medication or the wrong dose, or dispensing medication to the wrong patient
- Failure to follow a physician's orders
- Delaying patient care and/or failure to monitor a patient
- Incorrectly performing a procedure, or trying to perform a procedure without training
- Documentation error
- Failure to get informed patient consent.

LEGAL TERMS USES IN NURSING PRACTICE

- *Licensure:* All nurses who are in nursing practice have to passes a valid license, issued by the representative nursing council or Indian Nursing Council. There practice is controlled educational program.
- *Good Samaritan law:* In response to health professional, fear of malpractice claims, most states enacted 'Good Samaritan law' that exempt doctors and nurses from liability when they render first aid during emergency.
- *Good rapport:* Developing god rapport with the client is very important to prevent malpractice. A lawsuit is often circumvented when the nursing staff treats with warrants and caring. So nurse must never underestimate 'rapport' with the client in malpractice prevention. The ability to develop good rapport with clients is depends on the nurse having good interpersonal communication skills, e.g. listening.
- *Standard of care:* All professional practicing in the medical field are held to certain standard when administrating care comes from several sources including laws, organizational standard and institutional policies and procedures. It is always better to follow standards to avoid malpractice and do not attempt anything beyond the level of competence.

- *Standing orders:* Although a nurse legally diagnose illness or prescribe treatment, he or she may after assessing patients condition, apply 'standing order' or treatment guideline that have been established doctor as appropriate for the certain problem and the condition. Nurse do not take chance, if there is any doubt arise, it is always better to follow written order instead of oral orders.
- *Contract:* A contract is written or oral agreement between two people in which goods or services are exchanged. Section 13 to the Indian contract act defines the word that two or more people are said to consented when they agree upon the same thing in the same sense. Treating a patient without obtaining proper consent can lead to a chance of assault.
- *Consent for operation and other procedure:* A patient coming into the hospital still retain his/her right as a citizen and his entry only denotes his willingness to undergo an investigation or treatment of a serious nature, or an operation which needed anesthesia, requires the written consent of the patient if he has attain the age of 18 years or is a minor who has attain the age of 16 years.
- *Correct identity:* All patient in general hospitals wear identity band, in order to prevent the mistakes. It is very important that correct band is given to each patient and these are normally checked as the part of the admission procedure. Every patient before giving pre medication for an operation should be labeled approved by the hospital. The nurse or midwife has the great responsibility to make sure that all the babies born in the hospital are correctly labeled at birth and to ensure that no time they are placed in wrong cot or wrongly handled.
- *Counting of sponge, needle and instrument:* A Nurse advocate that sponge, instrument and needle count should be performed for all surgical procedures taking place in operation theater. When an instrument or needle left in patient's body, during surgery the operating room nurse will probably be liable for any patient's injury caused by the presence of foreign body. The nurse has to carry-out a final check before the body cavity is closed.
- *Accident or injury:* If a patient sustain injury while in hospital, she/he may bring an action against the hospital authority or against a person (member of medical, nursing or ancillary staff) to whom he/she attributes an injury. An action maybe brought away against the hospital even after the several years the accident occurred. It is therefore, necessary that at the time of incident an accurate and full record should be made on the special form provided.
- *Self discharge of the patient:* When the patient demands to discharge himself, the duty of nurse is to inform the medical officer concern with his care. It is probable that a senior administrative officer ask patient to sign a written statement that he is leaving against the medical advice.

If he refuses it, a note of this effect will have to be made and signed by two witnesses one of whom is usually an administrative officer and other is nurse incharge at that time.

- *Professional confidence:* Guarding the confidence of the patient is an ethical duty of the medical authority and nurses and it must take that it never should be discussed personal information received by the nature of their position, except with the senior members of the staff.
- *Documentation:* Documentation is by far the best one a lawsuit filled. Nurse should give themselves the credit from care they provide thoroughly documenting in the medical record. While documenting it is better to use formats of documentation for each activity specified by the respective institution or government.
- *Reporting:* In some situation, nurses have obligation or are required to report certain communicable diseases or criminal activity such as abuse, gunshot wound, attempted suicide or rape to the appropriate authority.

LEGAL HAZARDS OR ISSUES IN NURSING

A number of legal hazards or issues are related to nursing practice, including licensing, nurse practice acts, and standards of care. However, in these litigious times, the issue that most concerns those considering a career in nursing are negligence and malpractice.

- *Patient's advocate:* A nurse has a legal obligation to act as the patient's advocate in case of emergency. The nurse is to act as the liaison between the patient and the health care provider, such as a physician. The nurse will monitor the patient, ensuring that if any complications or abnormalities arise, a physician notified immediately. The nurse is legally obligated to keep the personal data and information of the patient private; not doing so is a violation of the code of ethics for nurses.
- *Administering medication:* Nurses are responsible for administering the correct doses and medications to patients. If the nurse gives a fatal dosage amount, she may face legal malpractice suits. It is also the responsibility to research the patient's records, or ask the patient and family members if there are any allergies or complications that may pose a risk if a certain medication is administered.
- *Informed consent:* When a nurse is administering treatment, she must explain what the effects and outcomes could be, and any other important information. It is the responsibility of the nurse to confirm that the patient or family member who will sign the informed consent form is coherent, and understands all the negatives and aspects of the treatment. The nurse, patient, or patient family member will

sign the informed consent form in front of a witness, a physician or another nurse. Not having this legal document signed and in front of a witness could be a legal issue for the nurse if complications arise during treatment.

- *Negligence:* It is the responsibility of the nurse to monitor the patient. If a patient calls for a nurse to come and assist him in going to the rest room for example, the nurse is to assist, or if the is busy with another patient, have another nurse assist the patient. Ignoring the patient or responding after a lengthy delay could be considered negligence, and if the patient is hurt from trying to move himself, the nurse could face legal suits. Also, it could be considered negligence if a physician orders the nurse to administer a prescription, and the nurse did not do so.
- *Duty:* Duty stands for a legal obligation owed by one person to another person. When nurses care for clients, they assume the duty to care for them in a competent and diligent manner. Nurses are expected to provide the degree of care ordinarily exercised by other nurses practicing in the same nursing specialty. Therefore, nurses are expected to adhere to standards of care—those imposed by the nurse's state board of nursing nurse practice act, the national nursing specialty standards of care and scope of practice, and the nurse's hospital, or other agency, protocols.
- *Breach:* A breach of duty takes place when there is failure to fulfill the duties established as being the responsibility of the nurse. In other words, nurses breach their duty when they do not meet the appropriate standard of care.
- *Causation:* Causation is the most difficult element to prove because it is the factual connection between what the nurse did and the injury to the client. Causation means that the nurse's breach of duty, or failure to meet the appropriate standard of care, caused the client's injury or adverse outcome.
- *Damages:* Damages are monetary payments designed to compensate the client for the injury or adverse outcome, and are intended to restore the plaintiff to the condition he or she was in prior to the injury. To recover damages, the client must establish that he or she suffered physical, financial, or emotional injury caused by the nurse's violation of the standard of care. Damages are usually compensatory or punitive.

HEALTH LAWS REGULATIONS AT CENTER LEVEL

The preamble to the constitution of India coupled with the directive principles of state policy strives to provide a welfare state with socialist patterns of society. It enjoins the state to make the "improvement of public health" a primary responsibility. Furthermore, articles 38, 42, 43 and 47 of the constitution provide for promotion of health of individuals as well as health care. The constitution of India also enumerates the separate and shared legislative powers of parliament and state legislatures in three separate lists: the union list, the state list and the concurrent list. The parliament and state legislatures share authority over matters on the concurrent list, which include criminal law and procedure; marriage, divorce and all other personal law matters; economic and social planning; population control and family planning; social security and social insurance; employment; education; legal and medical professions; and prevention of transmission of infectious or contagious diseases. Laws passed by parliament with respect to matters on the concurrent list supersede laws passed by state legislatures. The parliament generally has no power to legislate on items from the state list, including public health, hospitals and sanitation. However, two-thirds of the Rajya Sabha may vote to allow parliament to pass binding legislation on any state issue if 'necessary or expedient in the national interest'. In addition, two or more States may ask parliament to legislate on an issue that is otherwise reserved for the state. Other states may them choose to adopt the resulting legislation.

Issues in Regulation of Health Matters in India

Health regulation in India encompasses a variety of actors and issues. These include promulgation of legislation for health facilities and services, disease control and medical care, human power (Education, Licensing and Professional Responsibility), ethics and patients rights, pharmaceuticals and medical devices, radiation protection, poisons and hazardous substances, occupational health and accident prevention, elderly, disabled and rehabilitation family, women and child health, mental health, smoking/tobacco control, social security and health insurance, environmental protection, nutrition and food safety, health information and statistics and custody, civil and human rights to enumerate a few.

HEALTH LAWS REGULATIONS AT STATE LEVEL

Nursing regulation is the governmental oversight provided for nursing practice in each state. Nursing is regulated because it is one of the health professions that pose risk of harm to the public if practiced by someone who is unprepared and incompetent. The public may not have sufficient information and experience to identify an unqualified health care provider, and is vulnerable to unsafe and incompetent practitioners.

Through regulatory processes, the government permits only individuals who meet predetermined qualifications to practice nursing. The board of nursing is the authorized state entity with the legal authority to regulate nursing. Legislatures enact the nurse practice act for a state. The nurse practice act typically:

- Defines the authority of the board of nursing, its composition and powers
- Defines nursing and the boundaries of the scope of nursing practice
- Identifies types of licenses and titles
- States the requirements for licensure
- Protects titles
- Identifies the grounds for disciplinary action.

Boards of nursing are authorized to develop administrative rules and regulations that are used to clarify or make the statutes more specific. Rules and regulations must be consistent with the nurse practice act, cannot go beyond the law, and, once enacted, have the force and effect of law. Public comment periods are provided to allow nurses, students and the public to participate in the rule-making process by submitting written comments or participating in rule-making hearings.

The National Council of State Boards of Nursing (NCSBN) has a website that provides information about various practice acts for most states. The purpose of NCSBN is to provide an organization through which boards of nursing act and counsel together on matters of common interest and concern affecting the public health, safety and welfare, including the development of licensing examinations in nursing.

CONSUMER PROTECTION BILL AND ITS IMPACT IN NURSING PRACTICE

The Consumer Protection Act (CPA) was passed by the Government of India in 1986 to protect the interests of the consumer. Consumer means any person who buys any goods against consideration is a consumer. Similarly any person who hires services against consideration is also a consumer. In health care delivery, patient is a consumer. Government institutions do not come under the preview of CPA because the consumers pay only nominal amount of registration charges, so cannot fall within the ambit 'Consumer'.

Objectives of the Consumer Protection Act

- To provide for the better protection of the interests of the consumers
- To provide for the establishment of quasi judicial authorities for the settlement of consumer disputes

- The right to be protected against the marketing of goods and services which are hazardous to life and property
- The right to be informed about the quality, quantity, potency, purity, standard and price of goods or services as the case maybe so as to protect the consumer against unfair trade practices.
- The right to be assured, wherever possible access to variety of goods and services at competitive prices
- The right to be heard and be assured that consumer's interests will receive due consideration at appropriate forum
- The right to seek redressed against unfair trade practices or unscrupulous exploitation of consumer
- The right to consumer education.

Different Rights of Consumer Patients

- *Right for care:* The patient regardless of age, sex, disability, ethnicity, or religion has the right to accent treatment. It includes the patient's right to select his or her own physician.
- *Right to treatment:* The patient has the right to accent care as long as that care is within medical centers capacity. When the medical center can not provide the care a patient needs, the staff will inform the patient of other choices of care. It is necessary and medically advisable the medical center may transfer the patient to another facility.
- *Right to tespectful care:* The patient has the right to make decisions about medical care without an influence. The patient has also the right to receive from his or her physician the information regarding care prior to any treatment. Patients and when appropriate their families, are informed about the outcomes of care.
- *Right to research:* The patient has right to consent or refuse to participate in research studies or clinical trials affecting care and treatment.
- *Right to surrogate decision maker:* She/he has the right to designate within legal parameters.
- *Right to organ donation or anatomy gift:* She/he has the right to make a donation of his body or parts for transplantation. She/he has also right to make gift of his or her body parts thereof upon death for medical education or research.
- *Right to personal privacy:* Care discussion consultation, examination procedures and treatment shall be considered within respect of each patient's privacy. The personal privacy of each patient will be respected by the institution in as much as possible without compromise to their safety and clinical care.
- *Right to confidentiality:* She/he has a right to confidentiality of all communications and records about his or her care. Medical records

and all other information will be kept confidential law, written consent or allowed within limits of law.

- *Right to participate in care planning:* She/he has the right to make informed decisions regarding his/her care. She/he also is a part of treatment and care planning.
- *Right to respect of cultural and religious beliefs:* She/he has the right to continue to exercise his cultural and religious beliefs. She/he has the right to exercise that the health care team will respects his religious belief and personal value system.
- *Right to protective services:* She/he has a right to be free from all forms of abuse or harassment. She/he has the right to safe environment within management of infections and safe medical equipment, etc.
- *Right to billing explanation:* She/he has the right to be informed of services and related charges available in or through the facility to receive and itemized bill regardless of source of payment.

Negligence

Negligence is the conduct that falls below the standard of care. The standard of care is established by the law for the protection of consumers against and unreasonable practices which create risk or harm. Professional's person such as nurses, doctors having special skills and knowledge. Nursing Practice act describe and define the legal boundaries of nursing practice within each state. The responsibilities of the Indian Nursing Council, State Nursing Council and University have to regulate the standard of the nursing.

Common Sources of Negligence

Nurses should be aware of the common negligent acts that have resulted in lawsuits against hospital and nurses. The commonly occurring examples are outlined below:

- Medication errors that result in injury to client
- An intravenous therapy error resulting is infiltration or phlebitis
- Burn to clients caused by equipment, bathing, or spill of hot liquids and food
- Falls resulting in injury to client
- Failure to use aseptic technique where required
- Errors in sponge, instruments, or needle count in surgical cases
- Failure to give a report, or giving an incomplete report, to an oncoming shift
- Failure to adequately monitor a client's condition
- Failure to notify a physician of a significant change in a client's status.

Prevention of Error

Several suggestions are made for reducing error. Leaped suggests that many health care delivery systems, especially in hospital could be redesigned to significantly reduce the likelihood of error.

- Reduced reliance on memory by using checklists protocols and computerised decision aids for prescription writing.
- Improved information access with availability of computerized medical record at bedside.
- Error proofing - use of forcing function in computer programs so that a physician cannot enter an overdose or prescribe a medication to which the patient is allergic.
- Standardization of drug doses and time of administration, of information displays, equipment and supplies location in hospital.
- Training of doctors, nursing and other staff in safe practice.
- Read prescription carefully. Physician's prescriptions are at times illegible and lead to litigation and medication errors.
- Medication errors occur due to mistakes (knowledge-based or rule-based) and slips of action and lapses of memory. Focus on the task at hand. Knowledgeable and experienced nurses can easily identify the mistakes.
- Be careful while administering drugs/doses. Doctor should avoid trailing zeros, e.g. 10.0 mg which maybe read 100 mg.
- Beware of high-risk situations, e.g. elderly patients on multiple drugs.
- Review basic drug-related information from approved standard textbook.
- Avoid use of a drug for unproved unlabelled indications especially where risk of drug use is higher than expected benefits.
- Communicate effectively when patients, families, pharmacists question prescriptions.

FUNDAMENTAL CONDUCT IN NURSING LEGISLATION

- *Provision 1:* The nurse, in all professional relationships, practices with compassion and respect for the inherent dignity, worth, and uniqueness of every individual, unrestricted by considerations of social or economic status, personal attributes, or the nature of health problems.
- *Provision 2:* The nurse's primary commitment is to the patient, whether an individual, family, group, or community.
- *Provision 3:* The nurse promotes, advocates for, and strives to protect the health, safety, and rights of the patient.
- *Provision 4:* The nurse is responsible and accountable for individual nursing practice and determines the appropriate delegation of tasks

consistent with the nurse's obligation to provide optimum patient care.

- *Provision 5:* The nurse owes the same duties to self as to others, including the responsibility to preserve integrity and safety, to maintain competence, and to continue personal and professional growth.
- *Provision 6:* The nurse participates in establishing, maintaining, and improving healthcare environments and conditions of employment conducive to the provision of quality healthcare and consistent with the values of the profession through individual and collective action.
- *Provision 7:* The nurse participates in the advancement of the profession through contributions to practice, education administration and knowledge development.
- *Provision 8:* The nurse collaborates with other health professionals and the public in promoting community, national, and international efforts to meet health needs.
- *Provision 9:* The profession of nursing, as represented by associations and other members, is responsible for articulating nursing values, for maintaining the integrity of the profession and its practice, and for shaping social policy.

Nurses should also participate in civic causes that advocate for health-related legislation. There are many nurses who have demonstrated their dedication to migrant farm workers, people in refugee centers, or juvenile detention centers, and continue to educate the public on these vulnerable populations. Nurses individually and as a group should become familiar with the healthcare needs of their community and participate in their education. This can be accomplished through the participation in health fairs, school programs and community-based educational events and initiatives. Nurses should utilize their professional organizations to voice their concerns.

SERVICE AND INSTRUCTIONAL RULES

A registered nurse or licensed practical nurse at the discretion of the registered nurse may assign basic tasks to unlicensed persons. Basic tasks include non-injectable medications.

- The process of assignment requires the following steps:
  - The registered nurse develops a plan for teaching the basic task of nursing care.
  - The registered nurse or licensed practical nurse, at the discretion of the registered nurse, shall: Teach the basic tasks of nursing care to the unlicensed persons, including why the task is necessary.

- Assign the basic task of nursing care and document the assignment by summarizing which unlicensed persons will perform which tasks for each client.
- Give the unlicensed persons written or other retrievable instructions that can serve as a resource when the unlicensed person is performing the task.
- Periodically evaluate the performance of the unlicensed persons and the conditions of the clients. The interval for periodic evaluation is at the discretion of the registered nurse.

- Basic tasks of nursing care maybe taught to a group of unlicensed persons.
- The registered nurse retains the responsibility and accountability for determining the appropriateness of assigning basic tasks of nursing care to unlicensed persons.
- PRN medication and treatments maybe assigned to an unlicensed caregiver by a registered nurse provided the registered nurse leaves written parameters to clarify the physician's or nurse practitioner's PRN order and leaves guidelines which are so specific that the unlicensed caregiver uses no discretion in administering the PRN medication or treatment.
- Teaching basic tasks of client care which do not require client specific instructions is not considered assignment for the purposes of these rules.
- The registered nurse may delegate special tasks of nursing care, including the administration of subcutaneous injectable medications.
- The registered nurse may delegate the administration of medications by the intravenous route through a central venous catheter to one unlicensed person, specific to one client, provided the following conditions are met:
  - The delegation is done by a registered nurse who is an employee of a licensed home health, home infusion or hospice provider.
  - The medications which maybe delegated are limited to flushing the line with routine flushing solutions.
  - A registered nurse is available on call for consultation/intervention 24 hours each day.
- A registered nurse who is an employee of a licensed home health, home infusion or hospice provider may delegate the administration of a bolus of medication by pushing a button on a pre programd pump. This applies to any route of administration.
- The registered nurse may teach and delegate a task of nursing care to one unlicensed person, specific to one client, under the following conditions:
  - The client's condition is stable and predictable.

- He registered nurse considers the nature of the nursing care task to be provided, its complexity, the risks involved and the necessary skill needed to perform the task.
- The registered nurse assesses the client's condition and determines if the unlicensed person is capable to perform the task in the absence of direct registered nurse supervision.
- The registered nurse determines how frequently the client's condition shall be reassessed to determine the appropriateness of the continued delegation of the task to an unlicensed person.
- The registered nurse evaluates the ability of the unlicensed person to perform the nursing care task.
- The registered nurse documents the rationale for deciding that this task can be delegated to the unlicensed person.

The registered nurse may delegate a client specific task of nursing care to additional unlicensed persons provided the registered nurse limits the number of unlicensed persons to the number who will remain proficient in performing the task and can be safely supervised by the registered nurse.

- The registered nurse shall use the following process to delegate a special task of nursing care:
  - Assess the client's condition.
  - Evaluate the skills and ability of the unlicensed person.
  - Teach the task of nursing care including.
  - The proper procedure/technique.
  - The risks associated with performing the task.
  - Anticipated side effects.
  - The appropriate response to untoward or side effects.
  - Observe the unlicensed person performing the task to ensure that the unlicensed person performs the task safely and accurately.
  - Leave written instructions for performance of the task for the unlicensed person to use as a reference.
  - Instruct the unlicensed person that the task being taught and delegated is specific to this client only and is not transferable to other clients or taught to other care providers.
  - Assess the client and supervise the unlicensed person, at least every 60 days.
- The responsibility, accountability and authority for teaching and delegation of special tasks of nursing care to unlicensed persons shall remain with the registered nurse.
- It is expected that the registered nurse who delegates tasks of nursing care to unlicensed persons will also supervise the unlicensed persons. However, supervision may also be provided by another registered nurse who was not the delegator provided the supervising nurse is

familiar with the client, the skills of the unlicensed person and the plan of care. The acts of delegation and supervision are of equal importance for ensuring the safety of nursing care for clients. If the delegating and supervising nurses are two different individuals, the following shall occur:
  - The reasons for separation of delegation and supervision shall be justified from the standpoint of delivering effective client care, and not only for convenience.
  - The justification shall be documented in writing.
  - The supervising nurse agrees, in writing, to perform the supervision.
  - The supervising nurse is either present during teaching and delegation or is fully informed of the instruction, approves of the plan for teaching and agrees that the unlicensed person who is taught the task of nursing care is competent the perform the task.
- The registered nurse may transfer delegation and supervision to another registered nurse by using the following process:
  - Review the client's condition, teaching plan, competence of the unlicensed person, the written instructions and the plan for supervision.
  - Redo any parts of the delegation process which need to be changed as a result of the transfer.
  - Document the transfer and acceptance of the delegation/ supervision responsibility, the reason for the transfer and the effective date of the transfer, signed by both registered nurses.
  - Communicate the transfer to the persons who need to know of the transfer.

REGULATION OF LEGISLATION IN NURSING

Establishing a comprehensive regulatory system requires the completion of a number of steps. Ideally any new system should be considered as an integrated whole. In reality however few countries start from nothing; usually some work will already have been done and will need to be incorporated in some way into a new system. Whether starting a new system or modifying an existing one, it will be helpful to consider the following steps, if only to ensure that nothing has been left out. In practice, various elements of the process will need adjusting to accommodate the needs of country concerned and will assume greater or lesser importance depending upon the particular circumstances.

Determining a Policy

First of all a clear policy needs to be agreed by the body/bodies with responsibility for such. This maybe the nursing association, government, the nursing council/board or other body. Policy should be established through a process of formal and informal consultation if it is to be effectively put into practice. If the key players (who need to be carefully and comprehensively identified) are not involved in the process then the policy is likely to be unsuccessful. Consultation will not, of course, mean that everyone can have their own way; compromises will still have to be made but frank discussion of the options and the reasons for the final decisions will help those decisions to be better understood and accepted.

Ideally the total policy should relate to a comprehensive regulatory system even if implementation will take place on an incremental basis, depending on issues such as resources and infrastructure changes. In this way different elements can be worked on at different rates; for example, work could be done on preparing a code of conduct while also considering changes to license-to-practice requirements. If an existing system is used for a model, care should be taken to ensure that the final scheme is professionally, socially, economically and culturally appropriate to the setting in which it is to be used.

Determining A Strategy

Once the policy is agreed, a clear and explicit strategy and plan of action should be confirmed which encompasses all the elements of the policy from its inception to its final implementation. For ultimate success, it is vital that the implementation phase be given as much time and as many resources as the policy phase. The responsibility for implementing the total strategy and the separate phases/elements of the action plan should be clear, and lines of accountability should be explicit and visible. Good communication is essential to success, and time and effort should be given to ensuring that proposed changes are understood by all those who will be affected.

Identifying the Key Players

For policy change to be successful it is necessary to win as many hearts and minds as possible in advance of implementation. It is vital to consider everyone who may have a legitimate role. This may include, for example:

- Nursing associations/organizations
- Influential groups, e.g. managers, educationalists
- Government
- The public
- Patients' representatives
- Other professions
- Voluntary groups
- Other relevant/influential bodies

- Attention should also be given to identifying and cultivating influential individuals who maybe helpful in terms of achieving significant policy change, especially where there maybe some opposition.

Consultation (Formal and Informal)

Effective consultation processes are essential if the eventual policy is to have the goodwill and support of those affected. The ultimate operational success of the policy may well depend on the effectiveness of the consultation process. While it is clearly unlikely that all interested parties will be equally pleased with the policy outcomes, at least if an opportunity has been given for them to have their say and an explanation offered as to why certain decisions were made, goodwill will have been maintained.

If a policy-making body already exists, the requirements for formal consultation may already be well established. In some instances the process maybe set down within existing legislation and the organizations which have to be consulted will be explicitly defined. Alternatively, there maybe a general phrase to the effect that consultation must take place with all those organizations or individuals who maybe affected, actually or potentially, by any changes. Any formal consultation process should be regularly reviewed as "interested parties" are likely to change significantly overtime. The increased involvement of consumers and/or patient representatives is a good example of a significant change in the past decade.

In addition to honoring any formal consultation process, the informal processes are equally important, although they may not be as visible. Influential opinion formers, such as politicians, key health care managers and professionals, should be identified and lobbied by all appropriate means. Such activity is essential in terms of achieving significant policy change.

SUMMARY

In this unit we discuss that nurses need to understand the legalities involved in the delivery of safe health care. It is important to know the standards of care established within the institution because these will be the standards to which will be held accountable. Health care consumers have a right to quality care, and nurses have an obligation to deliver it. Caring for clients safely and avoiding legal difficulties require nurses to adhere to the expected standards of care and carefully document changes in client status.

Professional and Related Organizations

15 unit

INTRODUCTION

Professional organizations and associations in nursing are critical for generating the energy, flow of ideas, and proactive work needed to maintain a healthy profession that advocates for the needs of its clients and nurses, and the trust of society. Professionals create organizations to work collectively on behalf of issues that enhance their work and their involvement in communities, ensure continued learning and competence, and use political action to influence policymakers to support mission of organization. Professional organizations offer a supportive way to learn leadership skills, to test ideas, and to follow these ideas to completion.

TRAINED NURSES ASSOCIATION OF INDIA (TNAI)

The association had its beginning in the Association of Nursing Superintendents which was founded in 1905, at Lucknow. The organization was composed of nine European Nurses holding administrative posts in hospitals. The Association of Nursing Superintendents, therefore, sought the help and cooperation of nurses throughout the country. At the annual conference held in Bombay in 1908, a decision was taken to establish Trained Nurses Association. The association was inaugurated in 1909. The two organizations shared the same officers until 1910 when, at the first Trained Nurses Association (TNA) conference, held at Banaras (UP), the TNA members elected their own officers.

The trained nurses association of India is a national professional association of nurses. The present name and organization were established in 1922.

Aims of TNAI

- Upholding in every way the dignity and honor of the nursing profession
- Development and standardization of nursing education
- Improvement of living and working condition for nurses in India
- Promoting a sense of esprit de corps among all nurses
- Registration for qualified nurses.

Activities of TNAI

- TNAI gives scholarships for nurses who wish to go on for advanced study either here or abroad
- It helped to remove discrimination against male nurses
- Initiated much needed study and improvement of economic conditions for nurses
- The TNAI opposes strikes unless all other means of negotiating have failed to bring about satisfactory working conditions.

Membership of TNAI

It is possible to apply for a life membership. The official organ of the TNAI is The Nursing Journal of India which is published monthly. The cost of this is included in the annual subscription for membership in the association. It helps you to be informed of current events in nursing and offers opportunities to publish articles and voice opinions.

Policies and Practices of TNAI

The Trained Nurses Association of India has for many years been greatly concerned about the economic welfare of nurses and action which maybe taken to negotiate for better benefits and working conditions for the profession. The following facts have emerged during this time:

- The TNAI cannot be legally appointed as a negotiating bodies either at a Local, State or National level.
- The advice of the TNAI is listened to, with respect, and sometimes acted upon. But such advice is given on the initiative of the TNAI, but the TNAI does not have the right of representation in negotiations.
- The TNAI as a national body can give a broad support to local or state organizations of nurses.

The organization of the TNAI makes it possible for all nurses to participate at some level. In the beginning with the local unit, this is usually made-up of personnel in a specific institution, the level of organization moves to the district, state and national levels. Members of the TNAI are usually most active on the level of the local unit. Activities and conferences, however, are planned regularly by the state branches and provide opportunities for valuable professional participation and development of the individual member.

THE STUDENT NURSES ASSOCIATION (SNA)

The Student Nurses Association organized in 1920, is associated with and under jurisdiction of the TNAI. In addition to it provide the personal and professional development for the nursing student. The assistant secretary of the TNAI serves as advisor for the SNA.

Purposes and Functions of SNA

- To help the student nurses learn how the professional organization serves to uphold the dignity and ideals of the nursing profession
- To promote a close rapport with other student nurses
- To furnish student nurses advice in their courses of study leading up to professional qualifications
- To encourages leadership ability and help students to gain a wide knowledge of the nursing profession in all of its different branches
- To encourage both professional and recreational meetings, Games and Sports
- To encourage students nurses develop a cooperative spirit with other student nurses which will help them in future professional relationships.

Activities of SNA

- Fund raising for the TNAI
- Fund raising done for fine arts and sports competitions and conferences
- Special prizes given for outstanding achievement in specific areas of nursing education
- Unit activities include maintaining the diary of unit activities, giving quarterly reports, preparing articles for publication and distributing application forms for membership in the TNAI.

Membership of SNA

- Fees are minimal and easily met by the nursing student. Nursing students who participate in the student nurses association have a valuable opportunity to begin to develop leadership skills, competitive skills and an interest for the profession as a whole.

INTERNATIONAL COUNCIL FOR NURSES (ICN)

The International Council of Nurses (ICN) is a federation of more than 130 National Nurses Associations (NNAs), representing the more than 16 million nurses worldwide. Founded in 1899, ICN is the world's first and widest reaching international organization for health professionals. Operated by nurses and leading nurses internationally, ICN works to ensure quality nursing care for all, sound health policies globally, the advancement of nursing knowledge, and the presence worldwide of a respected nursing profession and a competent and satisfied nursing workforce.

Objectives of ICN

- To promote the development of strong national nurses associations
- To assist national nurses association to improve the standards of nursing and the competence of nurses
- To assist national nurses associations to improve the status of nurses within their countries
- To serve as the authoritative voice for nurses and nursing internationally
- Activities of ICN
- Makes policy statements on health and social issues
- Offers a great variety of seminars
- Maintaining and improving the status of nursing around the world.

Membership of ICN

All nurses can become members of the ICN but not as individuals. The individual nurse becomes a member if his/her national nurses association is a member of ICN. Nurses in India become members of ICN when they become members of the TNAI.

THE INDIAN NURSING COUNCIL (INC)

The Indian Nursing Council is a national regulatory body for nurses and nurse education in India. It is an autonomous body under the Government of India, Ministry of Health and Family Welfare, constituted by the Central Government under section 3(1) of the Indian Nursing Council Act, 1947 of Indian Parliament.

AIM of INC

- To establish a uniform standard of training for nurses midwives and health visitors.

- Functions of INC.
- To establish and monitor a uniform standard of nursing education for nurses midwife, auxiliary nurse midwives and health visitors by doing inspection of the institutions.
- To establish and monitor a uniform standard of nursing education for nurses midwife, auxiliary nurse midwives and health visitors by doing inspection of the institutions.
- To recognize the qualifications under section 10(2)(4) of the Indian Nursing Council Act, 1947 for the purpose of registration and employment in India and abroad.
- To give approval for registration of Indian and Foreign Nurses Possessing foreign qualification under section 11(2)(a) of the Indian Nursing Council Act, 1947.
- To prescribe minimum standards of education and training in various nursing programs and prescribe the syllabus and regulations for nursing programs.
- Power to withdraw the recognition of qualification under section 14 of the act in case the institution fails to maintain its standards under Section 14 (1)(b) that an institution recognised by a state council for the training of nurses, midwives, auxiliary vurse midwives or health visitors does not satisfy the requirements of the council.
- To advise the State Nursing Councils, Examining Boards, State Governments and Central Government in various important items regarding nursing education in the country.
- To regulate the training policies and programs in the field of nursing.
- To recognize Institutions/Organizations/Universities imparting Master's Degree/Bachelor's Degree/PG Diploma/ Diploma/Certificate Courses in the field of nursing.
- To Recognize Degree/Diploma/Certificate awarded by Foreign Universities/Institutions on reciprocal basis.
- To promote research in nursing.
- To maintain Indian Nurses Register for registration of Nursing personnel.
- Prescribe code of ethics and professional conduct.
- To improve the quality of nursing education.

STATE NURSING COUNCIL

The State Nursing Council is the provisions of nurses and midwives act and works as an autonomous body under the state government, Department of Health and Family Welfare. It is a regulatory body for nurses and education in nursing in state and it is monitored by Indian Nursing Council.

Functions of State Nursing Council

- To establish and maintain a uniform standard of nursing education for Nurses, Auxiliary Nurse Midwives and Health Visitors by doing periodical inspection of the institution.
- To give registration to Nurses and Midwives who had undergone their training from recognized institutions.
- To conduct undergraduate courses and to issue diploma and registration certificate.
- To conduct examinations for ANM, GNM, Post Basic Diploma Courses and Health Supervisor Courses.
- Power to withdraw the recognition of qualification in case the institution fails to maintain its standards.

COMMONWEALTH NURSES FEDERATION

Nurses and midwives form the majority of health care workers across all health care settings and particularly in the primary health care context. In rural settings and in developing countries the nurse or midwife maybe the only local source of health care.

The Commonwealth Nurses Federation (CNF) was formally organized in 1973 and operates in six regions of the world which are East, Africa, Atlantic, Australia, Pacific, South Asia and Europe.

The CNF has regular and constructive contact with major Commonwealth bodies in London including the Commonwealth Secretariat and the Commonwealth Foundation. The CNF is an accredited Commonwealth body, which allows involvement in annual Health Ministers' meetings, the biennial Commonwealth Peoples Forum held prior to the Commonwealth Heads of Government meeting and other Commonwealth meetings such as the civil society consultations. The TNAI is also affiliated with the Commonwealth Nurses Federation. It is made-up of nurses associations from commonwealth countries.

Aims of Commonwealth Nurses Federation

- To promote sharing, better communications and closer relationships between its member associations
- To provides expert professional advice
- To provide scholarships for advanced study
- To support in financial assistance for professional meetings and seminars
- To helps in running an office through which funds can be received and dispersed for the benefit of nursing in countries which are represented
- Work Program of Commonwealth Nurses Federation.

The CNF's Current Work Program Includes the Following

- Membership development
- Conducting in-country projects with national nursing organizations involving capacity building and training
- Communicating with member organizations through a newsletter and the website
- Conducting and facilitating research on nursing and midwifery within Commonwealth countries
- Involvement in the work of the Commonwealth Steering Committee for Nursing and Midwifery
- Participating in the work of the Commonwealth HIV/AIDS Action Group
- Collaboration with other international nursing and health bodies
- Participating in and contributing to Commonwealth Health Ministers' and Heads of Government meetings
- Participating in and contributing to Commonwealth Health Ministers and other Commonwealth meetings
- Promoting Commonwealth Day.

NURSES LEAGUE OF THE CHRISTIAN MEDICAL ASSOCIATION

The nurses league of the clinical medical association of India was founded in 1930. It became affiliated to the TNAI in 1936 and promotes membership in this organization.

Objectives

- Promote cooperation and encouragement among Christian Nurses
- Promote efficiency in nursing education and service
- Secure the highest standards possible in Christian nursing education through the Christian schools of nursing
- Considering the special work and problems of Christian nurses wherever employed.

Activities

- Activities include national and area conferences and retreats for its members. Development of leadership abilities is encouraged by participation in these meetings
- Each meeting also allows for sharing of problems common to the Christian nurse
- Provides expert professional advice

- Provides scholarships for advanced study
- Provides financial assistance for professional meetings and seminars.

Membership

- Membership fees are required and a life membership is available
- Nursing students maybecome associate members of the league
- Membership in the nurses league maybe a requirement for certain nursing positions under control of Christian employing authorities.

WORLD HEALTH ORGANIZATION (WHO)

The World Health Organization (WHO) is the body of the United Nations (UN) responsible for directing and coordinating health. As such WHO has come to play a vital role as an actor in the field of international public health and international public health policy. Since its inception in 1947 WHO has been at the forefront of many breakthroughs in the field including, most notably, what has come to be described as one of the greatest humanitarian achievements of the 20th century, the elimination of smallpox in 1979. However WHO's inability to control the spread of HIV/AIDS, particularly in Africa has cast doubt on its effectiveness. Though much of the media attention given to WHO concentrates on its role in controlling and ultimately eliminating infectious disease, which mandate is far broader.

The WHO has been active in nursing education and practice in a number of ways in India. It has offered guidance in setting up programs of nursing education. The WHO promotes public health in many ways around the world. It is currently known for the declaration of working towards 'Health for all by 2000 AD'. This declaration has given a tremendous push to developing primary health care and recognizing the very essential role of nursing in health care system.

Objectives of the World Health Organization (WHO)

- To create an interface between the developed and developing nations when pertaining to health issues.
- To patronize and support health programs in developing nations.
- To periodically formulate health policies that are readily endorsed by nations.
- To coordinate and oversee the procurement of health services.
- To immerse in disease inspection and analysis.
- To involve itself in promoting health and also to impart health education.
- To collaborate with governments and administrations all over the world to endorse health promotional programs.

- Activities of the World Health Organization.
- The most commendable achievements of the WHO are in the fight against and successful eradication of the world's most deadly communicable diseases.
- Coordination in efforts from all nations in the containment of such deadly diseases such as malaria, H_1N_1, tuberculosis, AIDS has been and continuously collaborated by the WHO.
- It also promotes and funds programs to prevent the occurrence of such diseases through vaccination and also to treat them through ground-breaking medicines.
- The WHO patronizes the distribution of secure drugs and medication throughout the world to fight against the outbreak of such communicable diseases.
- It also initiates a variant of health campaigns like propagating against the consumption of tobacco through smoking and other means.
- WHO experts are currently engaged in researching on a permanent vaccine against influenza, which is a very common chronic illness.
- WHO is also funding programs in member states so that they independently address the grievances associated within the nation and conduct extensive research on such subjects territorially.

RED CROSS SOCIETY

Indian Red Cross Society is constituted by the Government of India by Act XV of 1920 passed by the Indian Parliament. It is the instrument chosen by Indian Legislature to help carry-out the obligations assumed by India under international treaties known as Geneva Convention. The legislation imposes on Red Cross the duties to act for the voluntary relief to the Indian people and the Armed Forces, and to take suitable measures to ensure national and international relief to prevent and mitigate sufferings caused by disasters. All the activities of Indian Red Cross Society support these duties. Nationally and locally Indian Red Cross is governed by volunteers, most of its duties are performed by volunteers, and it is financed mostly by voluntary contributions.

Functions of National Red Cross Society

- Relief (National and International)
- Development of volunteer base
- Health, social welfare, nursing, first aid, maternity and child welfare.
- Help to disabled persons, weaker sections of society.
- Blood donation
- Junior and Youth Red Cross
- Information and dissemination.

Activities of Indian Red Cross Society (IRCS)

- The Indian Red Cross Society helped soldiers and war prisoners during crisis with neighboring countries.
- IRCS is always in the frontline to help people during natural calamities in situation such as cyclones, earthquakes, floods, famines.
- The general activities of Indian Red Cross are in the field of family welfare, antenatal and postnatal care, immunization, eradication of TB, polio and other like diseases.
- About four lakh units of blood are collected every year through Red Cross blood banks. Artificial limbs and other accessories such as wheelchairs and hearing aids are provided to needy and poor people.

ST JOHN'S AMBULANCE

St John Ambulance is a voluntary organization, that forms part of the 'Most Venerable Order of the Hospital of St John of Jerusalem', which was established by Queen Victoria in 1888. The St John Council, chaired by His Honour Chief Justice Professor JJ Cremona Emeritus, is the governing body of the organization. Under the Council there are three branches. These are The Training Association, First Aid and Nursing and The Rescue Corps.

The Training Association (also known as The Training Branch), was founded in 1882. This was the first branch of St John Ambulance which was formed outside of the United Kingdom. It aims is to teach First Aid to the general public and members of St John Ambulance. First Aid courses conducted by St John Ambulance are recognized and approved by the Occupational Health and Safety Authority.

Functions of St John's Ambulance

- It provide the care to the sick based on basic principles of health care in the sick room in the house and educate public by visiting houses and giving health advice
- It helps in training of nurses and volunteers in first aid and care of the sick
- It provides equipment required for care of the sick or giving first aid to the needy
- It provides ambulances to factories, industries, and mines
- It provides ambulances to factories, industries, and mines
- It also provides the ambulance at the time of accidents, floods, and when quick transport service is essential
- It provides health service to sick and wounded when there is peace in the world

- It provide highly accessible and effective ambulance services where contracted by Government.

UNITED NATIONS INTERNATIONAL CHILDREN'S EMERGENCY FUND (UNICEF)

The United Nations International Children's Emergency Fund (UNICEF) was created by the UN General Assembly during its first session in 1946 to help the emergency needs of children in post-war Europe. In 1950, its program was extended to provide long-range benefits to children of all developing countries. Later on, its name was changed to United Nations Children's Fund. However, its acronym UNICEF continued. UNICEF is governed by a 36-member Executive Board. The UNICEF has its headquarters in New York, and has more than 200 officers in developing countries.

Objective of the UNICEF

- The main objective of UNICEF is to look after children's welfare especially in developing countries by providing people with low cost community-based services in maternal and child-health, nutrition and immunization, etc.

Functions of the UNICEF

UNICEF provides services in primary health-care, nutrition, basic education, sanitation and women's development in developing countries. The main functions of UNICEF are broadly divided into the following categories:

- UNICEF works for the protection of children in respect of their survival, health, and well-being. This is done in cooperation with individuals, civic groups, governments and the private sector.
- It provides funds for training the personnel, including health and sanitation workers, teachers and nutritionists. Universal Child Immunizations against preventable diseases by 1990 was one of the leading goals of UNICEF.
- It provides technical supplies, equipment and other aids, ranging from paper for textbooks, to equipments and medicines to health clinics, to pipes and pumps for bringing clean water to villages.
- It assists governments to plan, develop and extend community-based services in the fields of maternal and child health's, nutrition, clean water and sanitation.
- It provides help to children and mothers in emergencies arising from natural calamities, civil strife's and epidemics.
- It makes effort to prevent diseases like TB, malaria, eye diseases, skin diseases, etc.

- UNICEF performs various other functions. As the sole agency for children, it speaks on behalf of children and upholds the Convention on the Rights of the Child and works for its implementation. UNICEF was awarded the Nobel Prize for peace in the year 1965 and the Indira Gandhi Prize for peace in 1989.

WORLD BANK

The World Bank was created at Bretton Woods in 1944 to lend to European countries to help them rebuild after World War II. It was the world's first multilateral development bank, and was funded through the sale of World Bonds. Its first loans were to France and other European countries, but soon lent money to Chile, Mexico and India to build power plants and railways. By 1975, the Bank also lent money to countries to help with family planning, pollution control and environmentalism.

The World Bank provides financial and technical assistance to emerging market countries. The World Bank is not actually a bank in the common sense. Instead, it consists of two development institutions—the International Bank for Reconstruction and Development (IBRD) and the International Development Association (IDA)-owned by 186 member countries.

The Bank is closely affiliated with three other organizations—the International Finance Corporation (IFC), the Multilateral Guarantee Agency (MIGA), and the International Centre for the Settlement of Investment Disputes (ICSID)—that support its goal of reducing worldwide poverty. The five organizations make-up the World Bank Group.

Objectives of the World Bank

The World Bank was established to promote long-term foreign investment loans on reasonable terms. The, purposes of the Bank, as set forth in the 'Articles of Agreement' are as follows:

- To assist in the reconstruction and development of territories of members by facilitating the investment of capital for productive purpose including:
  - The restoration of economies destroyed or disrupted by war
  - The reconversion of productive facilities to peaceful needs
  - The encouragement of the development of productive facilities and resources in less developing countries.
- To promote private investment by means of guarantee or participation in loans and other investments made by private investors.
- To supplement private investment by providing on suitable conditions finance for productive purpose out of its own capital funds raised by it and its other resources.

- To promote the long-range balanced growth of international trade and the maintenance of equilibrium in balances of payments by encouraging international investment for the development of the productive resources of members, thereby assisting in raising productivity, the standard of living, and conditions of labor in their territories.
- To arrange the loans made or guaranteed by it in relation to international loans through other channels so that the more useful and urgent projects, large and small alike, will be dealt with first.
- To conduct its operations with due regard to the effect of international investment on business conditions in the territories of members and in the immediate postwar years, to assist in bringing about a smooth transition from a wartime to peacetime economy.

Functions of the World Bank

World Bank performs the following functions:

- Granting reconstruction loans to war devastated countries
- Granting developmental loans to underdeveloped countries
- Providing loans to governments for agriculture, irrigation, power, transport, water supply, educations, health, etc.
- Providing loans to private concerns for specified projects
- Promoting foreign investment by guaranteeing loans provided by other organizations
- Providing technical, economic and monetary advice to member countries for specific projects
- Encouraging industrial development of underdeveloped countries by promoting economic reforms.

SUMMARY

In this unit we discuss about the characteristics of a profession, reviews the history of professional nursing organizations, and describes the advocacy activities of professional nursing organizations. Participation in professional organizations provides the benefit to nurses and to the profession. The profession provides a means through which united efforts can be made to elevate standards of nursing education and practice. It also offers a means of voicing nurse's opinions, developing their abilities and keeping informed of new trends.

4

Section

Administration and Ward Management

COURSE DESCRIPTION

Hrs. 45

Course Description

This course aims at giving the student an elementary understanding of basic principle of administration and its application to the management of ward and health unit.

General Objectives

Upon completion of the course the students will be able to:

- Describe the meaning and principle of administration
- Apply the principle of administration in practice of nursing in various health care settings
- Plan the nursing service in the ward and community health settings
- Describe the importance of good administration in the day-to-day nursing service in varied health care settings.

Course Content

Unit 16: Introduction to Management in Nursing

- Meaning and philosophy of administration and management and their significance.
- Elements and principles of administration.

Unit 17: Planning

Unit 18: Organization: Command, Coordination and Control, Delegation, Staffing and Budgeting

- Definition, aims principles and techniques
- Preparation of organizational chart of a hospital ward primary health center, sub center
- Policies of the hospital and of the various departments of the hospital.

Unit 19: Administration of a Hospital Unit and Ward

- Administration of ward/unit/health center, physical layout, safety measures, prevention of accident and infections, legal responsibilities of a nurse.

Personal Management

- Job description, job specification, job analysis, and job satisfaction.
- Staff development and staff welfare
- Leadership styles, democratic leadership.

Management of Equipment and Supplies

- Maintenance of supplies and equipment
- Handling over and taking over of inventory
- Indent and ordering of supplies and equipment
- Problem-solving: Process and approach, steps and methods of dealing with complaints of patients and other health team members
- Record and reports: Meaning, type of records and reports maintained in the ward, importance and use of records and reports. Records and reports maintained in Primary Health Center and Subcenter.

Introduction to Management in Nursing

16 unit

INTRODUCTION

In simple words, management means managing an activity. When we talk of managing an activity, we really mean to make the activity a success. In other words, we have in mind some goal and we decide about the ways of carrying out the activity so as to achieve the goal. Management is as old as human kind and existed since man has been organized into communities. Managers influence all phases of our modern organizations. Our society simply could not exist as we know it today or improve its present status without a steady stream of managers to guide its organizations. Peter Drucker makes this same point in stating that effective management is quickly becoming the main resource of developed countries and the most needed resource of developing ones. Essentially, the role of managers is to guide organizations toward goal accomplishment. All organizations exist for some purpose or objective, and mangers have the responsibility for combining and using organizational resources to ensure that the organizations achieve their purposes. Management moves organizations toward these purposes or goals by assigning activities that organization member perform. If these activities are designed effectively, the production of each individual worker represents a contribution to the attainment of organizational goals. Managers strive to encourage individual activity that will lead to reaching organizational goals and to discourage individual activity that hinders organizational goal accomplishment.

Meaning and Definition of Management

Different authorities define management differently but have strong unifying similarities in all the definitions. The term management can be used in several ways.

- According to *FW Taylor* (father of scientific management) 'Management is an art of knowing what is to be done and seeing that it is done in the best possible manner.' (Planning and controlling)
- According to *Henry Fayol* (father of modern management) 'Management is to forecast, to plan, to organize, to command, to coordinate and control activities of others'.
- According to *Joseph Massie* 'Management is the process by which cooperative group directs actions towards common goals'.
- According to *McFarland* 'Management is that process by which managers create, direct, maintain and operate purposive organization through systematic, coordinated and cooperative human efforts'.
- According to *Henry Sisk* 'Management is the coordination of all resources through the process of planning, organizing, directing and controlling in order to attain stated goals'.
- According to *Tho Harmann and William Scott* 'Management is a social and technical process that utilizes resources, influences human action and facilitates changes in order to accomplish an organization's goals'.
- According to *Rovert Kreitner* 'Management is a process of working with and through others to achieve organizational objectives in a changing environment, central to this purpose is the effective and efficient use of limited resources'.

Concepts of Management

Management involves characteristics of both art and science. While certain aspects of management make it a science, certain others which involve application of skills make it an art. Every discipline of art is always backed by science which is basic knowledge of that art. Similarly, every discipline of science is complete only when it is used in practice for solving various kinds of problems. Whereas under 'science' one normally learns the 'why' of a phenomenon, under 'art' one learns the 'how' of it. In the words of Robert H. Hilkert: 'In the area of management, science and art are the sides of the same coin'.

In the beginning of development of management knowledge, it was considered as an art. There was a jungle of management knowledge. Anyone used it to get things done in his own way. But later by codifying and systemizing the management, it became a science as well as being an art.

Management as an Art

Management as an art has the following characteristics:

- Just like other arts it has practical application. The knowledge of management should be learned and practiced by managers, just as medical or legal practitioners practice their respective sciences. In this sense, management is an art.

- The manager gains experience by continuous application of management knowledge. This experience helps them to develop more skills and abilities for translating management knowledge into practice.
- Application of management knowledge calls for innovativeness and creativity.
- The fourth reason to consider management as an art is that in many situations, theoretical knowledge of management may not be adequate or relevant for solving the problem. It maybe because of complexity or unique nature of the problem.

Management as a Science

Management as a science has the following characteristics:

- Its principles, generalizations and concepts are systematically. In this case the manager can manage the situation or organization in a systematic and scientific manner.
- Its principles, generalizations and concepts are formulated on the basis of observation, research, analysis and experimentation, as is the case with the principles of other sciences.
- Like other sciences, management principles are also based on relationship of cause and effect. It states that same cause under similar circumstance will produce same effect. Suppose if workers are paid more (cause), the produce more (effect).
- Management principles are codified and systematic, and can be transferred from one to another and can be taught.
- Management principles are universally applicable to all types of organizations.

Management: A Profession?

The following criteria identify the statues of a profession to management:

- Profession is a body of specialized knowledge.
- Professional knowledge in systemized and codified form can be learned through formal education system.
- A profession emphasizes on having a central body to formulate a code of behavior for its members.
- A profession calls for rendering competent and specialized services to clients.
- A profession maintains the scientific attitude and commitment for discovering new ideas and upgrading in order to improve quality of service and level of efficiency provided to clients.
- A profession requires members to exercise restraint and self-discipline.

Management knowledge meets the first two criteria because it has grown into a systematic body of knowledge and also it can be acquired and learned through the formal education.

There is no minimum qualification prescribed either for getting entry in the management profession or for becoming members of it. In practice, whosoever manages in known as manager, irrespective of qualifications? Peter Drucker in support of this view says that 'no greater damage could be done to our economy or to our society than to attempt to professionalize management by licensing managers, for instance, or by limiting access to management to people with a special academic degree'.

Regarding professional approach, a manager has to continuously strive for discovering new ideas, relationships and concepts and act in a dynamic and innovative manner to cope with the changing environment. Even so, managers are not respected as other professionals like doctors, advocates and chartered accountants.

Professional vs Family Management

Professionalization of Management

The following reasons are in support of the professionalization of management:

- In joint stock company, ownership has been separated from its management and control. This situation has really contributed to the development of management as a profession.
- Rapid expansion and growth of management universities and institutions is an indicative of management professionalization trend.
- In a high-tech industrial society, manifold changes have occurred in the role of managers.
- In the context of globalization of economic operations, many strategic areas have been developed which require professional expertise and specialized knowledge (e.g. strategic planning, etc.)
- Increased utilization of specialized management services (e.g. consultancy, human resource development, etc.) requires a team of professional managers.

Family Management

- Family management implies management and control of business operations by a group of members belonging to a particular family, regardless of their knowledge about management. Thus, the decisions and policies are largely influenced by family interest. Disputes and disagreements relating to family matters also tend to have a direct bearing on the functioning of the business organization. But in a professionally-managed enterprise, ownership is separated from management and control. Authority to manage and control business operations is delegated to professionally-qualified managers.

- A study covering 30 nations around the world points out that 75% of all firms in the world are family firms. In some of which, family inheritance has been continuing for centuries. The phenomenal progress of Ford Motors, IBM, etc. bears testimony to their quality of leadership and management. In the words of KK Birla, 'if people like Sir Jamshedji Tata or Rai Bahadur Gujarmal Modi were to start their business career again, I would any day put my rupee on them than on the best of the professionals'.

Management and Administration

There has been a controversy regarding the interpretation of these two terms. There are different views in this regard:

- According to first view (William Newman, Peter Drucker, etc.), there is no basic difference between the two terms, and they are interchangeable. If there is any difference, it may perhaps be in their usage in practice. The term administration is used for non-business activities, and management is used for business activities.
- According to second view (Kimball, Brech, other British writers, etc.), management is a more comprehensive term which includes administration. Management involves 'thinking' and administration involves 'doing'. Management is responsible for planning and organizing, and administration is responsible for directing and controlling. Whereas management refers to a high level of managerial activities such as goal-setting, policy formulation and strategy making, administration refers to an operative part concerned with lower level management activities such as execution of policies.
- According to third view (Sheldon, Speriegal, Milward, etc.), administration is a more comprehensive term which includes management. Administration involves "thinking" and management involves 'doing'. Administration is a top level function which concentrates on determination of plans, policies and objectives, whereas management is a lower level function which deals with the execution and direction of policies and operations. It does not mean that we need two separate sets of personnel, but each manager performs both the managerial as well as administrative functions. At top level more time is spent in administrative activity and as one move down, more time is spent in management activity.

PHILOSOPHY OF ADMINISTRATION

Nursing is an integral part of the organizational operation. We believe that the profession of nursing is both an art and science responding to the human condition.

- Clients have the right to the best possible health care regardless of their race, creed, color, sex, social status, capability to pay, and political belief.
- The clients are unique individuals with physiological, psychological, social and spiritual needs.
- Medical interventions require the coordinated efforts of all the various components of the health care delivery system since health and illness are multi-causal.
- A health care system should be dynamic to improve the delivery of health services.
- An integrated health service (including the Nursing Service) should be adequately operationalized to be responsive to the health needs of the clientele.
- Nursing personnel should be adequately prepared to assume their various roles in the promotion, maintenance and restoration of health.

ELEMENTS/FUNCTIONS OF ADMINISTRATION

Management has been described as a social process involving responsibility for economical and effective planning and regulation of operation of an enterprise in the fulfilment of given purposes. It is a dynamic process consisting of various elements and activities. These activities are different from operative functions like marketing, finance, purchase, etc. Rather these activities are common to each and every manger irrespective of his level or status.

Different experts have classified functions of management. According to George and Jerry, 'There are four fundamental functions of management, i.e. planning, organizing, actuating and controlling'. According to Henry Fayol, 'To manage is to forecast and plan, to organize, to command, and to control'. Whereas Luther Gullick has given a keyword 'POSDCORB' where P stands for Planning, O for Organizing, S for Staffing, D for Directing, Co for Coordination, R for Reporting and B for Budgeting. But the most widely accepted are functions of management given by KOONTZ and O'DONNEL, i.e. *Planning, organizing, staffing, directing and controlling.*

For theoretical purposes, it maybe convenient to separate the function of management but practically these functions are overlapping in nature, i.e. they are highly inseparable. Each function blends into the other and each affects the performance of others.

- *Planning:* It is the basic function of management. It deals with chalking out a future course of action and deciding in advance the most appropriate course of actions for achievement of pre-determined goals. According to KOONTZ, 'Planning is deciding in advance—

what to do, when to do and how to do. It bridges the gap from where we are and where we want to be'. A plan is a future course of actions. It is an exercise in problem-solving and decision-making. Planning is determination of courses of action to achieve desired goals. Thus, planning is a systematic thinking about ways and means for accomplishment of pre-determined goals. Planning is necessary to ensure proper utilization of human and non-human resources. It is all pervasive, it is an intellectual activity and it also helps in avoiding confusion, uncertainties, risks, wastages, etc.

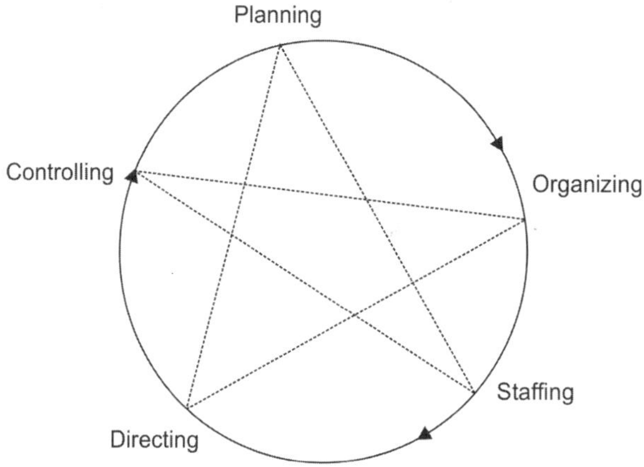

- *Organizing:* It is the process of bringing together physical, financial and human resources and developing productive relationship amongst them for achievement of organizational goals. According to Henry Fayol, 'To organize a business is to provide it with everything useful or its functioning, i.e. raw material, tools, capital and personnel's'. To organize a business involves determining and providing human and non-human resources to the organizational structure. Organizing as a process involves:
  - Identification of activities.
  - Classification of grouping of activities.
  - Assignment of duties.
  - Delegation of authority and creation of responsibility.
  - Coordinating authority and responsibility relationships.
- *Staffing:* It is the function of manning the organization structure and keeping it manned. Staffing has assumed greater importance in the recent years due to advancement of technology, increase in size of business, complexity of human behavior, etc. The main purpose o staffing is to put right man on right job, i.e. square pegs in square holes and round pegs in round holes. According to Kootz and O'Donell,

'Managerial function of staffing involves manning the organization structure through proper and effective selection, appraisal and development of personnel to fill the roles designed un the structure'. Staffing involves:

- Manpower planning (estimating man power in terms of searching, choose the person and giving the right place)
- Recruitment, selection and placement
- Training and development
- Remuneration
- Performance appraisal
- Promotions and transfer.

- *Directing:* It is that part of managerial function which actuates the organizational methods to work efficiently for achievement of organizational purposes. It is considered life-spark of the enterprise which sets it in motion the action of people because planning, organizing and staffing are the mere preparations for doing the work. Direction is that inert-personnel aspect of management which deals directly with influencing, guiding, supervising, motivating subordinate for the achievement of organizational goals. Direction has following elements:
  - *Supervision* implies overseeing the work of subordinates by their superiors. It is the act of watching and directing work and workers.
  - *Motivation* means inspiring, stimulating or encouraging the subordinates with zeal to work. Positive, negative, monetary, nonmonetary incentives maybe used for this purpose.
  - *Leadership* maybe defined as a process by which manager guides and influences the work of subordinates in desired direction.
  - *Communication* is the process of passing information, experience, opinion, etc. from one person to another. It is a bridge of understanding.
- *Controlling:* It implies measurement of accomplishment against the standards and correction of deviation if any to ensure achievement of organizational goals. The purpose of controlling is to ensure that everything occurs in conformities with the standards. An efficient system of control helps to predict deviations before they actually occur. According to Theo Haimann, 'Controlling is the process of checking whether or not proper progress is being made towards the objectives and goals and acting if necessary, to correct any deviation'. According to Koontz and O'Donell 'Controlling is the measurement and correction of performance activities of subordinates in order to make sure that the enterprise objectives and plans desired to obtain them as being accomplished'. Therefore controlling has following steps:
  - Establishment of standard performance.

- Measurement of actual performance.
- Comparison of actual performance with the standards and finding out deviation if any.
- Corrective action.

PRINCIPLES OF ADMINISTRATION

A principle refers to a fundamental truth. It establishes cause and effect relationship between two or more variables under given situation. They serve as a guide to thought and actions. Therefore, management principles are the statements of fundamental truth based on logic which provides guidelines for managerial decision-making and actions. These principles are derived:

- On the basis of observation and analysis, i.e. practical experience of managers
- By conducting experimental studies.

There are 14 Principles of Management Described by Henri Fayol

(a) *Division of labor*
  - Henry Fayol has stressed on the specialization of jobs.
  - He recommended that work of all kinds must be divided and subdivided and allotted to various persons according to their expertise in a particular area.
  - Subdivision of work makes it simpler and results in efficiency.
  - It also helps the individual in acquiring speed, accuracy in his performance.
  - Specialization leads to efficiency and economy in spheres of business.

(b) *Party of authority and responsibility*
  - Authority and responsibility are co-existing.
  - If authority is given to a person, he should also be made responsible.
  - In a same way, if anyone is made responsible for any job, he should also have concerned authority.
  - Authority refers to the right of superiors to get exactness from their subordinates whereas responsibility means obligation for the performance of the job assigned.
  - There should be a balance between the two, i.e. they must go hand in hand.
  - Authority without responsibility leads to irresponsible behavior whereas responsibility without authority makes the person ineffective.

(c) *Principle of one Boss*
- A subordinate should receive orders and be accountable to one and only one boss at a time.
- In other words, a subordinate should not receive instructions from more than one person because:
  - It undermines authority
  - Weakens discipline
  - Divides loyalty
  - Creates confusion
  - Delays and chaos
  - Escaping responsibilities
  - Duplication of work
  - Overlapping of efforts
- Therefore, dual subordination should be avoided unless and until it is absolutely essential.
- Unity of command provides the enterprise a disciplined, stable and orderly existence.
- It creates harmonious relationship between superiors and subordinates.

(d) *Unity of Direction*
- Fayol advocates one head one plan which means that there should be one plan for a group of activities having similar objectives.
- Related activities should be grouped together. There should be one plan of action for them and they should be under the charge of a particular manager.
- According to this principle, efforts of all the members of the organization should be directed towards common goal.
- Without unity of direction, unity of action cannot be achieved.
- In fact, unity of command is not possible without unity of direction.

Basis	Unity of command	Unity of direction
Meaning	It implies that a subordinate should receive orders and instructions from only one boss.	It means one head, one plan for a group of activities having similar objectives.
Nature	It is related to the functioning of personnel's.	It is related to the functioning of departments, or organization as a whole.
Necessity	It is necessary for fixing responsibility of each subordinate.	It is necessary for sound organization.
Advantage	It avoids conflicts, confusion and chaos.	It avoids duplication of efforts and wastage of resources.
Result	It leads to better superior subordinate relationship.	It leads to smooth running of the enterprise.

Therefore it is obvious that they are different from each other but they are dependent on each other, i.e. unity of direction is a prerequisite for unity of command. But it does not automatically come from the unity of direction.

(e) *Equity*

- Equity means combination of fairness, kindness and justice.
- The employees should be treated with kindness and equity if devotion is expected of them.
- It implies that managers should be fair and impartial while dealing with the subordinates.
- They should give similar treatment to people of similar position.
- They should not discriminate with respect to age, caste, sex, religion, relation, etc.
- Equity is essential to create and maintain cordial relations between the managers and sub-ordinate.
- But equity does not mean total absence of harshness.
- Fayol was of opinion that, 'at times force and harshness might become necessary for the sake of equity'.

(f) *Order*

- This principle is concerned with proper and systematic arrangement of things and people.
- Arrangement of things is called material order and placement of people is called social order.
- *Material order:* There should be safe, appropriate and specific place for every article and every place to be effectively used for specific activity and commodity.
- *Social order:* Selection and appointment of most suitable person on the suitable job. There should be a specific place for everyone and everyone should have a specific place so that they can easily be contacted whenever need arises.

(g) *Discipline*

- According to Fayol, 'Discipline means sincerity, obedience, respect of authority and observance of rules and regulations of the enterprise'.
- This principle applies that subordinate should respect their superiors and obey their order.
- It is an important requisite for smooth running of the enterprise.
- Discipline is not only required on path of subordinates but also on the part of management.
- Discipline can be enforced if:
  - There are good superiors at all levels.
  - There are clear and fair agreements with workers.
  - Sanctions (punishments) are judiciously applied.

(h) *Initiative*

- Workers should be encouraged to take initiative in the work assigned to them.
- It means eagerness to initiate actions without being asked to do so.
- Fayol advised that management should provide opportunity to its employees to suggest ideas, experiences and new method of work.
- It helps in developing an atmosphere of trust and understanding.
- People then enjoy working in the organization because it adds to their zeal and energy.
- To suggest improvement in formulation and implementation of place.
- They can be encouraged with the help of monetary and non-monetary incentives.

(i) *Fair remuneration*

- The quantum and method of remuneration to be paid to the workers should be fair, reasonable, satisfactory and rewarding of the efforts.
- As far as possible it should accord satisfaction to both employer and the employees.
- Wages should be determined on the basis of cost of living, work assigned, financial position of the business, wage rate prevailing, etc.
- Logical and appropriate wage rates and methods of their payment reduce tension and differences between workers and management creates harmonious relationship and pleasing atmosphere of work.
- Fayol also recommended provision of other benefits such as free education, medical and residential facilities to workers.

(j) *Stability of tenure*

- Fayol emphasized that employees should not be moved frequently from one job position to another, i.e. the period of service in a job should be fixed.
- Therefore employees should be appointed after keeping in view principles of recruitment and selection but once they are appointed their services should be served.
- According to Fayol. "Time is required for an employee to get used to a new work and succeed to doing it well but if he is removed before that he will not be able to render worthwhile services".
- As a result, the time, effort and money spent on training the worker will go waste.

- Stability of job creates team spirit and a sense of belongingness among workers which ultimately increase the quality as well as quantity of work.

(k) *Scalar chain*

- Fayol defines scalar chain as 'The chain of superiors ranging from the ultimate authority to the lowest'.
- Every orders, instructions, messages, requests, explanation, etc. has to pass through Scalar chain.

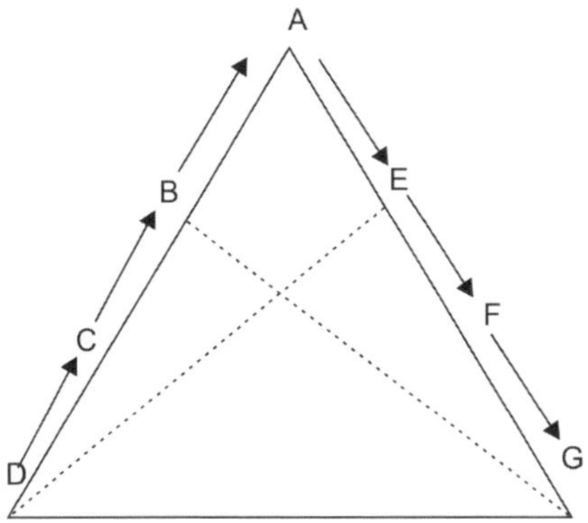

Fig. 16.1: Gang plank

- But, for the sake of convenience and urgency, this path can be cut shirt and this short cut is known as Gang Plank.
- A Gang Plank is a temporary arrangement between two different points to facilitate quick and easy communication as explained below:
  - In the figure given, if D has to communicate with G he will first send the communication upwards with the help of C, B to A and then downwards with the help of E and F to G which will take quite sometime and by that time, it may not be worth therefore a gang plank has been developed between the two.
- Gang Plank clarifies that management principles are not rigid rather they are very flexible. They can be moulded and modified as per the requirements of situations.
- Every orders, instructions, messages, requests, explanation, etc. has to pass through Scalar chain.

(l) *Subordination of individual interest to general interest*

- An organization is much bigger than the individual it constitutes therefore interest of the undertaking should prevail in all circumstances.

- As far as possible, reconciliation should be achieved between individual and group interests.
- But in case of conflict, individual must sacrifice for bigger interests.
- In order to achieve this attitude, it is essential that:
  - Employees should be honest and sincere.
  - Proper and regular supervision of work.
  - Reconciliation of mutual differences and clashes by mutual agreement. For example, for change of location of plant, for change of profit sharing ratio, etc.

(m) *Espirit De' Corps (can be achieved through unity of command)*
- It refers to team spirit, i.e. harmony in the work groups and mutual understanding among the members.
- Spirit De' Corps inspires workers to work harder.
- Fayol cautioned the managers against dividing the employees into competing groups because it might damage the moral of the workers and interest of the undertaking in the long run.
- To inculcate Espirit De' Corps following steps should be undertaken:
  - There should be proper coordination of work at all levels.
  - Subordinates should be encouraged to develop informal relations among themselves.
  - Efforts should be made to create enthusiasm and keenness among subordinates so that they can work to the maximum ability.
  - Efficient employees should be rewarded and those who are not up to the mark should be given a chance to improve their performance.
  - Subordinates should be made conscious of that whatever they are doing is of great importance to the business and society.
- He also cautioned against the more use of Britain communication to the subordinates, i.e. face to face communication should be developed. The managers should infuse team spirit and belongingness. There should be no place for misunderstanding. People then enjoy working in the organization and offer their best towards the organization.

(n) *Centralization and Decentralization:*
- Centralization means concentration of authority at the top level. In other words, centralization is a situation in which top management retains most of the decision-making authority.
- Decentralization means disposal of decision-making authority to all the levels of the organization. In other words, sharing authority downwards is decentralization.
- According to Fayol, 'Degree of centralization or decentralization depends on number of factors like size of business, experience of superiors, dependability and ability of subordinates, etc.'

- Anything which increases the role of subordinate is decentralization and anything which decreases it is centralization.
- Fayol suggested that absolute centralization or decentralization is not feasible. An organization should strike to achieve a lot between the two.

SUMMARY

In this unit, we have learnt about when we talk of managing an activity, we really mean to make the activity a success. In other words, we have in mind some goal and we decide about the ways of carrying out the activity so as to achieve the goal. Management is as old as human kind and existed since man has been organized in to communities. Theory and practice are related. To develop nursing as a profession the concept of theory must be addressed. If nursing theory does not drive the development of nursing, it will continue to develop in the footsteps of other disciplines such as medicine. The main purpose of management principles is to make available useful elements of a systematic theory of management, so as to improve the management practice. They provide a means of organizing knowledge and experience in management. Managers influence all phases of our modern organizations.

17 unit

Planning

INTRODUCTION

Planning is the most crucial and foremost function of management. It is an indispensable element which determines the overall functioning of the management system. A sound planning is imperative for the successful achievement of the goals in the desired direction. Planning spells out the answer to the questions like 'why', 'what', 'how', 'when', and 'where' of the different activities to be performed in the specific sequence. It involves setting of objectives and goals, designing appropriate strategy and course of action and framing plan and procedures, etc. for execution of the proposed activities under the project/programs.

DEFINITIONS OF PLANNING

Different authors have given different definitions of planning from time to time. The main definitions of planning are as follows:

- According to *Alford and Beatt*, 'Planning is the thinking process, the organized foresight, the vision based on fact and experience that is required for intelligent action'.
- According to *Theo Haimann*, 'Planning is deciding in advance what is to be done. When a manager plans, he projects a course of action for further attempting to achieve a consistent coordinate structure of operations aimed at the desired results'.
- According to *Billy E. Goetz*, 'Planning is fundamentally choosing and a planning problem arises when an alternative course of action is discovered.'
- According to *Koontz and O' Donnell*, 'Planning is an intellectual process, conscious determination of course of action, the basing of decision on purpose, facts and considered estimates'.
- According to *Allen*, 'A plan is a trap laid to capture the future'.

AIMS/OBJECTIVES OF PLANNING

Objectives/aims are the broad statements of overall intent of an organization or individual. They are usually stated in general terms. The purpose of writing objectives is to identify where you are going and to enable you to evaluate when you have arrived there. A meaningful stated goal is one that succeeds in communicating the intent of those generating the goal. It should be stated in such a way that it will be understood clearly by others. As a nurse in a health care institution, you need to be aware of the existence of several levels of goals: the institutional level, the nursing department level and the nursing unit level. The goal levels all need to relate to the health needs of the community, because these are the focus of health care.

Institutional Goals

- Based on the community's health needs, the institution forms goals and objectives. An institution that focuses thinking on goals for the future and activities that will move the organization toward these goals is referred to as a proactive institution. The managers of such institutions spend a great deal of time, money and energy on identifying possible future events and on preparing the institution to deal with them. Institutions that do not have specific or future oriented goals are reactive institutions. They spend their time reacting to events, that is, 'putting out fires' rather than 'preventing them'. A reactive facility would wait until such emergencies occurred and then would handle them as a crisis rather than as an anticipated event.

Nursing Department Goals

- The goals of the institution definitely affect those of nursing service, which must support and complement institutional goals. The astute manager of a nursing department must also be proactive about the national issues facing nursing, community needs for nursing, and the needs within the institution itself. This manager would formulate goals to help the nursing department meet the challenges of care in the future, because the ultimate nursing department goal is quality client care.

Nursing Unit Goals

- It is important that each employee understand the institutional and nursing department goals, because the group or unit goals develop from them. Each nurse should be able to contribute to the formation of unit goals in terms of philosophy of care, quality of care, and development of nursing expertise.

NATURE/CHARACTERISTICS OF PLANNING

The main characteristics or nature of planning is given below:

- *Planning is an intellectual process:* Planning is an intellectual process of thinking in advance. It is a process of deciding the future on the series of events to follow. Planning is a process where a number of steps are to be taken to decide the future course of action. Managers or executives have to consider various courses of action, achieve the desired goals, go in details of the pros and cons of every course of action and then finally decide what course of action may suit them best.
- *Planning contributes to the objectives:* Planning contributes positively in attaining the objectives of the business enterprise. Since plans are there from the very first stage of operation, the management is able to handle every problem successfully. Plan try to set everything right. A purposeful, sound and effective planning process knows how and when to tackle a problem. This leads to success. Objectives thus are easily achieved.
- *Planning is a primary function of management:* Planning precedes other functions in the management process. Certainly, setting of goals to be achieved and lines of action to be followed precedes the organization, direction, supervision and control. No doubt, planning precedes other functions of management. It is primary requisite before other managerial functions step in. But all functions are interconnected. It is mixed in all managerial functions but there too it gets precedence. It thus gets primary everywhere.
- *A continuous process:* Planning is a continuous process and a never ending activity of a manager in an enterprise based upon some assumptions which may or may not come true in the future. Therefore, the manager has to go on modifying revising and adjusting plans in the light of changing circumstances. According to *George R Terry,* 'Planning is a continuous process and there is no end to it. It involves continuous collection, evaluation and selection of data, and scientific investigation and analysis of the possible alternative courses of action and the selection of the best alternative'.
- *Planning pervades managerial activities:* From primary of planning follows pervasiveness of planning. It is the function of every managerial personnel. The character, nature and scope of planning may change fro personnel to personnel but the planning as an action remains intact. According to *Billy E Goetz,* 'Plans cannot make an enterprise successful. Action is required, the enterprise must operate managerial planning seeks to achieve a consistent, coordinated structure of operations focused on desired trends. Without plans, action must become merely activity producing nothing but chaos'.

PRINCIPLE OF PLANNING

The basic principles of the planning are briefly discussed below:

- *Objectives:* Objectives are to be framed in accordance with the overall goals and expected outcomes. The objectives should be stated clearly and precisely, which should be measurable and attainable in a given period of time. They should be SMART (Specific, Measurable, Action-oriented, Realistic and Time oriented.
- *Premising:* A consistent assumption based on forecasts of the future environmental conditions is vital, for realistic and effective planning.
- *Commitment:* It is related to the time period of planning for accomplishments of the objectives.
- *Coordinated approach:* It is pertinent that all the plans of the organization are integrated with each other and the strategic procedures, budget, etc. are properly tuned to implement the plans effectively.
- *Flexibility:* There should be adequate flexibility in the plan to deal with the unexpected circumstances due to situational factors. This implies the principal of flexibility with performance.
- *Efficiency:* The plan estimates should be developed in such a manner that the cost of planning in respect of all the resources viz. physical, financial, and human are minimized and they are utilized to their fully capacity.

TYPES OF PLANNING

- *Strategic planning:* Strategic planning involves analyzing competitive opportunities and threats, as well as the strengths and weaknesses of the organization, and then determining how to position the organization to compete effectively in their environment. Strategic planning has a long time frame, often three years or more. Strategic planning generally includes the entire organization and includes formulation of objectives. Strategic planning is often based on the organization's mission, which is its fundamental reason for existence. An organization's top management most often conducts strategic planning.
- *Tactical planning:* Tactical planning is intermediate-range planning that is designed to develop relatively concrete and specific means to implement the strategic plan. Middle-level managers often engage in tactical planning. Tactical planning often has a one- to three-year time horizon.
- *Operational planning:* Operational planning generally assumes the existence of objectives and specifies ways to achieve them. Operational planning is short-range planning that is designed to develop specific

action steps that support the strategic and tactical plans. Operational planning usually has a very short time horizon, from one week to one year.

STEPS/METHODS OF PLANNING PROCESS

Planning is a lengthy process which moves gradually and step by step approach is usually adopted. These steps are like stations in the journey of planning process. Usual steps in the planning process are as briefly explained below:

- *Classifying the problems:* The planning process starts with clear understanding and classifying business problems faced by a business unit. Identification of problems or opportunities by managers justifies the need for action. It is like the diagnosis of the health problem of a patient by his doctor. Planners have to understand the problems of the organization first and, then, prepare a plan to deal with the problems in the light of the prevailing business environment.
- *Determining the objectives:* In this second stage in the planning process, the planners decide the overall objectives to be achieved. Planning is always for achieving certain well defined objectives and naturally objectives must be spelt out precisely. Objectives act as pillars of the entire planning process. Business objectives maybe decided in terms of profit, sales, production or market reputation. Objectives maybe defined in quantitative or qualitative terms.
- *Collecting complete information and data:* The planners have to collect information relating to problems facing the business unit. Such information is necessary and useful for analyzing the problems in-depth and also for accuracy in planning. Information can be collected from internal and external sources. Reliable, updated and adequate data make planning process result-oriented.
- *Analyzing and classifying the information:* At this stage, the information collected is analyzed and interpreted systematically for drawing specific conclusions. This facilitates purposeful use of information, while preparing alternative plans. Irrelevant information can be discarded through such analysis.
- *Establishing planning premises:* Planning premises are various assumptions and predictions about the future business situation. Such premises act as background for planning activities. The planning premises are expected to supply relevant facts, information and data on the basis of which forecasts are prepared and future trends are indicated. Planning premises reduce uncertainties in the planning process. Planning premises are three in number viz., (a) Controllable permises, (b) Semi-controllable permises, and (c) Uncontrollable premises.

- *Determining alternative plans:* Here, the planners prepare and keep ready alternative plans suitable for use under different situations. The best among the available alternative plans is used for actual execution. The preparation of alternative plans is essential as one plan is normally not adequate under all types of situations. It is a type of standby arrangement useful for meeting any emergency situation.
- *Selecting operating plan and preparing derivative plans:* After study of the business environment and the alternative plans available, the planners select the best plan for actual execution. This decision is a delicate one and must be made with proper care. After the selection of operating plan, the planners have to prepare derivative plans. Such plans are related to different departments/activities and constitute sub-sections of the operating plan. The division of overall plan into derivative plans is necessary for effective execution.
- *Arranging timing and sequence of operations*: Timing involves fixation of starting and finishing time for each job or piece of work. Sequence of operations ensures proper flow of work. This step in planning process is important as it brings coordination in the activities of different departments. The timings and sequence of operations must be communicated to concerned departments, managers and staff for implementation of the plan.
- *Securing participation of employees:* Planning needs willing participation of all employees and departments. For this, information regarding the operative plan should be given to employees well in advance. Here, the internal communication system should be used extensively. For such participation, employees should be associated with the planning process.
- *Follow-up of the proposed plan:* The purpose of follow-up is to make periodical review of the execution process. It is useful for understanding actual progress and deficiencies in the process of execution of the plan. This also facilitates adoption of suitable remedial measures as and when required.

SUMMARY

In this unit we learnt about, planning is an exercise in forecasting and decision-making. It involves forecast of future conditions and an estimate of how the proposed plans would be affected by them. Thus planning involves two aspects. First it involves mental formulations of an idea of what is desired to be achieved. Up to this, it remains at the thinking level and is based on forecasts and estimates. Secondly it determines the mode of action to be pursued to achieve what has been thought up. At this stage, the idea takes a definite shape with a due regard to the ordinary and immediate circumstances facing the enterprise.

Organization: Command, Coordination and Control, Delegation, Staffing and Budgeting

18 unit

INTRODUCTION

An organization is a group of people working together, under formal and informal rules of behavior, to achieve a common purpose. Organization also refers to the procedures, policies, and methods involved in achieving this common purpose. Thus, organization is both a structure and a process. Organizational structure refers to the lines of authority, communication, and delegation; can be formal or informal. Organizational process refers to the methods used to achieve organizational goals. An organization's formal structure is depicted in its organizational chart that provides a "blueprint," depicting formal relations, functions and activities.

Meaning of Organization

The word organizing is derived from the word 'organism', which means that all subunits of a main unit have a definite relationship with the main unit. Organizing is the harmonious adjustment of special parts for accomplishing common purposes.

Organizing is a mechanism of management. The importance of organizing is as follows:

The word organizing is derived from the word 'organism', which means that all subunits of a main unit have a definite relationship with the main unit. Organizing is the harmonious adjustment of special parts for accomplishing common purposes.

Definition of Organization

- Organization is the process of identifying and grouping work to be performed defining and delegating responsibility and authority and establishing relationship for the purpose of enabling people to work most effectively together in accomplishing objectives.

- Organization thus is an arrangement for internal administration of the enterprise. It describes the part which each employee is intended to play in the operation of an enterprise and ensures that concerned endeavor of all of them will be conductive to the full implementation of the plans of the enterprise.

Principles of Organization

- *Principle of objective:* The organizational goal should be formulated for the institution as whole and organization should be framed to achieve that goal. Departmental goals should be developed so that ultimate common goal should be attained. If the common organizational goal is not decided, departments may set their own goals and there maybe occurrence of conflict about the common objective.
- *Division of work:* the organization should be framed in a manner such that every individual should get work according to his ability, skills and knowledge. The employees should do that work continuously to achieve specialization that particular work. This will increase his efficiency.
- *Authority and responsibility:* The amount of authority decreases as we go downward in the organizational level. For every given work or responsibility there must be provision of authority to get that work done. The manager can delegate his authority to his subordinates to complete the task but responsibility to complete that work cannot be delegated, only manager would be answerable for the given work not his subordinates.
- *Unity of command:* There should be unity of command in the organization. An employee should be controlled by one boss. He/she should get orders from one superior and should report to the same superior. If a person is under the control of more than one person then there would be confusions and conflicts. Unity of command would lead to better coordination and controlling.
- *Span of control:* There should be proper span of control. Span of control is the number of subordinate reporting directly to a manger. The number of subordinates should be in such manner so that supervision can be done effectively. If span is not planned appropriately efficiency of workers will be affected.
- *Scalar chain:* There should be proper chain of supervisor from top level to lower level in vertical direction. This also shows the direction of communication in the organization. This suggests that communication should pass through each position placed in the chain.

Importance of Organization

- *Benefit of specialization:* All activities are subdivided into various works or various jobs. The work is divided among groups of workers by division of labor. This helps in the completion of maximum work in minimum time. Thus, it gives benefit of specialization.

- *Transparency:* Organizing clarifies the working relations among employees. It specifies who is to report to whom. Due to this communication becomes specific and effective. It also helps in fixing accountability.
- *Optimum utilization of resources:* There is a different employee performing every job. By doing this, it can be ensured that no task is left undone or overdone. Therefore, there is optimum utilization of resources in the organization.
- *Adaptability:* Organizing makes a company capable of adapting any change which is connected with the post of employees. Whenever, a manager's post falls vacant, it is filled up by promotion, since every subordinate is aware of the working of his boss. Therefore, the subordinate has no difficulty in taking-up the vacant post of his immediate senior.
- *Effective administration:* The process of organizing clearly specifies the duties and tasks of every manager and also their extent of authority. Everybody knows to whom he is accountable, thereby making effective administration possible.
- *Development of personnel:* Delegation of authority is practiced under organizing. It provides opportunities to take decisions and delegate assignments to subordinate officers and employees. Consequently, it helps them to develop better personnel by helping them grow with experience at work.

COMMAND

Unity of command provides that an employee is responsible to only one supervisor, who in turn is responsible to only one supervisor, and so on up the organizational hierarchy. This is true even if the top of the organization is led by a group of people.

Advantages of Unity of Command

- *Better relationship:* Unity of command helps to develop a clear and better relationship among superior and subordinates.
- *Authority, responsibility and accountability:* Unity of command results in a clear and well-organized authority, responsibility and accountability between various levels of workforce of the organization.
- *Reduces duplication of work:* It helps to reduce and/or avoid duplication of work between the various levels of workforce of the organization.
- *Prompt or quick decisions:* The unity of command helps managers to take prompt or quick decisions properly.

- *Effective and efficient discipline:* The unity of command ensures an effective and efficient discipline within an organization.
- *Better coordination and team work:* The unity of command ensures better coordination, and team work in the organization.
- *Boosts morale and positive attitude:* It boosts morale and generates positive attitude among workers in the organization.
- *Higher productivity:* The unity of command leads to higher productivity of goods and services. This creates a better image or goodwill of the organization in the market.

COORDINATION

Coordinating is by definition the act of assembling and synchronizing people and activities so that they function harmoniously in the attainment of organizational objectives. Think about the situations in your own life when you have had to coordinate the multiple activities for an important event. An example in everyday life that demands coordination is a wedding. The music, flowers, ceremony and numerous other considerations must be coordinated so that each can contribute to make the wedding beautiful and joyful. The more assurance that all parties are cooperating and fulfilling their agreements, the more likely that they wedding will be a success with minimal complications.

Definition of Coordination

- In the words of Haimann, 'Coordination is the orderly synchronization of efforts of the subordinates to provide the proper amount, timing and quality of execution so that their unified efforts lead to the stated objective, namely the common purpose of the enterprise'.
- It maybe defined as balancing and keeping the teams together by ensuring a suitable allocation of working activities to the various members and seeing that they are performed with due harmony among the members themselves.

Types of Coordination

The coordination maybe divided on different bases, namely:

- *Scope:* It is on the basis of scope or coverage, coordination can be.
  - *Internal:* It refers to coordination between the different units of an organization within and is achieved by integrating the goals and activities of different departments of the enterprise.
  - *External:* It refers to coordination between an organization and its external environment comprising government, community, customers, investors, suppliers, competitors, research institutions,

etc. It requires proper match between policies and activities of the enterprise and the outside world.

- *Flow:* It is on the basis of flow, coordination can classified into:
  - *Vertical:* It implies coordination between different levels of the organization and has to ensure that all the levels in the organization act in harmony and in accordance with the goals and policies of the organization. Vertical coordination is assured by top management through delegation of authority.
  - *Horizontal or Lateral:* It refers to coordination between different departments and other units at the same level of the management hierarchy. For instance, coordination between production department and marketing department is horizontal or lateral coordination.
- *Procedural and substantive:* It is according to *Herbert A Simon,* procedural coordination implies the specification of the organization in itself, i.e. the generalized description of the behavior and relationship of the members of the organization. On the other hand, substantive coordination is concerned with the content of the organization's activities. For instance, in an automobile plant an organization chart is an aspect of procedural coordination, while blueprints for the engine block of the car being manufactured are an aspect of substantive coordination.

Techniques of Coordination

The main techniques of effective coordination are as follows.

- *Sound planning:* The unity of purpose is the first essential condition of coordination. Therefore, the goals of the organization and the goals of its units must be clearly defined. Planning is the ideal stage for coordination. Clear-cut objectives, harmonized policies and unified procedures and rules ensure uniformity of action.
- *Simplified organization:* A simple and sound organization is an important means of coordination. The lines of authority and responsibility from top to the bottom of the organization structure should be clearly defined. Clear-cut authority relationships help to reduce conflicts and to hold people responsible. Related activities should be grouped together in one department or unit. Too much specialization should be avoided as it tends to make every unit an end in itself.
- *Effective communication:* Open and regular communication is the key to coordination. Effective interchange of opinions and information helps in resolving differences and in creating mutual understanding. Personal and face to face contacts are the most effective means of communication and coordination. Committees help to promote unity of purpose and uniformity of action among different departments.

- *Effective leadership and supervision:* The effective leadership ensures coordination both at the planning and execution stage. A good leader can guide the activities of his subordinates in the right direction and can inspire them to pull together for the accomplishment of common objectives. Sound leadership can persuade subordinates to have identity of interest and to adopt a common outlook. Personal supervision is an important method of resolving differences of opinion.
- *Chain of command:* Authority is the supreme coordinating power in an organization. Exercise of authority through the chain of command or hierarchy is the traditional means of coordination. Coordination between interdependent units can be secured by putting them under one boss.
- *Indoctrination and incentives:* It indoctrinating organizational members with the goals and mission of the organization can transform a neutral body into a committed body. Similarly incentives maybe used to create mutuality of interest and to reduce conflicts. For instance, profit-sharing is helpful in promoting team-spirit and cooperation between employers and workers.
- *Liaison departments:* Where frequent contacts between different organizational units are necessary, liaison officers maybe employed. For instance, a liaison department may ensure that the production department is meeting the delivery dates and specifications promised by the sales department. Special coordinators maybe appointed in certain cases. For instance, a project coordinator is appointed to coordinate the activities of various functionaries in a project which is to be completed within a specified period of time.
- *General staff:* In large organizations, a centralized pool of staff experts is used for coordination. A common staff group serves as the clearing house of information and specialized advice to all department of the enterprise. Such general staff is very helpful in achieving inter-departmental or horizontal coordination. Task forces and projects teams are also useful in coordination.
- *Voluntary coordination:* When every organizational unit appreciates the workings of related units and modifies its own functioning to suit them, there is self-coordination. Self-coordination or voluntary coordination is possible in a climate of dedication and mutual cooperation. It results from mutual consultation and team-spirit among the members of the organization. However, it cannot be a substitute for the coordinative efforts of managers.

Principles of Coordination

Mary Parker Follett has laid out four principles for effective coordination:

1. *Direct personal Contact:* According to this principle coordination is best achieved through direct personal contact with people concerned.

Direct face to face communication is the most effective way to convey ideas and information and to remove misunderstanding.

2. *Early beginning:* The coordination can be achieved more easily in early stages of planning and policy-making. Therefore, plans should be based on mutual consultation or participation. Integration of efforts becomes more difficult once the uncoordinated plans are put into operation. Early coordination also improves the quality of plans.
2. *Reciprocity:* This principle states that all factors in a given situation are interdependent and interrelated. For instance, in a group every person influences all others and is in turn influenced by others. When people appreciate the reciprocity of relations, they avoid unilateral action and coordination becomes easier.
4. *Continuity:* Coordination is an on-going or never-ending process rather than a once-for-all activity. It cannot be left to chance, but management has to strive constantly. Sound coordination is not fire-fighting, i.e. resolving conflicts as they arise.

Benefits of Coordination

- *Higher efficiency and economy:* Coordination helps to improve the efficiency of operations by avoiding overlapping efforts and duplication of work. Integration and balancing of individual efforts provide a smooth and harmonious team work. Coordination is a creative force which makes possible a total result which is greater than the sum of individual achievements. This is the synergetic effect coordination. Coordination enables an organization to rake optimum use of its resources. The success of organized endeavor depends upon the quality of coordination. In fact, coordination is the first principle of organization as it expresses the principle of organization into. The quality of coordination is the crucial factor in the survival of an organization.
- *Good human relations:* Besides promoting the efficiency of operations, coordination improves the morale and job satisfaction of employees. Composite and orderly effort established through team spirit and executive leadership enables employees to derive a sense of security and personal contentment from their job. A well-coordinated organization can attract, retain and utilize better personnel. Coordination improves human relations by reconciling individual and organizational objectives.
- *Unity of direction:* Coordination helps to ensure unity of action in the face of disruptive forces. By welding together different departments and sections into one entity, coordination ensures the stability and growth of an organization. It enables the executives to see the enterprise as a whole instead of narrow sectional goals. Individual interests are subordinated to the common interest more easily and effectively.

- *Quintessence of management:* Coordination is an all inclusive concepts or the end result of the management process. Management is nothing more than coordination of all activities, efforts and forces that affect the organization from within and without. Coordination serves as a key to all managerial functions. According to Mary Parker Follett, 'the first test of a business administration should be whether you have a business with all its parts so coordinated, so moving together in their closely knit and adjusting activities, so linking, interlocking, inter-relating, that they make a working unit that is not a congenis of separate pieces, but a functional whole or integrated unit'.
- *Organizational effectiveness:* Coordination fosters loyalty and commitment among employees. This enhances the effectiveness and stability of the organization. According to McFarland, 'if job satisfactions are present, executives will tend to remain longer with the company. They will feel that they have a place in the organization. They will feel that they have earned that place. The presence of coordination becomes part of their job experience and hence can form a very useful part of their training'. Thus, coordination is the sine qua non of effective management.

CONTROL

Control is any process that guide activity towards some predetermined goals. Thus control can be applied is any field such as price control, distribution control pollution control, etc. Thus control process tries to find out deviations between planned performance and actual performance and to suggest corrective action wherever these are needed.

Definition of Control

- 'Controlling is determining what is being accomplish, that is evaluating the performance and, if necessary, applying corrected measures so that the performance takes place according to plan'.
- Control is checking event performance against predetermined standards contained in the plans, with a view to ensuring adequate progress and satisfactory performance.
- Controlling consists in verifying whether everything occurs inconformity with the plan adopted, the instructions issued and principles established. Its object is to point but weakness and errors in order to rectify them and prevent recurrence.
  - Control is forward looking.
  - Control is both executive process and from the point of view of the organization of the system, a result.
  - Control is a continuous process.
  - A control system is a coordinated—integrated system.

Importance of Control

Thus control is an integrated action of an organization or manager. It offers help in the following directions.

- *Adjustment in operations:* A control system acts as an adjustment in organizational operations. Every organization has certain objectives to achieve which become the basis for control.
- *Policy verification:* Various policies in the organization generate the need for control. For organizational functioning, managers set certain policies and other planning elements which later become the basis and reason for control.
- *Managerial responsibility:* In every organization, managerial responsibility is created through assignment of activities to various individuals. This process starts at the top level and goes to the lower levels.
- *Psychological pressure:* Control process puts a psychological pressure on the individuals for the better performance. The performance of the individuals is evaluated in the light of targets set for them.
- *Coordination in action:* Control system area designed such a way that they focus not only on the operating responsibility of a manager but also on his ultimate responsibility. This forces a manager to coordinate the activities of his subordinate in such a way that each of them contributes positively towards the objectives of the superior.
- *Organizational efficiency and effectiveness*: Proper control ensures organizational efficient and effectiveness various factors of control, namely, making managers responsible, motivating them for higher performance, and achieving coordination in their performance, control, ensures that their organization works efficiently.

Steps in Controlling

The various steps in control process which are necessary for its relationship to planning. These steps may broadly be classified into four parts.

a. *Establishment of control standards:* Every function in the organizations begins with plans which are goals, objectives or targets to be achieved. In the light of these standards are established which are criteria against which actual results are measured.
b. *Measurement of performance:* The second major step in control process is the measurement of performance. The step involves measuring the performance in respect of a work in terms of control standards.
c. *Comparing actual and standard performance:* The third major step in control process is the comparison of actual and standard performance. It involves two steps:
   (i) Finding out the extent of deviations and
   (ii) Identifying the causes of such deviations.

d. *Correction of deviations:* This is the last step in the control process which requires that actins should be taken to maintain the desired degree of control in the system or operation.

Essentials of Effective Control System

Control is necessary in every organization to ensure that everything is going properly. Every manager, therefore, should have an effective and adequate control system to assist him in making sure that events conform to plans.

In this tailoring of control system, there are certain requirements which should be kept in mind:

- *Reflecting organizational needs:* All control systems and techniques should reflect the jobs they are to perform.
- *Forward looking:* Control should be forward looking. Though many of the controls are instance, they must focus attention as to how future actions can be conformed with plans.
- *Promptness in reporting deviations:* The success of a thermostat lies in the fact that it points the deviation promptly and takes corrective actions immediately.
- *Pointing out exceptions at critical Points:* Control should point exception at critical points and suggest whether action is to be taken for deviations or not.
- *Objectives:* The control should be objective, definite and determinable in a clear and positive way.
- *Flexible:* Control system should be flexible so that it remains workable in the case of changed plans, unforeseen circumstances or failures.
- *Economical:* Control should be economical and must be worth its costs. Economy is relative since the benefits vary with the importance of the activity, the size of the operation the expense that might be incurred in the absence of control and the contribution the control system can make.
- *Simple:* Control system must be simple and understandable so that all managers can use it effectively.
- *Motivating:* Control system should motivate both controller and controlled.
- *Reflecting organizational pattern:* The control should reflect organizational pattern by focusing attention on positions in organization structure through which deviations are corrected.

Techniques of Control

To control the activities in the organization, managers can use variety of tools and techniques. They are broadly grouped under two heads.

1. *Traditional techniques:* Traditional techniques are those which have long been used by the managers. Some of the important techniques under this heads are budgetary control, financial statement and ratio analysis, auditing, break-even analysis and report writing, etc.

   "Budgetary control is a process of comparing the actual results with the corresponding budgeting data in order to approve accomplishments or to remedy differences by either adjusting the budget estimates or correcting the cause of the difference." The different budgets such as production budget, sales budget, overhead budget, labor budget, etc. clearly indicate the limits for expenses and also the results to be achieved in a given period. It ensures effective coordination of the work of the entire organization. It promotes cooperation and team spirit among the employees:

   - *Standard costing:* It is one of the techniques of cost control and it is being increasingly used by modern business concerns for the purpose of cost reduction and cost control. It involves a comparison of actual with the standards and the discrepancy is called variance.
   - *Break-even analysis:* It is useful in planning and control because it emphasizes the marginal cost and benefit concept. It helps to make profit estimation at the different levels of activity, ascertaining turnover for desire profit and estimating the impact of the variations of fixed and variable costs. It magnifies a set of relationships of fixed costs, variable cost, price, level of output and sales mix to the profitability of the organization.
   - *Financial statement analysis:* Such as found flow analysis, cash flow analysis and ratio analysis help to know the financial performance and financial position of the business unit. The liquidity, profitability and solvency position of the business unit can be ascertained and efforts can be taken to maintain these factors in an optimum proportion.
   - *Auditing:* It is the process of investigating financial and other operation of a business establishment. It maybe carried out by internal and external members. It helps to scrutinize the applicability and relevance of policy, procedure and method which have a tendency to become obsolete. This it helps in choosing a suitable working procedures and methods.
   - *Adoption of reporting system:* It helps to analyze a particular problem and to take necessary corrective action over it. Reports maybe prepared regarding taxation, legislation and its effect on profit, make or buy decisions, replacement of capital equipment, social pricing analysis, etc.

A manager can also exercise effective control over his subordinates by observing them while they are engaging in work. Personal observation helps the managers not only in knowing the workers attitude towards work but also correcting their work and method, if necessary.

2. *Modern techniques:* These are of recent origin, which provide information not readily available with traditional methods. These techniques help to give sharper focus and promise increasingly to improve the quality of control. Program Evaluation Review Technique (PERT) and Critical Path Method (CPM) are two major techniques coming under this head.

PERT has been, developed by an US Office in 1958 in connection with the Polaris Weapon System and is credited with reduction the completion time of the program by two years. CPM has been jointly developed by DU Point and Remington Rand USA in order to facilitate the control of large, complex industrial projects. These techniques are used to minimize total time, minimize to cost, minimize idle resources, etc. It is helpful in solving problems of scheduling the activities of on-time projects. These tools are widely being used in construction industry, planning and launching new projects, scheduling ship construction, etc. It ensures improved management of resources by facilitating better decision-making. It aims to have future oriented control mechanism for the organization.

- *Management information system (MIS):* It provides needed information to each manager at the right time, in right form which aids his understanding and stimulates his action. It is a refined form of traditional information collection and supply to the organization points.
- *Management audit:* It is an evaluation of management as a whole. It examines the total managerial process of planning, staffing, directing and controlling. To evaluate the management achievement, the organization plans, policies, procedures, organization structure, system of control personnel relation should be measure with its end results.

Budgetary control	Financial performance
Cost control	Cost performance
Production control	PERT, CPM, production, performance,
Inventory control	Stores function performance
Profit and Loss Control ROL control	Overall organizational objective performance.
External audit control	Statutory performance

DELEGATION

Delegation of authority is one vital organizational process. Delegation means assigning of certain responsibilities along with the necessary authority by a superior to his subordinate managers. Delegation does not mean surrender of authority by the higher level manager. It only means transfer of certain responsibilities to subordinates and giving them the necessary authority, which is necessary to discharge the responsibility properly. Even in the college, the principal delegates some of his authority to the vice-principal.

In delegation, an attempt is being made to have meaningful participation and cooperation from the subordinates for achieving certain well-defined results. Due to delegation, the routine responsibilities of the superior are reduced. As a result, he concentrates on more urgent and important matters. Secondly, due to delegation, subordinate becomes responsible for certain functions transferred to him. Delegation is a tool, which a superior manager uses for sharing his work with the subordinates and thereby raising his efficiency.

Definitions of Delegation of Authority

- According to *FC Moore,* 'Delegation means assigning work to the others and giving them authority to do so'.
- According to *OS Miner,* 'Delegation takes place when one person gives another the right to perform work on his behalf and in his name and the second person accepts a corresponding duty or obligation to do that is required of him.'
- According to *Louis Allen,* 'Delegation is the dynamics of management, it is the process a manager follows in dividing the work assigned to him so that he performs that part which only he, because of his unique organizational placement, can perform effectively, and so that he can get others to help him with what remains'.

Objectives of Delegation of Authority

- To reduce the excessive burden on the superiors, i.e. executives and managers functioning at different levels
- To provide opportunities of growth and self development to junior executives
- To create a team of experienced and matured managers for the organization. It acts as a technique of management and human resource development
- To improve individual as well as overall efficiency of the organisation.

Process of Delegation of Authority

Delegation process involves four distinct stages. The process of delegation moves through these stages. The following figure shows the stages in the process of *delegation of authority.*

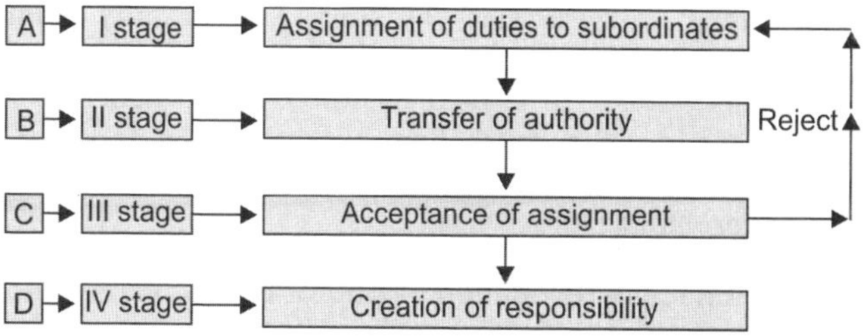

1. *Assignment of duties to subordinates:* Before delegating, the delegator has to decide precisely the duties which are to be delegated to the subordinate or a group of subordinates. The authority is delegated accordingly and the subordinate is told what is expected from him. The usual practice is to list the functions to be performed by the subordinate. If necessary, targets to be achieved by the subordinate are also spel out. Subordinates maybe assigned tasks either in terms of activities or results. The manager (delegator) must communicate clearly his expectations. Competent and responsible employees maybe given general guidelines about what needs to be accomplished. Their less competent and responsible counterparts need more specific guidelines. In brief, in the first stage of delegation process, duties are assigned to the subordinate.
2. *Transfer of authority to perform the duty:* In the second stage of delegation process, the authority is granted by the delegator to his subordinate (delegate). Authority must be delegated strictly to perform the assigned duty. The performance of duties suffers serious setback when required authority is not delegated along with the duty. In brief, the transfer of authority should be adequate considering the duties assigned to the subordinate.
3. *Acceptance of the assignment:* In this third stage of delegation process, the subordinate/delegate has to accept or reject the task assigned to him in the first stage along with the authority given in the second stage. If the delegates refuse, the delegator has to make fresh plan of delegation or may consider some other subordinate who is capable and is willing to accept the assignment. On the other hand, the process of delegation will move to the fourth and the last stage, if the first delegates accept the assignment of work accompanying the authority.

4. *Creation of obligation/accountability/responsibility:* The fourth stage in the, delegation of authority is the creation of obligation on the part of the subordinate to perform duties assigned to him in a satisfactory manner by using the authority given. When subordinate accepts a task and the authority is given, an obligation is created. He has to perform the assigned task by using the authority granted to him. A subordinate is also responsible/accountable for completing the assigned work. He is held answerable to a superior for the satisfactory performance of that work assigned. The delegator has to help his subordinate as and when necessary as he is responsible to his superior/organization.

Principles of Effective Delegation of Authority

- *Knowledge of objectives:* Before delegating authority, the subordinates should be made to understand their duties and responsibilities. In addition, knowledge of objectives and policies of the enterprise should be provided to them. This will enable them to discharge their roles purposefully in the process of delegation.
- *Parity of authority and responsibility:* This principle of delegation suggests that when authority is delegated, it should be commensurate with the responsibility of the subordinate. In fact, the authority and responsibility should be made clear to the subordinate so that he will know what he is expected to do within the powers assigned to them. There should be proper balance/parity or co-existence between the authority and responsibility. A subordinate will not function efficiently, if authority given to him is inadequate. On the other hand, if the excess authority is given, he may misuse the same. For avoiding this, the subordinates who are assigned duties should be given necessary/adequate authority enables them to carry-out their duties.
- *Unity of command:* This principle of delegation suggests that everyone should have only one boss. A subordinate should get orders and instructions from one superior and should be made accountable to one superior only. This means 'no subordinate should be held accountable to more than one superior'. When a subordinate is asked to report to more than one boss, it leads to confusion and conflict. Unity of command also removes overlapping and duplication of work. In the absence of unity of command, there will be confusion and difficulty in fixing accountability.
- *The scalar principle:* The scalar principle of delegation maintains that there should be clear and direct lines of authority in the organization, running from the top to the bottom. The subordinate should know who delegates authority to him and to whom he should contact for matters beyond his authority. They (subordinates) should also know

what is expected from them. This principle justifies establishment of the hierarchical structure within the organization.

- *Clarity of delegation:* The principle of clarity of delegation suggests that while delegating authority to subordinates, they should be made to understand the limits of authority so that they know the area of their operation and the extent of freedom of action available to them. Such clarity guides subordinates while performing their jobs.
- *Absoluteness of responsibility:* This principle of delegation suggests that it is only the authority which is delegated and not the responsibility. The responsibility is absolute and remains with the superior. He cannot run away from the same even after delegation. Even when the manager delegates authority to his subordinate, he remains fully accountable to his superiors because responsibility cannot be divided between a superior and his subordinate. No superior can delegate responsibilities for the acts of his subordinates. He is responsible for the acts and omissions of his subordinates.
- *Use of exception principle:* This principle of delegation indicates that when authority is delegated, it is expected that the subordinate will exercise his own judgment and take decisions within the purview of his authority. He is to be given adequate freedom to operate within his authority even at the cost of mistakes. He should refer the problems to the top level management only when he is unable to take decisions. Unnecessary interference in the work of delegates should be avoided. This normal rule can be given up under exceptional circumstances. Here, the superior can interfere in the work of his subordinate and even withdraw the delegated duties and authority. The superior takes this decision under exceptional circumstances.
- *Completeness of delegation:* This principle of delegation suggests that there should be completeness in the process of delegation. The process of delegation should be taken to its logical end. Otherwise, there will be confusion of authority and accountability.
- *Effective communication support system:* This principle suggests that there should be continuous flow of information between the superior and the subordinates with a view to furnishing relevant information to subordinate for decision-making. This helps him to take proper decisions and also to interpret properly the authority delegated to him. Delegation system may not work smoothly in the absence of effective communication between the superior and subordinates.
- *Reward for effective delegation:* This principle suggests that effective delegation and successful assumption of authority should be rewarded. This will facilitate fuller delegation and effective assumption of authority within the organization. Reward for effective delegation will provide favorable environmental climate for its fair introduction.

Advantages/Importance of Delegation of Authority

- *Relieves manager for more challenging jobs:* Delegation makes it possible for the managers to distribute their workload to others. Thus, managers are relieved of routine work and they can concentrate on higher functions of management like planning, organizing, controlling, etc.
- *Leads to motivation of subordinates:* Subordinates are encouraged to give their best at work when they have authority with responsibility. They take more initiative and interest in the work and are also careful and cautious in their work. Delegation leads to motivation of employees and manpower development.
- *Facilitates efficiency and quick actions:* Delegation saves time enabling tile subordinates to deal with the problems promptly. They can take the decisions quickly within their authority. It is not necessary to go to the superiors for routine matters. This raises the overall efficiency in an organization and offers better results in terms of production, turnover and profit.
- *Improves employee morale:* Delegation raises the morale of subordinates as they are given duties and supporting authority. They feel that they are responsible employees. The attitude and outlook of subordinates towards work assigned becomes more constructive.
- *Develops team spirit:* Due to delegation, effective communication develops between the superiors and subordinates. The subordinates are answerable to superiors and the superiors are responsible for the performance of subordinates. This brings better relations and team spirit among the superiors and subordinates.
- *Maintains cordial relationships:* The superiors trust subordinates and give them necessary authority. The subordinates accept their accountability and this develops cordial superior-subordinate relationships.
- *Facilitates management development:* Delegation acts as a training ground for management development. It gives opportunity to subordinates to learn, to grow and to develop new qualities and skills. It builds up a reservoir of executives, which can be used as and when required. Delegation creates managers and not mere messengers.
- *The advantages of delegation will not be available easily and automatically.* They will be available only when the process of delegation moves smoothly. Problems may develop, if the delegation is not introduced with proper planning and in proper spirit. For example, the authority given to subordinate is inadequate or the subordinate is not competent to discharge the responsibilities assigned or the superior fails to monitor the whole process of delegation effectively. In all such cases, the delegation will be ineffective and the expected advantages will not be available to the organization and also to concerned parties.

Obstacles/Barriers to Effective Delegation of Authority

- Obstacles/Barriers on the Part of Manager/Superior/Delegator:
  - *Unwillingness of the manager to delegate authority:* Some superiors/ managers tend to think that they can do the job better when they themselves handle the job. The attitude that *'I can do it better myself'* on the part of superior acts as an obstacle to delegation. Some managers (superiors) who are autocratic and power worshippers feel that delegation will lead to reduction of their influence in the organization. A manager may feel that if he has a competent subordinate and if he delegates authority to the subordinate, quite likely he will outshine him (manager) and maybe promoted.
  - *Fear of competition:* A manager may feel that if he has a competent subordinate and if he delegates authority to the subordinate, quite likely he will outshine him. Fear of subordinate's excellence may come in the way of delegation.
  - *Lack of confidence in subordinates:* A manager may hesitate to delegate authority, if he feels that his subordinate is not competent to deal with the problem and take decisions. Even *fear of losing control* over the subordinates acts as an obstacle to delegation. In addition, *fear of being exposed* due to personal shortcomings may act as an obstacle in the process of delegation.
  - *Lack of ability to direct:* Sometimes, a manager may experience difficulty in directing the efforts of his subordinates because of his inability to identify and communicate the essential features of his long-range plans and programs.
  - *Absence of controls that warn of coming troubles:* An organization might not have developed the controlling techniques to know in advance the serious problems lying ahead. It may happen due to concentration of power in the hands of few people. As a result, manager may resist delegation.
  - *Conservative and cautious temperament of the manager:* If a manager has a conservative and over-cautious approach, there will be psychological barrier in the way of delegation. A manager avoids delegation as he feels that something may go wrong even when the instructions given are clear and the subordinates are reliable.
  - *Desire to dominate subordinates:* Managers (Superiors) normally, have a desire to dominate the subordinates functioning under their control. They feel that their domination will reduce if the powers are delegated to subordinates. They also feel that due to delegation, the subordinates will know their managerial deficiencies. In order to maintain their superior status and in order to dominate the subordinates, they avoid delegation itself.

- Obstacles/Barriers on the Part of Subordinates (Why Subordinates Resist Delegation?):
  - *Too much dependence on the manager for decisions:* Some subordinates avoid responsibility even when the superior/manager is prepared to delegate authority. They want the manager to tackle problems and take decisions. A subordinate who is not confident about his performance/ability will certainly try to shirk responsibility even though his superior is prepared to delegate functions and authority.
  - *Fear of criticism:* Subordinates express unwillingness to accept delegated authority because of the fear of criticism in the case of mistakes. They fear that they maybe criticized by others if they commit mistakes. Such subordinates have the following feeling in their mind, '*Why should I stick my neck out for my boss*'?
  - *Lack of information:* A subordinate may hesitate to accept a new assignment, when he knows that necessary information to perform the job is not likely to be made available to him. He is reluctant to accept delegated functions and authority as he feels that he will not be able to perform well due to inadequate information available.
  - *Absence of positive incentives:* Positive incentives like recognition of work and rewards go a long way in building up the morale of subordinates. In the absence of such incentives in the form of recognition, appreciation or monetary benefit, a subordinate may not be prepared to accept delegation of authority.
  - *Absence of self-confidence:* A subordinate may lack self-confidence about his ability to take quick and correct decisions. He may not like to accept new challenging functions as he lacks self-confidence. Thus, lack of self-confidence on the part of subordinates is one obstacle which comes in the way of delegation of authority.
  - *Difficulty in decision-making:* A subordinate may not have the skill and the expertise to take quick and correct decisions. He prefers to go to his superior (boss) and ask for his guidance or opinion. Such psychology acts as a cause for non-acceptance of delegation. A subordinate avoids delegation due to such mental tension or inferiority complex.
  - *Poor superior-subordinate relations:* Absence of cordial relations in between the superior and the subordinates hampers the process of delegation of authority. The attitude of the superior towards subordinate may not be friendly but hostile. There maybe undue interference in the work assigned to the subordinate. Even the good work of subordinate may not be appreciated by the superior. Such situation creates unfavorable attitude of subordinate towards delegation. He avoids delegation as and when offered.

- *Undue interference by superior:* A superior should not interfere in the duties delegated to the subordinate. He may offer guidance as and when asked for. Some superiors interfere in the work of his subordinate and try to control him often and again. In the absence of legitimate freedom, the subordinate becomes uneasy and prefers to remain away from the process of delegation.
- *Fear of being exposed:* Some subordinates may have inferiority complex. They feel that they have limited capacity to accept the challenges which are bound to come out to delegation. They feel that their inability to deal with new problems will be exposed due to delegation. This fear acts as an obstacle to delegation.

STAFFING

Organizations require the services of a large number of personnel. These personnel occupy varies positions created through the process of organizing. Each position of the organization makes certain specific contributions to achieve organizational objectives. Hence, the person occupying the position should have sufficient ability to meet its requirement. Staffing is that part of the process of management which is concerned with obtaining, utilizing and maintaining a satisfactory and satisfied work force.

Definition

According to *Mc Farland* 'Staffing is the function by which managers build an organization through recruitment, selection and development of individuals as capable employees'.

According to *Harold Koontz and Cyril O'Donnell* 'Staffing is defined as filling positions in the organization structure through identifying workforce requirements, inventorying the people available, recruitment, selection, placement, promotion, appraisal, compensation and training of needed people'.

Philosophy

The Board recognizes that a professionally competent, dynamic and efficient staff dedicated to education is necessary to maintain a constantly improving educational program. The Board is interested in its personnel as individuals, and recognizes its responsibility for promoting the general welfare of the staff.

The Board is committed to providing a highly competent, well-trained staff, able to fit each discipline and area of responsibility into a balanced, well-run school program equal to or surpassing comparable American International Schools. The staff should show qualities of stability, creativeness and self-renewal.

Philosophy of Staffing in Nursing

- Nurse administrators of a hospital nursing department should adopt the following staffing philosophy.
- Nurse administrators believe that it is possible to match employees' knowledge and skills to patient care needs in a manner that optimizes job satisfaction and care quality.
- Nurse administrators believe that the technical and humanistic care needs of critically ill patients are so complex that all aspects of that care should be provided by professional nurses.
- Nurse administrators believe that the health teaching and rehabilitation needs of chronically ill patients are so complex that direct care for chronically ill patients should be provided by professional and technical nurse.
- Nurse administrators believe that patient assessment, work quantification and job analysis should be used to determine the number of personnel in each category to be assigned to care for patients of each type (such as coronary care, renal failure, chronic arthritis, paraplegia, cancer, etc.).
- Nurse administrators believe that a master staffing plan and policies to implement the plan in all units should be developed centrally by the nursing heads and staff of the hospital.
- Nurse administrators believe the staffing plan details such as shift–start time, number of staffs assigned on holidays, and number of employees assigned to each shift can be modified to accommodate the units' workload and workflow.

Objectives of Staffing in Nursing

- Provide an all professional nurse staff in critical care units, operating rooms, labor and emergency room.
- Provide sufficient staff to permit a 1:1 nurse-patient ratio for each shift in every critical care unit.
- Staff the general medical, surgical, obstetrics and gynecology, pediatric and psychiatric units to achieve a 2:1 professional- practical nurse ratio.
- Provide sufficient nursing staff in general, medical, surgical, obstetrics and gynecology, pediatric and psychiatric units to permit a 1:5 nurse patient ratio on a day and afternoon shifts and 1:10 nurse-patient ratio on night shift.
- Involve the heads of the nursing staffs and all nursing personnel in designing the department's overall staffing program.
- Design a staffing plan that specifies how many nursing personnel in each classification will be assigned to each nursing unit for each shift and how vacation and holiday time will be requested and scheduled.

- Hold each head nurse responsible for translating the department's master staffing plan to sequential eight weeks time schedules for personnel assigned to her/his unit.
- Post time schedules for all personnel at least eight weeks in advance.
- Empower the head nurse to adjust work schedules for unit nursing personnel to remedy any staff excess or deficiency caused by census fluctuation or employee absence.
- Inform each nursing employee that requests for specific vacation or holiday time will be honored within the limits imposed by patient care and labor contract requirements.
- Reward employees for long term service by granting individuals special time requests on the basis of seniority.

Functions in Staffing

- Identifying the type and amount of service needed by agency client
- Determining the personnel categories that have the knowledge and skill to perform needed service measures
- Predicting the number of personnel in each job category that will be needed to meet anticipated service demands
- Obtaining, budgeted positions for the number in each job category needed to service for the expected types and number of clients
- Recruiting personnel to fill available positions
- Selecting and appointing personnel from suitable applicants
- Combining personnel into desired configurations by unit and shift
- Orienting personnel to fulfill assigned responsibilities
- Assigning responsibilities for client services to available personnel.

Principles of Nursing Staffing

According to American Nurses Association (ANA) there are nine principles of nursing staffing.

Patient Care Unit Related

- Appropriate staffing levels for a patient care unit reflect analysis of individual and aggregate patient needs
- There is a critical need to either retire or seriously question the usefulness of the concept of nursing hours per patient day (HPPD)
- Unit functions necessary to support delivery of quality patient care must also be considered in determining staffing levels.

Staff Related

- The specific needs of various patient populations should determine the appropriate clinical competencies required of the nurse practicing in that area

- Registered nurses must have nursing management support and representation at both the operational level and the executive level
- Clinical support from experienced RNs should be readily available to those RNs with less proficiency.

Institution/Organization Related

- Organizational policy should reflect an organizational climate that values registered nurses and other employees as strategic assets and exhibit a true commitment to filling budgeted positions in a timely manner.
- All institutions should have documented competencies for nursing staff, including agency or supplemental and travelling RNs, for those activities that they have been authorized to perfor.
- Organizational policies should recognize the myriad needs of both patients and nursing staff.

Norms of Staffing Staff Inspection Unit (SIU)

Norms are standards that guide, control, and regulate individuals and communities. For planning nursing manpower we have to follow some norms. The nursing norms are recommended by various committees, such as; the Nursing Man Power Committee, the High-power Committee, Dr Bajaj Committee, and the staff inspection committee, TNAI and INC. The norms has been recommended taking into account the workload projected in the wards and the other areas of the hospital.

All the above committees and the staff inspection unit recommended the norms for optimum nurse-patient ratio. Such as 1:3 for Non Teaching Hospital and 1:5 for the Teaching Hospital. The Staff Inspection Unit (SIU) is the unit which has recommended the nursing norms in the year 1991–92. As per this SIU norm the present nurse-patient ratio is based and practiced in all central government hospitals.

Recommendations of SIU

- The norms for providing staff nurses and nursing sisters in government hospital is given in annexure to this report. The norm has been recommended taking into account the workload projected in the wards and the other areas of the hospital.
- The posts of nursing sisters and staff nurses have been clubbed together for calculating the staff entitlement for performing nursing care work which the staff nurse will continue to perform even after she is promoted to the existing scale of nursing sister.
- Out of the entitlement worked out on the basis of the norms, 30% posts maybe sanctioned as nursing sister. This would further improve

the existing ratio of 1 nursing sister to 3.6. Staff nurses fixed by the government in settlement with the Delhi nurse union in may 1990.

- The assistant nursing superintendent is recommended in the ratio of 1 ANS to every 4.5 nursing sisters. The ANS will perform the duty presently performed by nursing sisters and perform duty in shift also.
- The posts of Deputy Nursing Superintendent may continue at the level of 1 DNS per every 7.5 ANS.
- There will be a post of Nursing Superintendent for every hospital having 250 or beds.
- There will be a post of 1 Chief Nursing Officer for every hospital having 500 or more beds.
- It is recommended that 45% posts added for the area of 365 days working including 10% leave reserve (maternity leave, earned leave, and days off as nurses are entitled for 8 days off per month and 3 National Holidays per year when doing 3 shift duties).

Most of the hospital today is following the SIU norms. In this the post of the Nursing Sisters and the Staff Nurses has been clubbed together and the work of the ward sister is remained same as staff nurse even after promotion. The Assistant Nursing Superintendent and the Deputy Nursing Superintendent have to do the duty of one category below of their rank.

The Nurse-patient Ratio as per the SIU Norms

1.	General Ward	1:6
2.	Special Ward - (pediatrics, burns, neurosurgery, cardio thoracic, neuromedicine, nursing home, spinal injury, emergency wards attached to casuality)	1:4
3.	Nursery	1:2
4.	ICU	1:1 (Nothing mentioned about the shifts)
5.	Labor Room	1:l per table
6.	OT	Major - 1:2 per table Minor - 1:l per table
7.	Casualty:	
(a)	Casualty main attendance up to 100 patients per day thereafter	3 staff nurses for 24 hours, 1:1 per shift.
(b)	For every additional attendance of 35 patients	1: 35 3 staff nurses for 24 hours, 1:1/shift
(c)	Gyne/obstetric attendance	1: 15
(d)	Thereafter every additional attendance of 15 patients.	

Contd...

Contd...

8.	Injection room OPD	Attendance up to 100 patients per day 1 staff nurse 120–220 patients: 2 staff nurses 221–320 patients: 3 staff nurses 321–420 patients: 4 staff nurses
9.	OPD	
	Name of the Department	1
	• Blood bank	2
	• Pediatric	2
	• Immunization	1
	• Eye	1
	• ENT	1
	• Pre anesthetic	1
	• Cardio lab	1
	• Bronchoscopy lab	1
	• Vaccination anti rabbis	2
	• Family planning	1
	• Medical	1
	• Dental	1
	• Central sample collection center	1
	• Orthopedic	2
	• Gyne	2
	• X-ray	3
	• Skin	2
	• VD center	2
	• Chemotherapy	2
	• Neurology	1
	• Microbiology	2
	• Psychiatry	1
	• Burns	2

In addition to the 10% reserve as per the extent rules, 45% posts maybe added where services are provided for 365 days in a year/ 24 hours.

The Nurse-patient Ratio as per the norms of TNAI and INC (The Indian Nursing Council, 1985)

The norms are based on hospital beds.

- Chief Nursing Officer : 1 per 500 beds
- Nursing Superintendent : 1 per 400 beds or above
- DNS. : 1 per 300 beds and 1 additional for every 200 beds
- ANS. : 1 for 1000–150 beds or 3–4 wards
- Ward Sister : 1 for 25–30 beds or one ward. 30% leave reserve
- Staff Nurse : 1 for 3 beds in Teaching Hospital in general ward and 1 for 5 beds

in Non-teaching Hospital + 30% Leave reserve.

- Extra nursing staff to be provided for departmental research function.
- For OPD and Emergency : 1 staff nurse for 100 patients (1 : 100) + 30% leave reserve.
- *For intensive care unit: (ICU)* : 1 : 1 or (1:3 for each shift) + 30% leave reserve.
- It is suggested that for 250 beded hospital there should be one Infection Control Nurse (ICN).

For specialized departments, such as peration theater, labor room, etc. 1:25 +30% leave reserve. Norms are not based on Nursing Hours or Patient's Needs here.

Recruitment

Once a determination of human resources requirements has been made, the recruitment and selection process can begin. Very often, recruitment is misunderstood as filling in of vacancies. The real purpose of recruitment is not to fill-up a vacancy but to add a person to the staff whom the management expects to become important in the future scheme of things.

Definition of Recruitment

- '*Recruitment* is the process of searching for prospective employees and stimulating them to apply for jobs in the organization'.
- It is often termed 'positive' in that its objective is to increase the selection ratio, that is, the number of applicants per job opening.
- Recruitment or manpower selection process is the first step in the employment of labor and the methods through which labor is brought into industry has much to do with the ultimate success or failure of such employment. Despite tremendous unemployment it is not easy to find the right type of labor. Since workers were drawn from the rural population, in the early days of industrial evolution in India, factories found much difficulty in recruiting the necessary labor due to the reluctance of workers to leave their villages and work in distant towns cut off from their kith and kin.

Factors Affecting Recruitment

All organizations, whether large or small, do engage in recruiting activity, though not to the same extent. This differs with:

- The size of the organization
- The employment conditions in the community where the organization is located

- The effects of past recruiting efforts which show the organization's ability to locate and keep good performing people
- Working conditions and salary and benefit packages offered by the organization which may influence turnover and necessitate future recruiting
- The rate of growth of organization
- The level of seasonality of operations and future expansion and production programs
- Cultural, economic and legal factors, etc.

Sources of Recruitment

The sources of employees can be classified into two types, internal and external. Filling a job opening from within the firm has the advantages of stimulating preparation for possible transfer of promotion, increasing the general level of morale, and providing more information about job candidates through analysis of work histories within the organization. A job posting has a number of advantages. From the view point of the employee, it provides flexibility and greater control over career progress. For the employer, it should result in better matches of employee and job.

In most instances, the jobs are posted on notice boards, though some carry listings in the company newspapers. The posting period is commonly 1 week, with the final decision for hiring being completed within 4 weeks. Internal applications are often restricted to certain employees, the guidelines for one company including:

- 'Good' or 'better' on most recent performance review
- Dependable attendance record
- Not under probationary sanction
- Having been in present position for 1 year.

The present supervisor must at sometime be informed of his or her subordinate's interest in another job. Some require immediate notification, while others inform only if the employee becomes a prime candidate for the listed opening. The personnel unit acts as a clearing house in screening applications that are unrealistic, preventing an excessive number of bids by a single employee, and counseling employees who are constantly unsuccessful in their attempt to change jobs.

Inevitably, the firm must go to external sources for lower entry jobs, for expansion, and for positions whose specifications cannot be met by present personnel. Thus the firm has a number of outside sources available, among which are the following:

- *Advertising:* There is a trend toward more selective recruitment in advertising. This can be affected in at least two ways. First, advertisements can be placed in media read only by particular groups.

Secondly, more information about the company, the job, and the job specification can be included in the ad to permit some self-screening.

- *Employment agencies:* Additional screening can be affected through the utilization of employment agencies, both public and private. Today, in contrast to their former unsavory reputation, the public employment agencies in several states are well regarded, particularly in the fields of unskilled semiskilled and skilled operative jobs. In the technical and professional areas, however, the private agencies appear to be doing most of the work. Many private agencies tend to specialize in a particular type of worker and job, such as sales, office, executive or engineer.
- *Employee referrals:* Friends and relatives of present employees are also a good source from which employees maybe drawn. When the labor market is very tight, large employers frequently offer their employees bonus or prizes for any referrals that are hired and stay with the company for a specific length of time. Some companies maintain a register of former employees whose record was good to contact them when there are new job openings for which they are qualified. This method of recruitment, however, suffers from a serious defect that it encourages nepotism, i.e. persons of one's community or caste are employed, who may or may not be fit for the job.
- *Schools, colleges and professional institutions:* Offer opportunities for recruiting their students. They operate placement services where complete biodata and other particulars of the students are available. The companies that need employees maintain contact with Guidance Counsellors of Employment Bureaus and teachers of business and vocational subjects. The prospective employers can review Credentials and interview candidates for management trainees or probationers. Whether the education sought involves a higher secondary certificate, specific vocational training, or a college background with a bachelor's, masters' or doctoral degree, educational institutions provide an excellent source of potential employees for entry level positions in organizations. These general and technical/professional institutions provide blue collar applicants, white collar and managerial personnel.
- *Labor unions:* Firms with closed or union shops must look to the union in their recruitment efforts. Disadvantages of a monopolistically controlled labor source are offset, at least particularly, by savings in recruitment costs. With one fifth of the labor force organized into unions, organized labor constitutes an important source of personnel.
- *Casual applicants:* Unsolicited applications, both at the gate and through the mail, constitute a much used source of personnel. These can be developed through provision of attractive employment office facilities and prompt and courteous replies to unsolicited letters.

- *Professional organizations or recruiting firms or executive recruiters:* Maintain complete information records about employed executives. These firms are looked upon as 'head hunters', 'raiders' and 'pirates' by organizations which lose personnel through their efforts. However, these same organizations may employ 'executive search firms' to help them find talent. These consulting firms recommend persons of high caliber for managerial, marketing and production engineers' posts.
- Indoctrination seminars for colleges professors are arranged to discuss the problem of companies and employees. Professors are invited to take part in these seminars. Visits to plants and banquets are arranged so that the participant professors maybe favorably impressed. They may later speak well of a company and help it in getting the required personnel.
- *Unconsolidated applications:* For positions in which large numbers of candidates are not available from other sources, the companies may gain keeping files of applications received from candidates who make direct enquiries about possible vacancies on their own, or may send unconsolidated applications. The information maybe indexed and filed for future use when there are openings in these jobs.
- *Nepotism:* The hiring of relatives will be an inevitable component of recruitment programs in family owned firms, such a policy does not necessarily coincide with hiring on the basis of merit, but interest and loyalty to the enterprise are offsetting advantages.
- *Leasing:* To adjust to short term fluctuations in personnel needs, the possibility of leasing personnel by the hour or day should be considered. This practice has been particularly well developed in the office administration field. The firm not only obtains well trained and selected personnel but avoids any obligation in pensions, insurance, and other fringe benefits.
- *Voluntary organizations:* Such as private clubs, social organizations might also provide employees—handicaps, widowed or married women, old persons, retired hands, etc. in response to advertisements.
- *Computer data banks:* When a company desires a particular type of employee, job specifications and requirements are fed into a computer, where they are matched against the resume data stored therein. The output is a set of resumes for individuals who meet the requirements. This method is very useful for identifying candidates for hard to fill positions which call for an unusual combination of skills.

Selection

In order to initiate the procedure for selection, we must satisfy the three preliminary requirements depicted in the diagram. First, there must be the authority to select, which comes from the employment requisition, as developed through analysis of the work load and work force. Secondly, we must have a standard of personnel with which we can compare prospective employees. This is represented by the job specification, as developed through job analysis. A planned recruitment program provides us with these applicants.

The selection procedure is essentially a series of methods of securing pertinent information about the applicant. At each step we learn more about the prospect. The information obtained can then be compared with the job specification, the standard of personnel. If the applicant qualifies, he or she advances to the next step. Thus, the job specification and the job applicant are interrelated at each step in the selection procedure.

Selection Techniques

There is no shortcut to an accurate evolution of a candidate. The hiring procedures are therefore, generally long and complicated. Many employers make use of such techniques and pseudo sciences while coming to hiring decisions. However, in modern times, these are considered to be unreliable measures.

The following is a popular procedure though it maybe modified to suit individual situation:

- *Preliminary interview:* The more non selective the recruitment program, the more likely it is that a preliminary interview will be required. This initial interview is usually quite short and has as its object the elimination of the obviously unqualified. In many instances it is a stand-up interview conducted at a desk or railing. The more obvious facts and impressions are of the type generally obtained in an initial interview. Many firms do not bother to initiate any paperwork at this early stage. If the applicant appears to have some chance of qualifying for existing job openings, he or she is given the application blank to complete.
- *Application blank:* An application blank is a traditional, widely accepted device for getting information from a prospective applicant which will enable a management to make a proper selection. The blank provides preliminary as well as aid in the interview by indicating areas of interest and discussion. It is a good means of quickly collecting verifiable basic historical data from the candidate. It also serves as a convenient device for circulating information about the applicant to appropriate members of management and as a useful device for storing information for, later reference. Many types of application forms are generally called on the following items: biographical data, educational attainment, work experience, salary, personal items, and other items such as names and addresses of previous employers, references, etc.

- *Check of references:* The use of references is common in most selection procedures, for it involves only a little time and money, and minimum of effort. The procedure places reliance on the evaluation of former employers, friends and professional personnel, checks on references are made by mail or telephone, and occasionally in person, or by using a reference form.
- *Psychological tests:* The next step in the procedures outlined above is that of testing. If all organizations, large and small, are considered, it is apparent that most are not using psychological tests. However, there is a direct relationship between the size and firm and the use of tests in hiring. Most of the larger companies that can afford to have a more detailed and accurate selection procedure do utilize some form of employment testing. It is the smaller company that frequently does not bother with tests, but places greater reliance upon the interview.
- *Interviewing*: Interviewing is probably the most widely used single method of selection. A substantial amount of subjectivity, and therefore, unreliability, is to be expected from interviewing when used as a tool of evaluation.

  The interview consists of interaction between interviewer and applicant. If handled properly, it can be a powerful technique in achieving accurate information and getting access to material otherwise unavailable. Four kinds of interviews for selection have been identified. These are:

  (a) *Preliminary interview:* These interviews are preliminary screening of applicants to decide whether a more detailed interview will be worthwhile. The applicant is given job details during the interview to afford him freedom to decide whether the job will suit him. This method saves the company's time and money.

  (b) *Stress interview:* Stress interviews are deliberate attempts to create pressure to observe how an applicant performs under stress. Methods used to induce stress range from frequent interruptions and criticism of an applicant's opinion, to keeping silent for an extended period of time. The most important advantage of the stress interview is that helps to demonstrate important personality characteristics which would be difficult to observe in tension free situations. However, stress inducing must be done carefully by trained and skilled interviewers.

  (c) *Depth interview:* Depth interviews cover the complete life history of the applicant and include such areas as the candidate's work experience, academic qualifications, health interest, and hobbies. It is an excellent method for executive selection, performed by qualified personnel.

(d) *Patterned interview:* Patterned interviews are a combination of direct and indirect questioning of the applicant. The interviewer has certain clues and guidelines to areas which should be probed deeply and the interview also encourages the candidate to express the relevant information freely.

After the patterned interview is complete, the interviewer should evaluate the candidate on the basis of practical experience. According to *RN McCurry* and others, certain factors lead to accurate predictions of the candidate's suitability for a particular position. The factors are: (1) basic character traits, (2) motivation, and (3) emotional maturity. One advantage of a patterned interview is that systematic and chronological information is obtained, and hence this yields to statistical analysis.

Approval by the Supervisor

Following the outlined procedure, we should now be of the opinion that a candidate who has successfully completed all steps so far should be hired. In executing the personnel unit screening functions, the emphasis tends to be more on formal qualifications and general suitability. When the supervisor takes over, the emphasis tends to switch toward more specifically job oriented worker characteristics such as training and relevant past experience.

Physical Examination

The physical examination is an employment step found in most businesses. It can vary from a very comprehensive examination and matching of an applicant's physical capabilities to job requirements to a simple check of general physical appearance and well-being. In the selection procedure the physical examination has at least three basic objectives. First, it serves to ascertain the applicant's physical capabilities. The second objective of the examination is to protect the company against unwarranted claims under workers' compensation laws, or against lawsuits for damages. And the final objective is to prevent communicable diseases from entering the organization.

Induction

Induction is concerned with the problem of introducing or orienting a new employee to the organization. In as much as various firms report that over half of their voluntary resignations occur within the first 6 months, proper orientation can do much to reduce this problem and its accompanying costs.

BUDGETING

Budget is derived from the French word 'Budgette' meaning a small leather bag. Today this word is used to convey a much wider and comprehensive meaning. Budget besides including the ideas of 'Plans estimate' 'Forecasts', etc. connects the future to the present as well as the past. While planning or preparing the budget for the future one has to always take guidance from the past experience and know the present. Budgeting maybe regarded as the most important tool of management which enables them to obtain a synthesis of the past, present and future. In simple words 'Budget' is an instrument used by management in planning its future activities. It is a means by which management charts its course for any given period of one month, six months, one year or five years. It includes an estimate of revenue, services and costs or expenses involved. In general it maybe stated as an estimate of anticipated requirements so arranged in a systematic manner to cover some or entire activities of an organization spread over a period of time.

Definition of Budget

- 'Budget' is a structured plan for managing income and expenses
- 'Budget' is an estimate of future needs arranged account to an orderly basis, covering some or all the activities of an enterprise for a definite period of time
- 'Budget' is a detailed plan of operations for some specified future period, followed by a system of record which will serve as a check upon the plan
- 'Budget' is thus a standard with which to measure the actual achievements of people, department, and organization.

Purposes of Budgeting

- It allows for feedback, concerning the extent to which actual spending conforms the budgetary spending
- It makes possible the early identification of problem areas and thus facilitates the development of effective solution
- It provides a means of measuring and recording financial successes in relation to the goals and objectives of the organization
- It supplies the mechanism for translating financial objectives into projected monthly spending pattern
- It enhances financial planning and decision-making
- It clearly identifies controllable cost areas
- It offers a useful format for communicating financial objectives to all concerned parties.

Importance of Budgeting

- Budget is needed for planning the future course of action and has a control over all activities in the organization
- Budget is facilitates co-coordinating operation of various departments and sections for realizing organizational objectives
- Budget serves as a guide for action in the organization
- Budget helps one to weigh the values and to make decision when necessary on whether one is of a greater value in the program than the other.

Principle of Budgeting

- Budget should provide sound financial management by focusing on requirement of the organization
- Budget should focus on objectives and policies of the organization
- Budget should ensure the most effective use of scarce financial and non-financial resources
- Budget process requires consistent delegation for which fixed duties and responsibilities are required to be allocated to managers
- Budgeting should include coordinating efforts of various departments establishing a frame of reference for managerial decisions
- Setting budget target requires an adequate checks and balance against the adoption of too high or too low estimate
- Budget must be appropriate to the nature of business or service
- Budget is prepared under the direction and supervision of the administrator or financial officer.
- Budgets are to be prepared and interpreted consistently throughout the organization in the communication of planning process
- Budget necessitates a review of the performance of the previous year and an evaluation of its adequacy both in quality and quantity
- While developing a budget, the provision should be made for its flexibility.

Classification of Budgeting

Budget consists mainly three sections: manpower budget, capital expenditure budget and operating budget.

- *Manpower budget:* It includes wages and other benefits provided for regular and temporary workers.
- *Capital expenditure budget:* It includes purchases of land, buildings and major equipments of considerable expense and long life.
- *Operating budget:* It includes the cost of supplies, minor equipment, repairs and overhead expenses.

Types of Budget

- *Incremental budget:* It is one based on estimated changes in present operation, plus a percentage increase/inflation, all of which is added to previous year budget.
- *Open ended budget* is a financial plan in which each operating manager presents a single cost estimate for what is considered optimal activity level for each program in the unit, without indicating how the budget should be scaled down if less funding is available.
- *Fixed ceiling budget:* It is a financial plan in which the uppermost spending limit is set by the top executive before the unit and divisional managers develop budget proposals for their areas of responsibility.
- *Flexible budget:* It consists of several financial plans, each for a different level of program activity. It is based on the fact, that operating conditions rarely conform to expectations.
- *Roll Over Budget:* It is one that forecasts program, revenues and expenses for a period greater than a year, to accommodate program that are larger than annual budget cycle.
- *Performance budget:* It is based on functions, which allocate functions, not divisions, e.g. direct nursing care, in service education, quality improvement, nursing research.
- *Program budget:* It is one where costs are computed for a total program, i.e. group total costs for each service program, e.g. MCH, FP.
- *Zero based budget:* Requires the nurse manager to examine, justify each cost of every program both old and new, in every annual budget preparation.
- *Sunset budget:* It is designed to 'self-destruct' within a prescribed time period to ensure the cessation of spend in by a predetermined date.
- *Sales budget:* It is the starting point in a budgetary program, since sales are basic activities which give shape to all other activities.
- *Production budget:* It aims at securing the economical manufacture of products and maximizing the utilization of production facilities.
- *Revenue and expense budget:* It is expressed in financial terms and takes the nature of a performa income statement for the future.
- *Production budget:* It is the budget that aims at securing the economical manufacture of products and maximizing the utilization of production facilities.
- *Capital expenditure budget:* It is prepared for assuring planned timely capital investment in the business to ensure the availability of capital at the right time over longer period.
- *Cash budget:* It is arrived at through a projection of future cash receipts and cash disbursements of the firm over various intervals of time. It reveals the timing and amount of expected cash inflows and outflows over the period studied.

POLICIES OF THE HOSPITAL

- Hospital-wide policies/procedures are developed for significant organizational issues that are interdepartmental or mandated to be hospital wide by accreditation agencies or state/federal legislation.
- The Hospital Policy Committee shall be:
  - Composed of representatives from hospital administration, nursing services, professional and support services, human resources and the business and reimbursement division.
  - Chaired by a member of the hospital administration staff. The chair shall maintain a current distribution list for all policies, distribute policies for review, and insure timely completion of the process.
- Committee members shall be selected annually by the hospital administrator with recommendations from the administrative staff.
- The committee will identify the appropriate entity for policy development, and insure that input is solicited and incorporated into a final policy statement. Once completed, the committee shall submit the policy, with verification of review, to the clinical board for final approval. Following approval, the policies shall be signed by the hospital administrator and distributed.
- Documentation of the review process and revised policies shall be maintained in an historical file for legal and reference purposes in hospital administration.
- The policy committee shall meet monthly unless otherwise directed.
- Policies shall be:
  - Reviewed in committee, obtaining committee input as needed.
  - Submitted to individuals/departments for additional comments and revisions as needed. The chairperson shall review and compile comments/revisions; final policy will be determined by committee majority.
  - Submitted to the hospital administrator for final comments, revisions and written approval and will be effective upon such approval.
- Requests for policy introductions, revisions, or deletions, maybe made by medical staff committees, hospital committees, hospital departments, medical center departments, or individuals on the hospital policy committee.
- All hospital policies will be reviewed at least every three years and/or as needed.
- Department specific policies and procedures shall be reviewed and revised at least every three years and as needed, to ensure compliance with institutional practice.

- Clinical and administrative staffs monitor and evaluate the quality of patient care and clinical performance, including proactive risk assessment of selected high-risk processes. Assess the intended and actual implementation of the process to identify variations or potential "failure modes", and report information to the clinical board for action.
- Communication of identified failure modes and potential impact on patient care/safety among departments/services when opportunities for improvement are multidisciplinary.
- Identified problems are tracked to assure improvement or resolution through redesign of the process.
- Information from departments/services related to tested and implemented process findings of discrete performance improvement activities are used to detect trends, opportunities to improve, or potential problems.
- The objectives, scope, organization, and effectiveness of the redesigned processes are evaluated annually and revised as necessary to ensure effectiveness is maintained overtime.

SUMMARY

In this unit, we have learnt about the plan should be communicated to all persons concerned in the organization. Its objectives and course of action must be clearly defined leaving no ambiguity in the minds of those who are responsible for its execution. Planning and budgeting is effective only when the persons involved work in a team spirit and all are committed to the objectives, policies, programs, strategies envisaged in the plan.

Administration of a Hospital Unit and Ward

19 unit

INTRODUCTION

The nursing unit is an integral part of the hospital complex. The hospital is divided into the blocks and each block is divided in wards. A ward is that area of the hospital where all amenities—physical, social and special medical care are made available to make the patient feel at home till they are discharged. In other words, a ward is temporary home for the patients admitted there. Evidently, there is a need to ensure a healthy environment to help in early recovery of the patients and to win their confidence. In each ward there is a nursing unit to take care of the patients for all the 24 hours.

ADMINISTRATION OF THE HOSPITAL UNIT/WARD

The nursing superintendent is responsible to the administration for planning organization and development of nursing services in the hospital. He/she is the administrative incharge of the nursing department of the hospital and will ensure smooth functioning of all the nursing services in the hospital and mini units. There are following function maintaining by the nursing superintendent.

- To implement hospital/center policies in the various nursing units.
- Recommend personnel and material requirement for nursing and various nursing service departments of the hospital.
- Take regular rounds of the hospital wards.
- Responsible for high standards of nursing care and behavior towards all patients admitted in the hospital.
- To organize, direct and supervise day, evening and night nursing services for competent nursing care.
- To continuously analyze and evaluate the nursing services.

- Initiate and encourage research in nursing services.
- Evaluate confidential reports of her subordinate staff and recommend for higher studies, etc.
- To educate the supporting staff by programs conducting continuing nursing education for the nursing staff of the hospital.
- To provide awareness regarding cleanliness as part of infection control.

PHYSICAL LAYOUT OF THE HOSPITAL

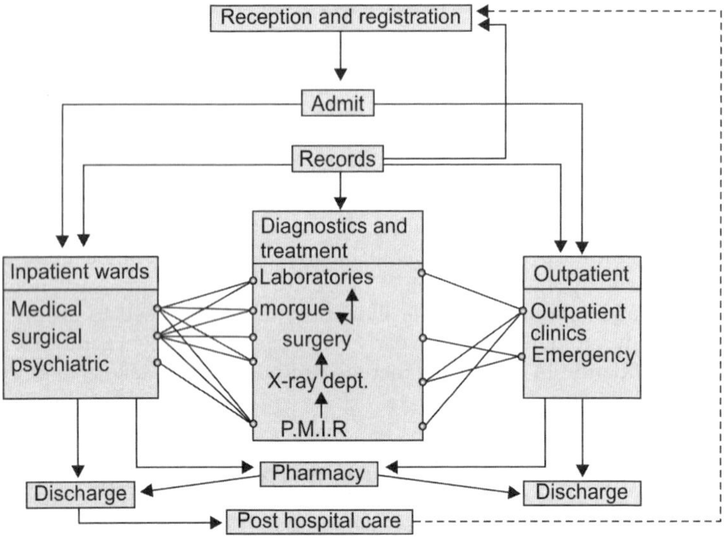

Fig. 19.1: Major clinical relationships

SAFETY MEASURES IN THE HOSPITAL

Healthcare waste management policies or plans should include provision for the continuous monitoring of workers health and safety to ensure that correct handling, treatment, storage, and disposal procedures are being followed. Essential occupational health and safety measures include the following:

- Proper training of workers
- Provision of equipment and clothing for personal protection
- Establishment of an effective occupational health program that includes immunization, post-exposure prophylactic treatment, and medical surveillance.

Training in health and safety should ensure that workers know of and understand the potential risks associated with healthcare waste, the value of immunization against viral hepatitis B, and the importance of consistent use of personal protection equipment.

Workers at risk include healthcare providers, hospital cleaners, maintenance workers, operators of waste treatment equipment, and all operators involved in waste handling and disposal within and outside healthcare establishments.

Workers Protection

The production, segregation, transportation, treatment, and disposal of healthcare waste involve the handling of potentially hazardous material.

- Protection against personal injury is therefore essential for all workers who are at risk. The individuals responsible for management of healthcare waste should ensure that all risks are identified and that suitable protection from those risks is provided.
- A comprehensive risk assessment of all activities involved in healthcare waste management, carried out during preparation of the waste management plan, will allow the identification of necessary protection measures.

Protective Clothing

The type of protective clothing used will depend to an extent upon the risk associated with the healthcare waste, but the following should be made available to all personnel who collect or handle healthcare waste:

- Helmets, with or without visors depending on the operation
- Face masks depending on operation
- Eye protectors (safety goggles) depending on operation
- Overalls (coveralls) obligatory
- Industrial aprons obligatory
- Leg protectors and/or industrial boots obligatory
- Disposable gloves (medical staff) or heavy-duty gloves (waste workers) obligatory.

Industrial boots and heavy-duty gloves are particularly important for waste workers. The thick soles of the boots offer protection in the storage area, as a precaution from spilled sharps, and where doors are slippery.

If segregation is inadequate, needles or other sharp items may have been placed in plastic bags; such items may also pierce thin-walled or weak plastic containers. If it is likely that healthcare waste bags will come into contact with workers legs during handling, leg protectors may also need to be worn.

Personal Hygiene

Basic personal hygiene is important for reducing the risks from handling healthcare waste, and convenient washing facilities (with warm water and soap) should be available for personnel involved in the task. This is of particular importance at storage and incineration facilities.

Immunization

Viral hepatitis B infections have been reported among healthcare personnel and waste handlers, and immunization against the disease is therefore recommended. Tetanus immunization is also recommended for all personnel handling waste.

Management Practices

- Many of the management practices recommended to a reduction in risk for personnel who handle healthcare waste; these are summarized as follows:
  - *Waste segregation:* careful separation of different types of waste into different and distinct containers the risk linked to each waste package.
  - *Appropriate packaging:* prevents spillage of waste and protects workers from contact with waste.
  - *Waste identification (through distinct packaging and labelling):* allows for easy recognition of the class of waste and of its source.
  - *Appropriate waste storage:* limits the access to authorized individuals only, protects against infestation by insects and rodents, and prevents contamination of surrounding areas.
  - *Appropriate transportation:* reduces risks of workers being exposed to waste.
  - *Special precautions for clearing up spillages of potentially hazardous substances:* For clearing up spillages of body fluids or other potentially hazardous substances, particularly if there is any risk of splashing, eye protectors and masks should be worn, in addition to gloves and overalls. Respirators (gas masks) are also needed if an activity is particularly dangerous, for example if it involves toxic dusts, the clearance of incinerator residues, or the cleaning of contaminated equipment.
  - *Response to injury and exposure:* A program of response should be established that prescribes the actions to be taken in the event of injury or exposure to a hazardous substance. All staff who handles healthcare waste should be trained to deal with injuries and exposures. The program should include the following elements:
    - Immediate first-aid measures, such as cleansing of wounds and skin, and irrigation (splashing) of eyes with clean water.

- An immediate report of the incident to a designated responsible person.
- Retention, if possible, of the item involved in the incident; details of its source for identification of possible infection.
- Additional medical attention in an accident and emergency or occupational health department, as soon as possible.
- Medical surveillance.
- Blood or other tests if indicated.
- Recording of the incident.
- Investigation of the incident, and identification and implementation of remedial action to prevent similar incidents in the future.

In case of a needle stick injury, bleeding of the wound should be encouraged and the area should be washed under clean running water. The remaining elements of the accident response plan should then be followed.

The purpose of incident reporting should not be seen as punitive; active support by managers should encourage prompt and accurate reporting.

Cytotoxic Safety

The senior pharmacist of the healthcare establishment should be designated to ensure safe use of cytotoxic drugs. Large oncological hospitals may appoint a full-time Genotoxic Safety Officer, who should also supervise the safe management of cytotoxic waste. The following key measures are essential in minimizing exposure:

- Written procedures that specify safe working methods for each process.
- Data sheets based on the suppliers specifications, to provide information on potential hazards.
- Established procedure for emergency response in case of spillage or other occupational accident.
- Appropriate education and training for all personnel involved in the handling of cytotoxic drugs.

These measures are unlikely to be needed in rural or urban district hospitals of middle- and low-income countries, which do not typically use genotoxic products, either cytotoxic or radioactive. In countries where the safe use of cytotoxic and radioactive materials is difficult to ensure, it maybe advisable for use of those substances to be limited to a small number of specialized (e.g. oncological) hospitals, that are better able to implement appropriate safety measures.

In hospitals that do use cytotoxic products, specific guidelines on their safe handling should be established for the protection of personnel.

These guidelines should include rules on the following waste handling procedures:

- Separate collection of waste in leak-proof bags or containers, and labelling for identification.
- Return of outdated drugs to suppliers.
- Safe storage separately from other healthcare waste; ¥ provisions for the disposal of contaminated material, for the decontamination of reusable equipment, and for the treatment of spillages.
- Provisions for the treatment of infectious waste contaminated with cytotoxic products, including excreta from patients and disposable linen used for incontinent patients.
- Hospital staff should ensure that the families of patients undergoing chemotherapy at home are aware of the risks and know how they can be minimized or avoided.
- Minimal protective measures for all waste workers who handle cytotoxic waste should include protective clothing, gloves, goggles, and masks.

PREVENTION OF ACCIDENTS

Hospitals are supposed to be institutions that will help people recuperate, treat any illness that they have, and ease away any pain. Unfortunately, there are circumstances when hospitals can bring people even more misfortune. There are a few common accidents that also happen within the hospital vicinity and put people's life at risk or more prone to danger. Needless to say, hospitals should be the safest places you can go to but in reality, there are still threats and harms you can encounter inside.

Hospitals have a very busy and hectic environment. There are patients and medical professionals moving around all the time. There are deliveries being made left and right. Equipment is transferred from one room to another. On top of it all, there is a cleaning routine that happens all around the hospital 24/7. With such busy and hectic environment, accidents and work injuries are inevitable. It can be sustained by visitors, patients, and even the doctors themselves—everyone is at risk. Here are some of the most common accidents and injuries you need to watch out for if you work or if you visit the hospital:

Faulty Equipment

- Despite how advanced and modern medical equipment is nowadays, it is not 100% perfect. There are still chances of it becoming faulty and there will be times when it will fail to operate properly. Patients are more at risk of injuries brought about by faulty equipment. Therefore, it is a must for medical practitioners to always check if the equipment is fully operational and well-functioning.

Slipping and Tripping

Another common accident that can happen in hospitals is slipping and tripping on wet floors. Because there is a cleaning routine that happens 24/7, it is inevitable that there will be wet floors in some areas. Furthermore, areas where there are water systems such as the operating room and the restroom can have water spillage on the floor which can make anyone stepping on that floor slip or trip.

Food Poisoning

Hospitals have their own nutritionists and dieticians who plan the menu for each patient and the food they serve in the canteen. Unfortunately, for some hospitals, food poisoning can still occur despite having such people to plan the menu. The environment and sources of ingredients are factors that come into play which can result to food poisoning.

Hospital Infection

Because almost everyone you will encounter in the hospital is infected with some virus or bacteria, you are at high-risk of acquiring an infection as well. This is more prevalent in hospitals where proper sanitation and proper disposal of used medical devices are not priority. This is why hospitals must employ a 24/7 cleaning routine and ask all staff and medical practitioners as well as visitors and patients to always wash their hands.

Even hospitals are not 100% safe from any injuries. People working and visiting hospitals can still incur injuries. This is why we need to keep hospitals clean at all times, check all equipment, keep the floor dry at all times, and make sure that food served are always clean and fresh.

PREVENTING TRANSMISSION OF INFECTION

Preventive practice focuses on interrupting the transmission of an infectious agent and includes four major elements. Practices will vary according to practice setting, the level of care that is being provided, and the inherent risk to the client and client population if transmission occurs. The four major elements to preventive practice are:

Handwashing

Handwashing is the single most important infection prevention and control practice. It is vital that nurses follow handwashing protocols that are appropriate for their clients and facility.

Protective Barriers

Examples of protective barriers include gloves, masks, eyewear, gowns and plastic aprons. The appropriate barrier should be used when blood, secretions or bodily fluids are likely to come in contact with the nurse's skin or mucous membranes, or could penetrate clothing.

Care of Equipment

This involves the appropriate disposal of waste, contaminated laundry and sharps; and the cleaning, sterilization and disinfection of equipment, instruments and devices. Nurses should follow manufacturer and facility protocols in all instances.

Health Practices of the Nurse

Nurses who believe they have been contaminated with an infectious agent should contact their primary health care provider or an occupational health department for follow-up and advice. The nurse should assess the risk of transmitting the infectious agent to others and take appropriate precautions. Nurses should also know and review their immunization status with their primary health care provider.

LEGAL RESPONSIBILITIES OF A NURSE

Nurses have to abide by laws and regulations when practicing nursing. All of the regulations and legal aspects of nursing are taught and explained to nurses throughout nursing school. Not abiding by the code of ethics could cost the nurse his or her nursing license and result in a malpractice suit.

Nurse Practice Act

Every state has a nurse practice act, which states all the guidelines and laws for the nurses who are licensed to practice in the state. The act includes the limitations and training specifications of each nurse. This means that each nurse has been trained in a specific area of nursing; therefore, the nurse must practice in that area only. If a nurse is not trained to administer medication or treatment to a patient, the nurse is not permitted to do so. The nurse must consult with a physician or other nursing authority when a situation arises that the nurse is not certified to handle. Any wrong doing is a violation of this act, and the nurse may lose his or her nursing license, as well as having a suit filed against him or her or the health care agency or hospital.

Patient Advocate

A nurse has the legal responsibility to be the advocate for the patient in all health care instances, including emergencies. The nurse will be the liaison between the physician and the patient. The nurse has the legal duty to monitor the patient and watch for any abnormalities or complications that may occur. If any occur, the nurse must access a physician to provide immediate care for the patient.

Administering Medication

Any nurse who is certified to administer medication to a patient must do so accurately and timely. The nurse has the legal responsibility to interpret the charts and files of a patient and to understand what allergic reactions patients may or may not have to a certain medication. If a nurse does not administer the correct dosage or medication to a patient, the patient could suffer major health risks or even death. This is grounds for a malpractice suit against the nurse and health care facility.

Patient Neglect

The nurse will provide care for the patient he or she is monitoring at all times. If the patient needs assistance with any issues, such as hygiene, the nurse has the legal responsibility to assist the patient. If a nurse does not monitor and provide care to the patient, this can be considered patient neglect, which is unethical and illegal. The patient may try to move and use the restroom on his or her own and maybe physically injured in the process. Some patients may harm themselves while under the influence of medication, which should not happen if the nurse is paying proper attention to his or her patient.

Consent Forms

Nurses have the legal responsibility to explain all treatment, medications and lab results to patients or authorized family members of patients. Before a patient may undergo surgery, he or she will need to sign a consent form. If the nurse is administering the treatment, such as anesthesia, it is the nurse's legal obligation to explain the negatives and positives of the anesthesia. The patient or family member must then sign a consent form acknowledging that the patient understands the procedure. If this form is not signed and complications occur, the nurse may face legal consequences.

JOB DESCRIPTION

- *Post title:* Advanced Nurse Practitioner

- *Department:* Nursing
- *Location:* All ridge sites
- *Grade:* Equivalent to Band 8A agenda for change
- *Hours:* Full or part time
- *Accountable to:* Business manager and clinical services development nurse manager.
- *Responsible to:* Clinical services development nurse manager for clinical issues and business manager for managerial issues.

Job Purpose

- To act as an autonomous practitioner working independently and in conjunction with other health care professionals to assess, diagnose and treat the conditions of patients attending within primary care initiating direct referrals as appropriate.
- To provide expert professional advice to patients, carers and colleagues and ensure the maintenance of clinical excellence.
- To develop new and innovative concepts, models, methods and practices to deliver new and improved primary care services to meet the needs of the practice and PCT population.
- To provide education and training to other staff and students.
- To undertake research as part of the role.

Primary Duties and Areas of Responsibilities

Key Role Clinical Nursing Practice

The advanced nurse practitioner works autonomously and is accountable for own professional actions.

- Undertakes clinical nursing practice at an advanced level using expert knowledge and clinical skills to deliver holistic care to people accessing primary health care services.
- Assesses diagnoses and treats patients attending primary health care services with a range of acute, non acute and chronic medical conditions.
- Assesses diagnoses and treats patients in surgery or own home who require acute medical attention and refer to appropriate agency.
- Directly admits patients to secondary care hospital in acute medical need.
- Refers patients to other medical specialities for assessment if deemed appropriate.
- Refers patients as appropriate to other members of the multidisciplinary team, secondary care and to other statutory and voluntary organizations including referral for X-ray.

- It has undertaken X-ray training as required by hospitals trust.
- Undertakes and interprets a range of diagnostic tests and routine clinical procedures, e.g. cytology, venepuncture, blood pressure monitoring, etc.
- Makes critical judgments of the highest order to satisfy the expectations and demands of the job, e.g. first contact with patients presenting acutely and manages care in the presence and absence of protocols.
- Makes decisions where precedents do not exist, where appropriate without recourse to others, e.g. direct referral of patients to hospital consultants without prior reference to other medical colleagues.
- Advises and supports others where standard protocols do not apply.
- Works within professional guidelines and codes of conduct.
- Works within all relevant practice policies and procedural guidelines, e.g. infection control, chaperoning, risk management.
- Extended and supplementary prescriber.

Key Role Care and Program Management

- Develops and manages highly specialized programs of care and care packages and provides highly specialized advice concerning care normally beyond the scope of normal nursing practice, e.g. establishes differential diagnoses, management/treatment plans and makes referrals as appropriate. Makes fast track referrals.
- Communicates highly sensitive condition related information to patients, relatives and carers.
- Initiates the process of diagnosis with patients suspected to have a chronic disease, e.g. diabetes, COPD, asthma, IHD referring to other clinical staff as appropriate.
- Contribute to practice targets both local and national within the disease management agenda, e.g. QOF, prescribing incentive scheme, NSFs, National benchmarking.
- Contributes to disease registers.
- Audits outcomes of care against standards and initiate changes as necessary.
- Undertakes annual review of patients' understanding and ability to self-manage.
- Refers to other members of the extended primary health care team as appropriate, e.g. chiropodist, dietician, specialist nurses.

Key Role Strategic Development of Primary Care Services

- Contributes to the strategic development of primary care and public health services to meet patient and population needs within the practice and across the wider organization. Works/liaises across multi-professional and agency boundaries.

- Works at the forefront of practice innovation. Determines how to deal with ambiguous or unique problems to develop and advance primary care services for the benefit of patients, carers and communities.
- Recognition and involvement in the ridge medical practice as a teaching unit and help drive the nursing element of training.
- Develop links within the PCT and other local and national bodies relevant to primary care nursing initiatives, e.g. national wipp project.

Key Role Health Improvement

- Initiates and carries out programs of health screening and ensures other team members are aware of health agendas and screening programs.
- Introduces innovation in practice to meet on going health need demands of the practice.
- Works to introduce new developments that will improve health outcomes for patients and is able to demonstrate through written and presentation these developments, i.e. sexual health agenda.
- Shares innovation with others.
- Supports practitioners in profiling the practice population in order to initiate contribute and promote improved health and prevent disease in individuals and groups.
- Represents individuals and families interests when they are not able to do so themselves.
- Makes referrals to statutory and voluntary agencies as appropriate.

Key Role Communication

- Provides and receives highly complex, sensitive or contentious information and frequently deals with situations which are hostile or emotive.
- Uses developed communication, negotiation, conflict management skills which require empathy, reassurance and persuasive skills where there can be significant barriers to acceptance which need to be overcome.
- Regularly communicates service related information to partners, business manager, salaried GP's, nursing and administrative staff, patients, relatives and carers.
- Makes operational judgments, manages conflicting views and reconciles inter and intra professional differences of opinion.
- Builds and communicates therapeutic working relationships with a wide array of statutory and voluntary organizations for the benefit of patient care and facilitates good working relationships.

- Develops and delivers presentations to large groups, e.g. local and national conferences, clinical meetings, empowers staff to develop presentation skills in order to promote good practice.

Key Role Manage/lead Self/others

- Develops a leadership role within the practice.
- Encourage and motivate others to be forward thinking in ideas that address the health needs of the practice that will be innovative whilst managing and developing new ways of working, e.g. Implanon clinic, teenage heath clinic.
- Develops and leads on evidence based practice.
- Promotes effective communication and relationships within the team.
- Partakes in clinical supervision for own development.
- Actively participates in clinical and practice meetings.
- Develops own knowledge and practice to meet objectives/changes in service.
- Integrates theory into practice and establishes formal links with educational institutions.
- Assists in the mentorship and assessment of trainee nurse practitioners.
- Acts as mentor for pre registration students and other staff within the practice.
- Leads on setting standards and promotes best practice.
- Operates high standards of probity.

Key Role Influence and Develop Policy

- Responsible for establishing how policies should be interpreted and translated within the practice.
- Implements local/national, PCT and practice policies, proposes developments and improvements to service delivery.

Key Role Manage and Use Information

- Makes effective use of the clinical system by ensuring the consistent and accurate entering of data and use of read codes.
- Facilitates the use of up to date information technology in order to collate accurate and timely information as and when required by the practice.
- Ensures a satisfactory call and recall system of patients.
- Assist in the development of practice protocols for the surgery and clinical protocols for the clinical team.

- Identifies monitors and reviews deficiencies in procedures and implements remedial action.

Key Role Research and Development

- Continuous involvement in research/evaluation and/or development work which maybe as part of one or more formal research programs or activities.
- Actively contributes to practice/service/team audit/research activity as required.
- Instigates audit activity as required, e.g. new services.
- Identifies, applies and disseminates research findings relating to clinical practice.

Working Conditions

- Frequent exposure to body fluids, blood, wounds, fleas and lice.
- Occasional exposure to aggressive behavior.
- Frequent use of VDU equipment.
- Frequent requirement to travel between different locations.

Terms and Conditions of Service

- *Salary:* £ per annum.
- *Method of payment:* Monthly by Bank credit transfer
- *Hours of work:* To be discussed.
- *Superannuation:* This post is optionally super annuable.
- *Health assessment:* This post is subject to a satisfactory pre-employment health assessment.
- *Terms and conditions:* All terms will be agreed by the practice and maybe amended from time to time. Successful applicants will be required to complete a Criminal Records Bureau (Disclosure) application form.

Rehabilitation of Offenders Act 1974

Because of the nature of this work, this post is exempt from the provisions of section (42) of the Rehabilitation of Offenders Act 1974 (exemptions) Order 1975. Applicants for this post are not entitled to withhold information about convictions which for other purposes are 'spent' under the provisions of the act and in the event of employment, any failure to disclose such convictions could result in disciplinary action or dismissal. Any information given will be completely confidential and will be considered only in relation to an application for a position to which this order applies.

Data Protection Act

All members of staff are bound by the requirements of the data protection act 1998 and any breaches of the act or of the confidential nature of the work of this post could lead to dismissal.

General

- *Health and safety/risk management:* The post holder must comply at all times with the PCT's health and safety policies, in particular by following agreed safe working procedures and reporting incidents using the PCT's risk incident reporting system.
- *Equality and diversity:* The post holder must cooperate with all policies and procedures designed to ensure equality of employment. Co-workers, patients and visitors must be treated equally irrespective of gender, ethnic origin, age, disability, sexual orientation, religion, etc.
- *Training and personal development:* The post holder must take responsibility in agreement with his/her line manager for his/her own personal development by ensuring that continuous professional development remains a priority. The post holder will undertake all mandatory training required for the role.
- *Respect for Patient Confidentiality:* The post holder should respect patient confidentiality at all times and not divulge patient information unless sanctioned by the requirements of the role.

JOB SPECIFICATION

Job title: Advanced nurse practitioner.

Main purpose of post: An autonomous practitioner working independently of and in conjunction with other health care professionals to assess, diagnose and treat the conditions of patients attending within primary care initiating direct referrals as appropriate.

Attributes	Essential	Desirable	How identified
Qualifications	• RN/RM • MSc in nurse practitioner studies, plus supplementary post graduate level courses: Extended and supplementary nurse prescriber. • Teaching and assessing in clinical practice. • Counseling skills.		Nursing council registration check Professional portfolio

Contd...

Contd...

Attributes	Essential	Desirable	How identified
Special knowledge/experience/competences	• Minimum of 3 years post MSc nurse practitioner studies experience within the clinical field. • Demonstrate the application of evidenced based practice. • Able to demonstrate a depth and breadth of current issues and policies within the NHS and have the ability to translate into practice • Experience in leadership role and change management. • Autonomous practitioner working independently and in conjunction with other health care professionals. • Very high level of clinical skills and competency relevant to the role. • Understanding and experience of interagency working and adult/child protection. • Evidence of teaching/mentoring students/groups • Evidence of continued professional development. • Experience of clinical governance and risk assessment		Application form Interview References
Practical and intellectual skills	• Able to communicate highly complex, highly sensitive and/or contentious information, including where there are barriers to understanding. • Demonstrate high level of self-awareness, i.e. strengths and weaknesses, personal qualities and skills. • IT skills. • Able to organize and present seminars, workshops or teaching sessions.		Application form Interview

Contd...

Contd...

Attributes	Essential	Desirable	How identified
	• Able to communicate with a wide range of people at all levels of the organization. • Demonstrate leadership behavior in a variety of settings, i.e. strategically and corporately. • Competent prescriber. • Evidence of innovation in practice.		
Analytical and Judgmental Skills	• Able to understand highly complex situations/ information, e.g. working with patients with acute, non acute and chronic illnesses and using a range of skills to decide the best course of action from a range of options and consider the implications of each of these. • Be able to manage clinical uncertainty • Be able to manage conflict.		
Planning and organizational skills	• Able to plan and organize own time and workload and cope with last minute changes. • Organizing others work patterns to meet changing demands in practice.		
Training and education	• Provide education and training to other staff and students. • Work with educational institutions in developing and delivering educational programs • Conduct research in specialist area. • Willingness to undergo education/training for both practice and service need. • Willingness to work towards professional and performance objectives (appraisal).		Application form Interview References

Contd...

Contd...

Attributes	Essential	Desirable	How identified
Deposition/ Personal	• Demonstrates motivation, reliability and commitment to team working and development of others. • Flexibility, commitment and adaptability. • Can demonstrate an ability to value others opinions.		Application form Interview References
Physical Skills	• Fitness to do the job. Able to work within Manual Handling Policy. • Advanced keyboard skills. • Highly developed physical skills requiring dexterity and accuracy. • Hepatitis-B immune or willing to undergo immunization course.		Health screening
Mental and emotional effort	• Frequent periods of concentration. Work pattern unpredictable and multi-tasking required. • Occasional requirement for prolonged concentration. • Occasionally required to work outside normal working hours. • Able to deal with exposure to distressing circumstances, or highly emotional events. • Able to cope with exposure to aggressive behavior.		

JOB ANALYSIS

Job analysis is the foundation for all assessment and selection decisions. To identify the best person for the job, it is crucial to fully understand the nature of that job. Job analysis provides a way to develop this understanding by examining the tasks performed in a job, the competencies required to perform those tasks, and the connection between the tasks and competencies.'

Definitions of Job Analysis

- *Harry L Wylie* 'Job analysis deals with the anatomy of the job..... This is the complete study of the job embodying every known and determinable factor, including the duties and responsibilities involved in its performance; the conditions under which performance is carried on; the nature of the task; the qualifications required in the worker; and the conditions of employment such as pay, hours, opportunities and privileges'.

- In the words of *Dale Yoder,* 'A Job is a collection of duties, tasks and responsibilities which are assigned to an individual and which is different from other assignment'.
- According to *Michael J Jucius,* 'Job analysis refers to the process of studying the operations, duties and organizational aspects of jobs in order to derive specification or, as they are called by some job description'.
- In the words of *Edwin B Flippo,* 'Job analysis is the process of studying and collecting information relating to the operations and responsibilities of a specific job'.
- *According to Blum,* 'A job analysis is an accurate study of the various components of a job. It is concerned not only with an analysis of the duties and conditions of work, but also with the individual qualifications of the worker'.
- According to *John A Shubin,* 'Job analysis is the methodical compilation and study of work data in order to define and characterize each occupation in such a manner as to distinguish it from all others'.
- In the words of *Scott, Clothier and Spriegel,* 'Job analysis is the process of critically evaluating the operations, duties and relationship of the job'.
- In simple words Job analysis is a formal program which examines the tasks, duties and responsibilities contained in an individual unit of work.

Steps Involved in Job Analysis or Job Analysis Process

Job analysis is a process of collecting information related to various aspects of the job. It collects and analyzes the information associated with job description and specifications. Following steps are involved in job analysis:

- *Information collection:* This is the first step of job analysis under which required information related to various aspects of jobs are collected. Information is obtained through different methods such as interview, observation, questionnaire, critical incidents, etc. It is associated with preparation of plans and programs and assignment of responsibilities to the concerned person.
- *Review background information:* This is the second step of job analysis process under which the previously collected information is reviewed to design organizational charts, current position descriptions and

specifications, procedures, manuals and process charts. These help in detailed assessment of job.

- *Selection of representative position to be analyzed:* Analyzing all jobs at a time is complex and costly affair. So, only a representative sample of jobs is selected for the purpose of detailed analysis. Under it, the job analyst investigates to determine which organization managers or employees require job analysis. He should also determine for what purpose the job must be analyzed.
- *Analysis of jon by collecting data:* Under this step of job analysis process, a job analyst obtains the data and information related to the selected jobs. The information is collected on the job activities, required employee behaviors, working conditions, human traits and qualities, abilities of performing the job and other various dimension of the job. Data can be collected either through questionnaire, observation or interviews.
- *Develop job description:* In this step of job analysis, a job description schedule is developed through the information collected in the above step. This is the written statement which describes the prominent characteristics of job along with duties, location and degree of risk involved in each job.
- *Develop job specification:* Developing the job specification is the last step of job analysis process under which a detailed specification statement is prepared showing minimum requirement of each job. A job specification summarizes the personal qualities, traits, skills, knowledge, and background required to perform specific task. It also involves the physical and psychological attributes of the incumbent.

Importance of Job Analysis

- *Organizational structure and design:* Job analysis helps the organization to make suitable changes in the organizational structure, so that it matches the needs and requirements of the organization. Duties are either added or deleted from the job.
- *Recruitment and selection:* Job analysis provides information about what the job entails and what human characteristics are required to perform these activities. This information, in the form of job descriptions and specifications, helps management decide what sort of people to recruit and hire.
- *Performance appraisal and training/development:* Based on the job requirements identified in the job analysis, the company decides a training program. Training is given in those areas which will help to improve the performance on the job. Similarly when appraisal is conducted we check whether the employee is able to work in a manner in which we require him to do the job.

- *Job evaluation:* Job evaluation refers to studying in detail the job performance by all individual. The difficulty levels, skills required and on that basis the salary is fixed. Information regarding qualities required, skilled levels, difficulty levels is obtained from job analysis.
- *Promotions and transfer:* When we give a promotion to an employee we need to promote him on the basis of the skill and talent required for the future job. Similarly when we transfer an employee to another branch the job must be very similar to what he has done before. To take these decisions we collect information from job analysis.
- *Career path planning:* Many companies have not taken up career planning for their employees. This is done to prevent the employee from leaving the company. When we plan the future career of the employee, information will be collected from job analysis. Hence, job analysis becomes important or advantageous.
- *Labor relations:* When companies plan to add extra duties or delete certain duties from a job, they require the help of job analysis, when this activity is systematically done using job analysis the number of problems with union members reduce and labor relations will improve.
- *Health and safety:* Most companies prepare their own health and safety, plans and programs based on job analysis. From the job analysis company identifies the risk factor on the job and based on the risk factor safety equipments are provided.
- *Acceptance of job offer:* When a person is given an offer/appointment letter the duties to be performed by him are clearly mentioned in it, this information is collected from job analysis, which is why job analysis becomes important.

JOB SATISFACTION

A job specification describes the knowledge, skills, education, experience, and abilities you believe are essential to performing a particular job. The job specification is developed from the job analysis. Ideally, also developed from a detailed job description, the job specification describes the person you want to hire for a particular job.

A job specification cuts to the quick with your requirements whereas the job description defines the duties and requirements of an employee's job in detail. The job specification provides detailed characteristics, knowledge, education, skills, and experience needed to perform the job, with an overview of the specific job requirements.

Components of a Job Specification

- *Experience:* Number of years of experience in the job you are seeking to fill. Number of years of work experience required for the selected candidate. Note whether the position requires progressively more complex and responsible experience, and supervisory or managerial experience.

- *Education:* State what degrees, training, or certifications are required for the position.
- *Required skills, knowledge and characteristics:* State the skills, knowledge, and personal characteristics of individuals who have successfully performed this job. Or, use the job analysis data to determine the attributes you need from your "ideal" candidate. Your recruiting planning meeting or email participants can also help determine these requirements for the job specification.
- *High level overview of job requirements:* In less than ten bullet points, cite the key components and requirements of the job you are filling. A job specification is useful for recruiting as it helps you write your job postings and your website recruiting material. The job specification is also useful for distribution in social media, for screening resumes, and for interviewers.

Ways to Increase the Employee's Satisfaction

There are seven simple ways to inspire employees and increase satisfaction:

a. *Employee orientation:* One of the best ways to have satisfied employees is to make sure they are pleased from the get-go. Offering a thorough orientation will ensure expectations are realistic and that new staffers do not come in with rose-colored glasses that will quickly fade. Proper on boarding encourages positive attitudes and can reduce turnover.
b. *Positive work environment:* An upbeat workplace is a necessity. If the workspace is not positive, you can not expect the workers to be. Encouraging one another, avoiding micromanagement, giving positive feedback and ensuring criticism is constructive are all ways to keep the environment a place where employees can do more than survive—they can thrive.
c. *Provide competitive benefits:* Fair wages are important, but competitive benefits are also critical to keeping your workforce satisfied. If your benefits package is thin, employees may look for other opportunities with firms that are more generous. Beyond insurance, benefits such as flex time, paid holidays and personal days are important factors to employee satisfaction.
d. *Workforce engagement:* Employees that do not find their work interesting or do not feel they are contributing to the mission of the firm will not be engaged. For employees to be satisfied, they must feel like they are part of something bigger than just what their individual

work tasks are. Include staffers in goal setting and how they fit in the corporation fabric to increase engagement and satisfaction.

e. *Develop skills:* Everyone needs something to working toward. Stagnation is unfulfilling. Employees have more potential than their current level of functionality. Encouraging employees to fulfill that potential will increase engagement and satisfaction. Whether it is training opportunities, mentoring, online courses or external training, encourage staff to always be improving their skills.
f. *Recognition and rewards:* Employees need not be a public show to mean something to employees. Encourage supervisors and managers to acknowledge employees deeds on a daily basis. Also implement a formal program company-wide to recognize top achievers in every job category. Healthy competition can boost morale, encourage hard work and increase satisfaction and retention.
g. *Track job satisfaction:* Do not sit back and just hope that employees are satisfied—put some data behind it. Offer anonymous online surveys or mobile surveys to effectively track how employees feel about benefits, recognition, supervisor feedback and other aspects that contribute to employee satisfaction.

Staff Development and Staff Welfare

The key responsibilities for Staff Health and Welfare Division is to provide quality and timely health and welfare services; consultations, referral and advice to the nursing staff and their dependents designed to assist staff to avoid interruption on their jobs and to prevent conditions (physical, mental or social) that will keep staff away from giving their full attention to their work. This is principally done through preventive; early detection, curative, counseling and welfare services. The division's health center provides emergencies and first aid care in addition to limited health care services. The division is responsible for overseeing specialized medical evacuations, pre-employment physicals, workability examinations, and work-related injury and illness assessments.

Activities of Staff Welfare

- Develop, review, establish and implement health, safety and welfare policies, systems, and strategies that assure a safe, health and conductive working environment.
- Provide medical consultations, nursing care; clinical laboratory services and treatment; and ensure a safe working environment for the staff as per current regulations and guidelines.
- Provide information and counsel on health, safety and welfare to assist employees in their work lives thereby providing an environment that optimizes work performance and productivity.

- Ensure timely implementation of quality health and welfare services within approved policies, guidelines and procedures.
- Develop, review existing practices and propose new policies and strategies health and welfare in hospital.
- Provide a safe working environment and minimize occupational hazards to all persons working with the hospital.
- Promote and provide preventive health care programs (including vaccinations; immunizations, etc.) and undertake periodic health assessment of staff and their recognized dependants for early detection and prevention of illnesses.
- Develop and provide a comprehensive social welfare package including counseling; stress management; post recovery and settling in services.
- Undertake research and investigation in the different kinds of occupational hazards befalling staff from time to time and take appropriate measures to correct them and set in motion mechanisms to prevent their recurrence.

Staff Development Programs

To enhance growth, development and competence of professional and general grades staff and to meet new service requirements through organizing and coordinating short courses delivered in classroom, e-learning and blended modes, seminars, workshops, overseas training courses and attachment and local part-time courses at tertiary institutes covering a wide range of topics and areas of concern including:

Training on Rehabilitation and Medical Social Services

- Understanding and managing different mental problems of children and adolescents assessing and managing the rehabilitation needs of mentally incapacitated persons and implementing the statutory duties of mental health ordinance.
- Understanding and implementing the medical fee waiving mechanism.
- Strengthening the understanding on infection control and common infectious diseases for staff of residential care home for persons with disabilities.
- Understanding and managing the standardized assessment tool for residential services for people with disabilities.

Training on services for offenders

- Understanding the operation and skills required for community-based rehabilitation, including probation service and community service orders scheme, etc.
- Understanding correctional home services for young offender.

Training on children and families welfare services

- Multi-skills training on working with individual and families in crisis or encountering physical, psychosocial and interpersonal problems.
- Knowledge and skills in handling domestic violence, child abuse and sexual violence cases and providing counseling to victims, batterers/abusers and their family members.
- Knowledge and skills in working with young children.

Training on elderly services

- Understanding the physiological, psychological, emotional and social needs of the elderly and acquiring skills in providing counseling to elders.
- Understanding dementia and taking care of the demented elders.
- Multi-skilled training in taking care of elders.

Training on Youth Services

- Volunteer service management.
- Understanding the physiological, psychological and emotional problems of young people and acquiring relevant counseling skills.
- Understanding the developmental and preventive educational programs and the service strategies and skills in dealing with young people and their families.

LEADERSHIP STYLE

Leadership can be defined as a multifaceted process of identifying a goal or target, motivating other people to act, and providing support and motivation to achieve mutually negotiated goals (Porter-O'Grady, 2003). In the daily life of a senior nurse, this could refer to coordinating the day/night shift and the team of nurses and support staff on duty under the direction of that nurse.

The successful operation of the shift, staff morale and managing difficult or challenging situations depends largely on the senior nurse's leadership skills.

It is important to appreciate that leadership roles are different from management functions. In Stephen Covey's (1999) book The Seven Habits of Highly Effective People, he quoted Peter Drucker as saying: 'Management is doing things right; leadership is doing the right things. Management is efficiency in climbing the ladder of success; leadership is about determining whether the ladder is leaning against the right wall.' This suggests that management is about tasks, whereas leadership is about perception, judgment, skill and philosophy. We could infer from this that it is much more difficult to be an effective leader than an effective manager.

Characteristics of an Effective Leader

- Leaders are often described as being visionary, equipped with strategies, a plan and desire to direct their teams and services to a future goal.
- Effective leaders are required to use problem-solving processes, maintain group effectiveness and develop group identification.
- They should also be dynamic, passionate, have a motivational influence on other people, be solution-focused and seek to inspire others.
- Senior nurses must apply these characteristics to their work in order to win the respect and trust of team members and lead the development of clinical practice.
- By demonstrating an effective leadership style, these nurses will be in a powerful position to influence the successful development of other staff, ensuring that professional standards are maintained and enabling the growth of competent practitioners.
- Leadership for senior nurses is primarily about the following: making decisions; delegating appropriately; resolving conflict; and acting with integrity. The role also involves nurturing others and being aware of how people in the team are feeling by being emotionally in tune with staff.

Political Context

- Nurse leaders need to be able to respond to an ever-changing healthcare environment, including organizational expectations and changes to local and national policy. I do not know of any clinician or manager who would dispute that nursing roles are changing.
- These roles have become more specialists, autonomous, accountable and focused on outcome, with both positive and negative consequences for the profession. Consumers and purchasers of healthcare services have greater expectations of higher standards, particularly in relation to nursing care.
- Nurse leaders must demonstrate resilience in responding to change and supporting others to embrace this in a positive way.
- Effective leaders should be capable of reframing the thinking of those whom they are leading, enabling them to see that changes are not only imperative but achievable.
- Senior nurses need to find ways of becoming involved in organizational decision-making on issues impacting on clinical care such

as: developing policy; workforce planning; departmental business planning; and clinical and corporate governance.

Leadership Activities of Senior Nurses

- Senior nurses should be able to develop other staff by enabling them to apply theory to practice and encouraging them to test new skills in a safe and supportive environment.
- This, again, is an example of where leadership activities combine with developmental ones to create competent practitioners through practice-based learning.
- These nurses should adopt a supportive leadership style with mentorship, coaching and supervision as core values. Constable and Russell (1986) showed that high levels of support from supervisors reduced emotional exhaustion and buffered negative effects of the job environment. Consequently, it would be particularly beneficial for supervisors to provide emotional support to nurses and give them adequate feedback about performance to increase self-esteem (Bakker et al 2000).
- Senior nurses should also apply leadership skills in encouraging staff to use critical reflection to facilitate new understanding.
- In the ward environment, there can be tensions between professional disciplines. Resolving these and building effective relationships between multidisciplinary team members is a test of senior nurses' leadership abilities. With nurses becoming more autonomous decision-makers, this must inevitably lead to revising the relationship between professional roles.
- Senior nurses also have a leadership role in facilitating their organization's staff support and development program, which should aim to reduce stress, burnout, sickness and absenteeism among colleagues. Supervisors have a significant influence on employees' personal and professional outcomes. Bakker et al (2000) reported that senior nurses can buffer the effects of a demanding work environment on staff nurses by thoughtfully maintaining a leadership style that supports staff needs.
- A successful leader will see each person as an individual, recognizing their unique set of needs, as not everyone will perform at the same level or respond in the same way to environmental stressors or workplace pressure. Leaders need to support staff in ways in which individuals recognize as being useful.
- In the same way, staff will be motivated by different factors. Leaders must focus on the needs of individual staff and use motivational strategies appropriate to each person and situation. They must seek to inspire demotivated staff and maintain the motivation of those

who are already motivated. Leadership seeks to produce necessary changes in demotivated staff by developing a vision of the future and inspiring staff to attain this.
- Leadership is the driving force of the work environment and directly affects staff motivation and morale.

Mentorship

Different people are motivated in different ways, so leaders must use strategies that individuals find motivating to empower them and highlight the importance of the nursing role. One method of achieving this is through structured mentorship. I believe that mentorship should foster ongoing role development and be based on the acquisition and mastery of new skills.

Senior nurses should take time every shift (5–30 minutes) to be involved in some form of mentoring activity, which should then be recorded in staff members' 'learning log'.

The learning log is a simple, task-specific recording method used as documented evidence that mentorship has been given on a particular area of work activity. The staff member participates in the completion of their log, which briefly records:
- The nature of the activity being coached.
- Strengths and weaknesses in performing the activity; coaching intervention; Future goals.

It is important that staff members do not feel micromanaged. Learning logs must be viewed as a mentorship tool, rather than a management one. The log is merely used to remind and refresh the mentor and staff member about what has been achieved between the last formal clinical supervision session and the next. The learning log will be used for reflection purposes to form the basis of a more comprehensive supervision discussion.

Leaders, in their capacity as mentors, must ensure that more junior staff has the freedom to seek information, through an open exchange of opinions and ideas. Staff should also be given the opportunity to show initiative, thus promoting confidence in decision-making and underpinning knowledge and competence in their own skills. The goal of mentorship should be to create a stable and supportive environment which encourages professional growth through effective role modeling.

DEMOCRATIC LEADERSHIP

Democratic leadership is an approach to management in which certain democratic principles are encouraged, such as self-determination, inclusiveness, equal participation and deliberation. While the manager in a group maybe the only one with formal authority, other members of the group can serve leadership functions by influencing other members' beliefs and behaviors. Characteristics of democratic leadership include distribution of responsibility, empowering group members and aiding group decision-making.

Definition

'Democratic leadership in an organization involves the redistribution of power and authority between employees and managers to provide employee involvement in decision-making'.

Features of Democratic Leadership

Democratic leadership attempts to manage with democratic principles, such as self-determination, inclusiveness, equal participation and deliberation. The following three features characterize democratic leadership:

- *Distribution of responsibility:* A manager that leads democratically will distribute responsibility among his group to facilitate participation in decision-making.
- *Empowering group members:* Leaders must empower their members so that the members can accomplish their responsibilities. Empowerment includes providing training and education necessary for delegated task completion.
- *Aiding group decision-making process:* A major role of a democratic leader is to ensure democratic deliberation in making group decisions. This means that a leader should act as a facilitator and mediator between group members and ensure that a psychologically healthy and respectful environment is maintained.

Advantages

Let's talk about some of the advantages. Democratic leadership techniques generally will do a better job creating job satisfaction because it fosters a sense of participation, control and autonomy. Greater employee participation in decision-making may also lead to greater innovation and creative solutions to problems that will better serve an organization.

Disadvantages

A democratic approach to management may not be as efficient as a more traditional centralized and authoritarian form of direction. Consequently, it maybe more costly to the organization in time and resources. Accountability may sometimes present a problem. When responsibility is diffused among several different individuals or groups, accountability for mistakes or failures maybe harder to determine. Some organizations or tasks may simply not be compatible with the type of employee participation required for democratic leadership. For example, consider the effects of democratic leadership in a military unit during combat.

MAINTENANCE OF SUPPLIES AND EQUIPMENT

The maintenance of medical equipment requires a wide range of technical abilities, and the costs and time required to train a technician increase markedly with the level of skill that has to be attained. Experience in many developing countries has revealed that training of technicians to a high level of skills is very expensive.

Therefore, the approach for the training of technicians, to do front-line maintenance, for medical equipment in health facilities requires less time, costs, and delivers benefits to a larger population, supporting primary health care, by servicing large volume of essential medical equipment in widely distributed health facilities in the capital city and other parts of regional administrations.

Medical equipment maintenance and operation training service, includes provision of services like training, maintenance and repair of medical equipment, focusing on building sustainable technical capacity, implementing transparent and pragmatic systems, while focusing on the preventative care and safe usage of medical equipment.

Maintenance Service Process

The medical equipment maintenance and operation training services are rendered to various hospitals, clinics, diagnostic laboratories, biomedical research centers and other related institutions utilizing medical equipment. The services are provided both at the service center and at the client's site, as required. The service provision is basically categorized as follows:

Full-fledged and Packaged Consultancy Service: Procurement of Medical Equipment:

- Based on the specifications and the standards set out by concerned governmental bodies, the envisaged center will participate on the pre and post tendering activities.
- Acquisition and translation of manuals and other vital medical documents/materials.
- Developing and implementing procedures and rules designed to better care for the medical equipment, create accountability, clarity

and transparency in the care and usage of medical equipment; implement a plan to prevent unauthorized repair and usage.

Installation, Testing and Commissioning

- Handling of erection or erection supervision activities (Installation, testing, commissioning and operation, and safety training), as required.
- Maintenance contract for scheduled and unscheduled maintenance comprehensive inventory including:
  - Development of detailed historical maintenance records which show history, current status, location, responsible staff member for oversight, scheduled (Preventive) maintenance needs, online and updated supplier contact information, etc.
  - Proper cleaning, calibration and other regular scheduled maintenance work.
  - Critical/emergency equipment response program (on-call service including emergency response procedures).
  - Equipment repair; if an extremely specialized and sophisticated piece of equipment, if cannot be handled by and local technicians.
  - Quality assurance/quality control plan customized for a hospital or clinic.
  - Work order system: request which will be acted upon in under 24 hours including an urgency criteria, etc.

INDENT AND ORDERING OF SUPPLIES AND EQUIPMENT

Hospital supplies and equipments are dealt with under material management. Supplies are those items that are used up or consumed; hence the term consumable is used for supplies. The supplies in hospital include drugs, surgical goods (disposables, glass wares), chemicals, antiseptics, food materials, stationeries, the linen supply, etc. The term equipment is used for more permanent type of article and maybe classified as fixed and movables. Fixed equipment is not a structure of the building, but it is attached to the walls or floors (egg; sterilizer,) Movable equipment includes furniture, instruments, etc.

Purchase of Supplies and Equipment

The purchase of supplies and equipments in a hospital is carried out through:

- General store
- Dietary department and
- Pharmacy department

When planning for the purchase of articles, budgeting is done not only for the actual price of articles but also for the additional costs that are involved such as:

- Transport charges (local delivery reduce the transport charge)
- Incidental costs
- Cost of chemicals and other consumable to be used with the equipment (e.g. ECG paper for an ECG machine)
- Operating cost (hiring a technician)
- Cost of maintenance service: 10–20% of hospital equipment may remain idle if serving is not done periodically
- *Cost of technology obsolesces:* when a better quality appears in market there is tendency to discard the old model
- Replacement cost of equipment.

Selection of Article

While buying articles it has to meet the standards. Indian Standards Institution is the national agency set up to bring standardization of articles in India. Articles that meet the criteria specified by the Indian Standard Institution will be marked by ISI markings. The articles bought should provide safety to the patient and personnel. Faulty instruments and equipments cause not only inconvenience in the patient care, but also it may cause the loss of life.

Purchasing Article

- The material used for any equipment should be durable, non-corroding, non toxic and safe for use
- Should have standard shapes and dimensions to fit into various situations
- Reparability and spare part availability of the article
- Interchangability of the article
- All surgical instruments used in a hospital should be sterilisable and they should stand the tests for leakage, hydraulic pressure tests for bursting, etc.
- Should have accuracy in measurements
- Should have ease of operation.

The Central Supply Service

Most hospitals have a central department where equipments and supplies are stored and from which they are distributed to the units. The type of materials that is kept in the central supply room varies from hospital to hospital. In some hospital the central soppy room deals with only the sterile supplies and ward trays. In other hospitals all types of equipment such as oxygen, suction, ward trays, catheters, syringes, etc. are stored here.

Linen supply: Methods of handling linen supply include:

- *Departmentalized system:* Here the supply of linen for each department of the hospital is marked for that department. The head of the department is responsible for making a linen standard for his own department.
- *Centralized linen supply:* Under centralized system, linen is issued on exchange basis, that is clean linen is exchanged for soiled linen.

Factors to be Considered

Type of service provided by the hospital: a maternity hospital requires more equipment related to gynecologic procedures than a cardiac hospital.

- *Age of patients:* Children need different type and amount of equipments than adults.
- Sex: Men and women sometime require different type of equipment.
- *Degree and type of illness:* Neurologic patients sometimes require more bedsides, rubber mattress and linen than patients with other type of illness.
- *Cost of items:* Cost of items will limit the purchase of number of equipment.

General Utility Services in the Hospital

Electric Supply and Installations

- A hospital must have a steady electrical supply at a stable voltage. Voltage fluctuations play havoc with sophisticated electronic equipment, endoscope, sterilizers, X-ray equipments, etc. While planning hospital departments, provision should be made for voltage stabilization in areas with heavy concentration of electrical and electronic equipment. This is preferred over using voltage stabilizers with individual equipment. There should be an emergency generator capable of supplying power to all emergency areas of the hospital. This generator should be of right capacity and kept in working order by periodic test runs.
  - Water supply
  - Since safe water supply is not always assured, hospitals must have their own purification system. Also there should be plumbing system
  - Disposal of waste –liquids and solids
  - Disposal of waste both solid and liquid is a totally neglected area. A hospital incinarator good for the waste management

- Refrigeration, air conditioning, ventilation and environment control
- Air conditioning is required for protection of sophisticated electronic equipment, X-ray, machines, etc.
- Transport.

Lifts are needed for vertical transport. There should be separate lifts for patients, visitors, staff and supply. Patients lift should accommodate a standard hospital bed. Sides of the lift must be protected to prevent damage by trolleys. Lift surfaces and flooring should be capable of easy cleaning and disinfection. Ventilation, communication and emergency escape system should be provided on all lifts. As for horizontal transport also trolleys and ramps with gentle gradient are useful.

- Supply of medical gases, compressed air, hot water, vacuum suction and gas plants
- Piped supply of medical gases, compressed air, vacuum suction, hot water, steam, necessitates thoughtful planning at all stages to consider problems of:
  - Easy uninterrupted safe supply
  - Fire and explosion hazards
  - Easy of servicing and maintenance without disrupting hospital services
  - *Laundry:* A hospital laundry has 2 separate areas, with provision for decontamination and sterilizing of soiled linen.
  - *Fire hazard:* There should be consideration of ventilation, exhaust systems and adequate earthing of all electrical installation.
  - *Communication:* Public telephone and internal telephones are required in each hospital.
  - Repairs workshop
  - There should be provision for repair and maintenance of necessary equipments used in the hospital.

Materials Used in Hospitals

Hospital material medical side	Hospital material management side
• Perfusion materials • Surgical disposables • Instruments • Drugs, medicine, oxygen, linen • Biomedical equipment • Disinfecting items • Computers, telephone and fax • Food and beverage materials • Anesthetic equipment	• Computer, fax, telephone, stationary items • Public address items overhead projector • Audiovisual systems

Contd...

Contd...

• Electro medical equipment • Glass ware, dental machines • Surgical dressing utensils • Artificial limbs, bandages, cots for patient, furniture • Engineering items and many others	

Essential Equipments (50 Bedded District Hospital)

Scope of Services

- *Essential clinical services:* Medicine, surgery, pediatrics, OBG, and acute psychiatry (when necessary)
- *Optional clinical services:* Oral surgery, orthopedic surgery, otolaryngology, neurology and psychiatry.
- *Essential clinical support:* Anesthesia, radiology and clinical laboratory
- *Optional clinical support services:* Pathology and rehabilitation including physiotherapy.

Essential Medical Equipment

- Diagnostic imaging equipment: It include X-ray and ultrasound equipment. X-ray equipment can be stationary in one room or mobile laboratory equipment:
  - Microscope
  - Blood counter
  - Analytical balance
  - Calorimeter (spectrophotometer)
  - *Centrifuge:* A small centrifuge that can accommodate six 15 ml tubes should be available.
  - *Water bath:* Used for stabilizing temperature at 25, 37, 42, or 56 degree Celsius.
  - *Incubator/oven:* A small hot air oven to carry-out standard cultivations and sensitisations.
  - *Refrigerator:* An ordinary household refrigerator with a freezer unit, for storing preparations, vaccines, blood, etc.
  - *Istillation and purification apparatus:* It should be made of metal that resists acid, and alkali and should be free standing.

Electrical Medical Equipment

- Portable electrocardiograph
- Defibrillator (external)

- *Portable anesthetic unit:* 2 small esthetic units should be obtained, complete with a range of masks.
- *Respirator:* It should be applicable for prolonged administration during postoperative care.
- *Dental chair unit:* A complete unit should be available to carry-out standard dental operations.
- *Suction pump:* One portable and one other suction pump are required.
- *Operating theater lamp:* One main lamp with at least 8 shadows lamp and an auxiliary of 4 lamp units.
- *Delivery table:* It should be standard and manually operated.
- *Diathermy unit:* A standard coagulating unit which is operated by hand or foot switch, with variable poor control.

Other Equipment

- autoclave: for general stabilization
- Small sterilisers: for specific services, e.g. Stabilizer
- Cold chain and other preventive medical equipment
- Ambulance

Small, Inexpensive Equipment and Instruments

  - Equipment and instrument, such as BP apparatus, oxygen manifolds, stethoscope, diagnostic sets and spotlights.

HANDLING OVER AND TAKING OVER OF INVENTORY

Inventory is an administrative tool designed to control supplies and equipment by listing the names, description, number and location of supplies.

Purposes of Inventory

- To determine if standards are maintained
- To serve as a basis for the revision of standards and systems
- To recommend proper action on obsolete and surplus materials
- To determine the operational status of equipment
- To prepare plan for repair and replacements
- To determine the proper location of supplies, materials, and equipment
- To gather factual information to serve as basis for sound procurement planning.

Kinds of Inventory

- *Perpetual inventory:* Recording is done as soon as supplies were used and replenished, thus, indicating the number of supplies on hand at a time.
- *Physical inventory:* It is the actual count made at designed intervals to correct accumulative errors resulting from loss, breakages or deterioration. Fixed equipments are usually inventoried annually, movable equipment, monthly; instruments, weekly; and narcotics, daily:
  - A, ward nurse implement 24 hour class three turns duty institution, the officer on duty to perform duties nursing patients all class.
  - Everyday, all the briefings collective handover nursing personnel to participate, usually less than 15 minutes. Detailed report by night nurses heavy endanger patients condition, the new diagnosis and nursing care and other relevant matters. The head nurse according to the report, briefly summarized as necessary to decorate the days work.
  - The collective handover everyday all class all needs to transfer on time.
  - Those on duty besides completing this before in various work outside, need good finishing used items, keep therapeutic room, nurse's station for the next clean, and do the necessary preparations.
  - The psychological situation, with the illness change, on or surgical patients and special inspection patient's preparations and the matters needing attention. The total number of the patients, the new admission, discharge, operation, delivery, dying, death, and first-aid drug devices, special treatment and special specimen to return, etc.

PROBLEM-SOLVING

Problem-solving is a process that includes the components of critical thinking and decision-making. It tries to identify and correct the underlying problem in situations. Problem-solving requires that a lot of time and energy be spent on identifying the real problem. The most common cause of failure to solve a problem is the improper identification of the problem.

A Problem is part of a situation that has some kind of barrier, so that it cannot complete its function or cannot reach its purpose. A situation is just what a circumstance is; it is neither good nor bad. Situations need to be evaluated clearly, without identifying them as problems or non-problems. Until a situation is recognized objectively, the problem solver will be swayed by prejudice (Shibata, 1998).

Definition

'Problem-solving is a mental process that involves discovering, analyzing and solving problems. The ultimate goal of problem-solving is to overcome obstacles and find a solution that best resolves the issue'.

The best strategy for solving a problem depends largely on the unique situation. In some cases, people are better off learning everything they can about the issue and then using factual knowledge to come-up with a solution. In other instances, creativity and insight are the best options.

Steps and Methods of Problem-Solving

In order to correctly solve a problem, it is important to follow a series of steps. Many researchers refer to this as the *problem-solving cycle,* which includes developing strategies and organizing knowledge. While this cycle is portrayed sequentially, people rarely follow a rigid series of steps to find a solution. Instead, we often skip steps or even go back through steps multiple times until the desired solution is reached.

- *Identifying the problem:* While it may seem like an obvious step, identifying the problem is not always as simple as it sounds. In some cases, people might mistakenly identify the wrong source of a problem, which will make attempts to solve it inefficient or even useless.
- *Defining the problem:* After the problem has been identified, it is important to fully define the problem so that it can be solved.
- *Forming a strategy:* The next step is to develop a strategy to solve the problem. The approach used will vary depending upon the situation and the individual's unique preferences.
- *Organizing information:* Before coming-up with a solution, we need to first organize the available information. What do we know about the problem? What do we *not* know? The more information that is available, the better prepared we will be to come-up with an accurate solution.
- *Allocating resources:* Of course, we do not always have unlimited money, time and other resources to solve a problem. Before you begin to solve a problem, you need to determine how high priority it is. If it is an important problem, it is probably worth allocating more resources to solving it. If, however, it is a fairly unimportant problem, then you do not want to spend too much of your available resources into coming-up with a solution.
- *Monitoring progress:* Effective problem-solvers tend to monitor their progress as they work towards a solution. If they are not making good progress toward reaching their goal, they will re-evaluate their approach or look for new strategies.

- *Evaluating the results:* After a solution has been reached, it is important to evaluate the results to determine if it is the best possible solution to the problem. This evaluation might be immediate, such as checking the results of a math problem to ensure the answer is correct, or it can be delayed, such as evaluating the success of a therapy program after several months of treatment.

RECORDS

Records are hospital administrative tools used in collecting data directed towards the attainment of the objective of its sections and department. They are the sources of cumulative and relevant information that maybe used as basis for patient management and the effective programming of activities for research and decision-making. "The nurse has a duty to maintain confidentiality of all patient information" (ANA code of ethics 2001). The records are used in client conferences, clinics, rounds, client studies, and written papers. It is the responsibility of the student or health professional to protect the client's privacy by not using a name or any statements in the notations that would identify the client.

Definition

'Records are written or computer based, the process of making an entry on a client's record is called *recording, charting, or documenting.* A clinical record, also called a chart or client record is a formal, legal document that provides evidence of a client's care'.

Purposes of Client Records

- *Communication:* The record serves as the vehicle by which different health professionals who interact with a client communicate with each other.
- *Planning client care:* Each health professional uses data from the client's record to plan care for that client.
- *Auditing Health agencies:* An audit is a review of client records for quality assurance purpose.
- *Research:* The information contained in a record can be a valuable source of data for research. The treatment plans for a number of clients with the same health problems can yield information helpful in treating other clients.
- *Education:* A record can frequently provide a comprehensive view of the client, illness, effective treatment strategies, and factors that affect the outcome of the illness.
- *Reimbursement:* It is for a facility to obtain payment through medicare, the client's clinical record must contain the correct diagnosis.

- *Legal documentation:* The client's record is a legal document and is usually admissible in a court as evidence.
- *Health care analysis:* It assists health care planners to identify agency needs.

Essential Points in Keeping Records

- Records should be accurate, adequate and up to date.
- Records should be clear, brief and concise.
- Records should provide relevant facts for evaluation and study.
- Records and reports maybe temporary or permanent, and policies should be provided for their disposition.
- Record forms must be maintained at all times.
- Confidential records and reports should be safeguarded. The word 'confidential' should either be stamped of written preferably in red ink.
- Records must be kept in dry storage.
- Records should be filed chronologically by subjects to facilitate accessibility and effective use of data.
- A properly-trained responsible person should be incharge of records and reports.

Documentation Systems

Source Oriented Record

- It is a traditional client record, each person or department makes notations in a separate section or sections of the client's chart, For example, the admissions department has an admission sheet, the physician's has order sheet, a physician's history sheet, and progress notes, nurse's notes.

Narrative Charting

It is a traditional part of the source—oriented record. It consists of written notes that include routine care, normal findings, and client problems.

- *Advantage:* Source-oriented records are convenient because care providers from each discipline can easily locate the forms on which to record data and it is easy to trace the information specific to one's discipline.
- *Disadvantage:* Information about a particular client problem is scattered throughout the chart, so it is difficult to find chronological information on a client's problems and progress. This can lead to decreased communication among the health team, an incomplete picture of the client's care, and a lack of coordination of care.

Problem-oriented Medical Record (POMR)

The data are arranged according to the problems the client has rather than the source of information. Members of the health care team contribute to the problem list, plan of care, and progress notes.

Basic Components of POMR

- *Database:* Consists of all information known a but the client when the client first enters the health care agency. It includes nursing assessment, the physician's history, social and family data, and baseline diagnostic tests.
- *Problem list:* Problems are listed in the order in which they are identified, and the list is continually updated as new problems are identified and others resolved.
- *Plan of care:* Care plans are generated by the person who lists the problems. Physicians write medical care plans; nurses write nursing care plans.
- *Progress notes:* It is a chart entry made by all health professionals involved in a client's care; they all use the same type of sheet for notes. For example, the **SOAP** format is frequently used.

S – Subjective data consist of information obtained from what the client says. It describes the client's perceptions of and experience with the problem.

O – Objective data consist of information that is measured or observed by use of the senses (e.g. Lab test, X-ray results).

A – Assessment is the interpretation or conclusions drawn about the subjective and objective data. "A" should describe the client's condition and level of progress rather than merely restating the diagnosis or problem.

P – Plan is the plan of care designed to resolve the stated problem.

The **SOAP** format has been modified to **SOAPIER:**

I – Interventions refer to the specific interventions that have been performed by the caregiver.

E – Evaluation includes client responses to nursing interventions and medical treatments.

R – Revision reflects care plan modifications suggested by the evaluation.

Advantage of POMR

- Encourages collaborative.
- The problem list in the front of the chart alerts caregivers to the client's needs and makes it easier to track the status of each problem.

Disadvantage

- Caregivers differ in their ability to use the required charting format.
- It takes constant vigilance to maintain an up-to-date problem list.
  - *PIE charting (Problem, intervention, evaluation):* Each client problem is labeled and numbered for easy reference. When interventions are implemented to manage the client's problem, the problem number is identified.
  - *Focus charting:* It is intended to make the client and client concerns and strengths the focus of care. The progress notes are organized into (D) data which reflects the assessment phase of the nursing process. (A) action which reflects planning and implementation and includes immediate and future nursing action. (R) response which reflects the evaluation phase of the nursing process and describes the client's response to any nursing and medical care.
  - *Charting by exception (CBE):* It is a documentation system in which only abnormal or significant findings or exceptions to norms are recorded.
  - *Computerized documentation:* Nurses use computers to store the client's database, add new data, create and revise care plans, and document client progress.

General Guidelines for Recording

As the client's record is a legal document and maybe used to provide evidence in court, many factors are considered in recording:

- *Date and time:* Document should be fill the date and time in each recording. This is essential not only for legal reasons but also for client safety. It is accurate according to the 24-hours clock wise or in the conventional manner (am, pm).
- *Timing:* The follows the hospital policy about the frequency of documenting, and adjusts the frequency as a client's condition indicates. No recording should be done before providing nursing care.
- *Legibility:* All entries must be legible and easy to read to prevent interpretation errors.
- *Permanence:* All entries made in dark ink so that the record is permanent and changes can be identified.
- *Correct spelling:* It is essential for accuracy in recording. Incorrect spelling gives a negative impression to the reader and, thereby, decreases the nurse's credibility.
- *Signature:* In each recording on the nursing notes is signed by the nurse making it. The signature includes the name and title.

- *Accuracy:* The client's name and identifying information should be stamped or written on each page of the clinical records. Before making any entry, check that it is the correct chart. Do not identify charts by room number only, check the client's name. Notations on records must be accurate and correct. Accurate notations consist of facts or observations rather than opinions or interpretation. It is more accurate, for example, to write that the client 'refused medication' (fact) than to write that the client 'was uncooperative' (opinion).
- When describing something, avoid general words, such as large, good, or normal, e.g. chart specific data such as '2 cm × 3 cm bruise' rather than 'large bruise'. When a recording mistake is made, draw a line through it and write the words mistaken entry above or next to the original entry, with your initials or name. Do not erase, or use correction fluid. Write on every line but never between lines.
- *Sequence:* All document events in the order in which they occur, such as record assessments, then the nursing interventions, and then the client's responses. Update or delete problems as needed.
- *Appropriateness:* Records only information that pertains to the client's health problems and care. Recording irrelevant information maybe considered an invasion of the client's privacy.
- *Appropriateness:* Records only information that pertains to the client's health problems and care. Recording irrelevant information maybe considered an invasion of the client's privacy.
- *Completeness:* It is not that all the data a nurse obtains about a client can be recorded; however, the information that is recorded needs to be complete and helpful to the client and health care professionals. Nurse's record need to reflect the nursing process, record assessment, dependent and independent nursing interventions, client problems, client comments and responses to interventions and tests, progress toward goals.
- *Conciseness:* Recording needs to be brief as well as complete to save time in communication.
- *Accepted terminology:* Use only commonly accepted abbreviations, symbols, and terms are specified by the agency. Many abbreviations are standard and used universally.
- *Legal prudence:* Accurate, complete documentation should give legal protection to the nurse; the client's other caregivers, the health care facility, and the client. 'Complete charting for example, by using the steps of the nursing process as a framework, is the best defense against malpractice'.

REPORTS

Reports are prepared accounts of important activities of the nursing service within a particular period. They must always be dated.

Definition: 'Is oral, written, or computer-based communication intended to convey information to others'. The purpose of reporting is to communicate specific information to a person or group of people.

Types of Reports

- *Change-of–shift reports:* It is a report given to all nurses on the next shift. Its purpose is to provide continuity of care for clients by providing the new caregivers a quick summary of client needs and details of care to be given.
- *Telephone reports:* Health professionals frequently about a client by telephone. Nurses inform primary care providers about a change in a client's condition.
  - The nurse receiving a telephone report should document the date and the time, the name of the person giving the information, and the subject of the information received.
  - The person receiving the information should repeat it back to the sender to ensure accuracy.
  - When giving a telephone report to a primary care provider, begin with name and relationship to the client. For example, 'This is Maher Battat, RN, I'm calling about your client, Shamsa Mendes. I'm her nurse on the 7 pm to 7 am shift'.
  - Telephone reports usually include the client's name and medical diagnosis, etc. The nurse should have the client's chart ready to give any further information.
  - Telephone orders, physicians often order a therapy for a client by telephone. While the primary care provider gives the order, write the complete order down and read it back to ensure accuracy. Question about any order that is ambiguous, unusual, or contraindicated by the client's condition.
- *Incident or occurrence reports:* These are used to document any unusual occurrence or accident in the delivery of client care, such as falls or medication errors. These reports are used for quality improvement and should not be used for disciplinary action against staff members. Incident reports improve the management and treatment of patients by identifying high-risk patterns and initiating in-service programs to prevent future problems.

Important Points to Consider in Making Reports

- Reports, whether written or oral, must be up to date, clear, and concise
- Channels of communication should be properly observed
- Reports should be accomplished in forms adopted by the hospital
- Reports should be factual and may include recommendation for action

- Verbal reports made in an emergency situation should be confirmed in writing and duly signed by the person making the report.

Records and Reports Maintained in Primary Health Center and Subcenter

There are certain records maintain by the nurses in PHC and subcenters:

- Register (a) Pregnant women at earliest contact (b) Infants zero to one year of age (c) Women aged 15–44 years (d) Under and above five children (e) Adolescents
- Eligible Couple Register including Contraception
- Maternal and Child Health Register:
  - Antenatal, intranatal, postnatal
  - *Under-five register:*
    - Immunization
    - Growth monitoring
- Above five child immunization
- Number of HIV/STI screening and referral
- Births and deaths register
- Drug register
- Equipment furniture and other accessories register
- Communicable diseases/epidemic register/register for syndromic surveillance
- Passive surveillance register for malaria cases.
- Register for records pertaining to Janani Suraksha Yojana
- Register for maintenance of accounts including untied funds.
- Register for water quality and sanitation
- Minor ailments register
- Records/registers as per various National Health Program guidelines (NLEP, RNTCP, NVBDCP, etc.)

Reporting Format for Syndromic Surveillance (Form S) under Integrated Disease Surveillance Project

- The healthworker is required to transfer the information from the 'Register for Syndromic Surveillance' to Form S (Reporting Format for Syndromic Surveillance). The information in the registers of the AWW, village volunteers and non-formal providers will also be transferred to the Form S, at the subcenter. Each reporting unit will be assigned a Unique Identifier or ID Number which will be filled in by the District Surveillance Unit and the Healthworker should leave this space blank. The Healthworker will fill the information on reporting week (copy the information from the 'Register for Syndromic Surveillance').

- Form S will be provided in triplicate (three copies). The first and second pages of Form S (colors Yellow and Green respectively), will be separated from the third page (color–Blue).
- The third page (Blue color page) will be retained by the Healthworker and the first and second pages (Yellow and Green) will be given/ sent to the Medical Officer of the supervising PHC on the Monday, following the end of a particular reporting week.

SUMMARY

In this unit we discuss about the ward/unit administration and healthcare services are the result of a number of materials used in the process. As hospital administrator's nurses should also know about the materials. Medical items such as perfusion materials, surgical disposables, instruments, electrical, civil and engineering items for maintenance, housekeeping materials, linen, biomedical equipment, drugs, food items, etc. pay an effective role in improving the quality of health care services.

5

Section

Health Economics

COURSE DESCRIPTION

Hrs. 20

This course will help student to understand the basic concept of economics, health economics, the relationship between health and economic development, demand and supply, concept of cost and financing system of health care services in India. This will enable them to appreciate financial aspects of health care services.

General Objectives

Upon completion of this course, the students will be able to:

- Explain the meaning of economics and health economics
- Analyze the relationship between health and economic development
- Explain the concept of demand and supply
- Describe the structure of health care industry and characteristics of market for health care services
- Analyze the concept of cost in health care
- Discuss financing system of health care services in India.

Course Content

Unit 20: Introduction to Economics

- Definition and meaning, dimensions of economics, positive and normative economics.

Unit 21: Introduction to Health Economics

- Concept of health economics
- Focus of health economics
- Areas of health economics
- The economics of health and health care service Health and economic development
- Causes of health problems in India.

Unit 22 Costs of Health Care

- Concept of cost, types of costs
- Opportunity cost, total fixed and variable cost, average marginal and sunk costs, cost benefit, cost effectiveness.

Unit 23: Demand and Supply in Health Care

- Concept of demand, need, supply input, output, production function, industry and market
- Structure of health care industry
- Characteristics of health care services market
- Demand side and supply side.

Unit 24: Financing of Health Care in India

- Financing system and allocation
- Sources of financing of health care services
- Health plans and outlays, the relative role of state and central government on financing of health care services
- Factors influencing the state's ability to finance health care services.

Introduction to Economics

20 unit

INTRODUCTION

Economics was formerly called political economy. The term political economy means the management of the wealth of the state. Adam Smith, the father of modern economics, in his book entitled 'An Enquiry into the Nature and Causes of the Wealth of Nations' (Published in 1776) defined economics as a study of wealth. Smith considered the acquisition of wealth as the main objective of human activity. According to him the subject matter of economics is the study of how wealth is produced and consumed. Later economists held that apart from man they said study of wealth has no meaning economics is concerned not only with the production and use of wealth but also with man, it deals with wealth as serving the purpose of man. Wealth is only a means to the end of human welfare.

MEANING OF ECONOMICS

The word 'Economics' originates from the Greek work *'Oikonomikos'* which can be divided into two parts:

1. *'Oikos'*, which means 'Home', and
2. *'Nomos'*, which means 'Management'.

Thus, economics means 'Home Management'. The head of a family faces the problem of managing the unlimited wants of the family members within the limited income of the family. In fact, the same is true for a society also. If we consider the whole society as a 'family', then the society also faces the problem of tackling unlimited wants of the members of the society with the limited resources available in that society. Thus, economics means is the study of the way in which mankind organizes itself to tackle the basic problems of scarcity. All societies have more wants than resources. Hence, a system must be devised to allocate these resources between competing ends.

DEFINITION OF ECONOMICS

Several definitions of economics have been given. For the sake of convenience let us classify the various definitions into four groups:
1. Science of wealth
2. Science of material well-being
3. Science of choice making and
4. Science of dynamic growth and development.

Science of Wealth

Some earlier economists defined economics as follows: 'An inquiry into the nature and causes of the wealth of the nations' *by Adam Smith.* 'Science which deals with wealth' by *JB Say.*

The definition of economics, as science of wealth, had some merits. The important ones are:
- It highlighted an important problem faced by each and every nation of the world, namely creation of wealth.
- Since the problems of poverty, unemployment, etc. can be solved to a greater extent when wealth is produced and is distributed equitably; it goes to the credit of Adam Smith and his followers to have addressed to the problems of economic growth and increase in the production of wealth.
- The study of economics as a 'Science of Wealth' has been criticized on several grounds. The main criticisms levelled against this definition are:
- Adam Smith and other classical economists concentrated only on material wealth. They totally ignored creation of immaterial wealth like services of doctors, chartered accountants, etc.
- The advocates of Economics as 'science of wealth' concentrated too much on the production of wealth and ignored social welfare. This makes their definition incomplete and inadequate.

Science of Material Well-being

Under this group of definitions the emphasis is on welfare as compared with wealth in the earlier group. Two important definitions are as follows:
- According to Alfred Marshall define 'Economics is a study of mankind in the ordinary business of life. It examines that part of individual and social action which is most closely connected with the attainment and with the use of the material requisites of well-being. Thus, it is on the

one side a study of wealth and on the other and more important side a part of the study of the man'.

- According to *AC Pigou* define 'The range of our inquiry becomes restricted to that part of social welfare that can be brought directly or indirectly into relation with the measuring rod of money'.

  In the first definition economics has been indicated to be a study of mankind in the ordinary business of life. By ordinary business we mean those activities which occupy considerable part of human effort. The fulfillment of economic needs is a very important business which every man ordinarily does. Professor *Marshall* has clearly pointed that.

  - Economics is the study of wealth but more important is the study of man. Thus, man gets precedence over wealth. There is also emphasis on material requisites of well-being.
  - Obviously, the material things like food, clothing and shelter, are very important economic objectives.

  The second definition by *Pigou* emphasizes social welfare but only that part of it which can be related with the measuring rod of money. Money is general measure of purchasing power by the use of which the science of economics can be rendered more precise.

  Marshall's and *Pigou's* definitions of economics are wider and more comprehensive as they take into account the aspect of social welfare. But their definitions have their share of criticism. Their definitions are criticized on the following grounds.

  - Economics is concerned with not only material things but also with immaterial things like services of singers, teachers, actors, etc. *Marshall and Pigou* chose to ignore them.
  - Robbins criticized the welfare definition on the ground that it is very difficult to state which things would lead to welfare and which will not. He is of the view that we would study in economics all those goods and services which carry a price whether they promote welfare or not.

Science of Choice Making

- According to *Robbins* define 'Economics is the science which studies human behavior as a relationship between ends and scarce means which have alternative uses'.

  The definition deals with the following four aspects:

  a. *Economics is a science:* Economics studies economic human behaviour scientifically. It studies how humans try to optimise (maximize or minimize) certain objective under given constraints. For example, it studies how consumers, with given income and prices of the commodities, try to maximize their satisfaction.

b. *Unlimited ends:* Ends refer to wants. Human wants are unlimited. When one want is satisfied, other wants crop-up. If man's wants were limited, then there would be no economic problem.
c. *Scarce means:* Means refer to resources. Since resources (natural productive resources, man-made capital goods, consumer goods, money and time, etc.) are limited economic problem arises. If the resources were unlimited, people would be able to satisfy all their wants and there would be no problem.
d. *Alternative uses:* Not only resources are scarce, they have alternative uses. For example, coal can be used as a fuel for the production of industrial goods, it can be used for running trains, and it can also be used for domestic cooking purposes and for so many purposes. Similarly, financial resources can be used for many purposes. The man or society has, therefore, to choose the uses for which resources would be used. If there was only a single use of the resource then the economic problem would not arise.

Science of Dynamic Growth and Development

- Although the fundamental economic problem of scarcity in relation to needs is undisputed it would not be proper to think that economic resources-physical, human, financial are fixed and cannot be increased by human ingenuity, exploration, exploitation and development. A modern and somewhat modified definition is as follows:
  - According to *Paul A Samuelson* define 'Economics is the study of how men and society choose, with or without the use of money, to employ scarce productive resources which could have alternative uses, to produce various commodities overtime and distribute them for consumption now and in the future amongst various people and groups of society'.
  - The above definition is very comprehensive because it does not restrict to material well-being or money measure as a limiting factor. But it considers economic growth overtime.

DIMENSION OF ECONOMICS

Economic theory, as it stands today, has several dimensions. Of these, two are most important. These are *microeconomics* and *macroeconomics.*

Microeconomics

Microeconomics is that branch of economics which is concerned with the decision-making of a single unit of an economic system. How does an individual (or a family) decide on how much of various commodities and services to consume? How does a business firm decide how much of its product (or products) to produce? These are the typical questions discussed in microeconomics. Determination of income, employment, etc. in the economic system as a whole is not the concern of microeconomics. Thus, microeconomics can be defined as the study of economic decision-making by microunits.

Importance of Microeconomics

- *Determination of demand pattern:* The study of microeconomics has several uses. It determines the pattern of demand in the economy, i.e. the amounts of the demand for the different goods and services in the economy, because the total demand for a good or service is the sum total of the demands of all the individuals. Thus, by determining the demand patterns of every individual or family, microeconomics determines the demand pattern in the country as a whole.
- *Determination of the pattern of supply:* In a similar way, the pattern of supply in the country as a whole can be obtained from the amounts of goods and services produced by the firms in the economy. Microeconomics, therefore, determines the pattern of supply as well.
- *Pricing:* Probably the most important economic question is the one of price determination. The prices of the various goods and services determine the pattern of resource allocation in the economy. The prices, in turn, are determined by the interaction of the forces of demand and supply of the goods and services. By determining demand and supply, microeconomics helps us in understanding the process of price determination and, hence, the process of determination of resource allocation in a society.
- *Policies for improvement of resource allocation:* As is well-known, economic development stresses the need for improving the pattern of resource allocation in the country. Development polices, therefore, can be formulated only if we understand how the pattern of resource allocation is determined. For instance, if we want to analyze how a tax or a subsidy will affect the use of the scarce resources in the economy, we have to know how these will affect their prices. By explaining prices and, hence, the pattern of resource allocation, microeconomics helps us to formulate appropriate development policies for an underdeveloped economy.
- *Solution to the problems of microunits:* Finally, it goes without saying that, since the study of microeconomics starts with the individual consumers and producers, policies for the correction of any wrong decisions at the microlevel are also facilitated by microeconomics.

    For example, if a firm has to know exactly what it should do in order to run efficiently, it has to know the optimal quantities of outputs produced and of inputs purchased. Only then can any deviation from these optimal levels be corrected. In this sense, microeconomics helps the formulation of policies at the microlevel. In every society, the economic problems faced by different economic agents (such as individual consumers, producers, etc.) can be analyzed with the help of microeconomic theories. This shows that **economics is a social science** which aims at analyzing the economic behavior of individuals in a social environment.

Limitations of Microeconomics

- *Monetary and fiscal policies:* Although total demand and total supply in the economy is the sum of individual demands and individual supplies respectively, the total economic picture of the country cannot always be understood in this simplistic way. There are many factors affecting the total economic system, which are outside the scope of microeconomics. For example, the role of monetary and fiscal policies in the determination of the economic variables cannot be analysed completely without going beyond microeconomics.
- *Income determination:* Microeconomics also does not tell us anything about how the income of a country (*i.e.* national income) is determined.
- *Business cycles:* A related point is that, it does not analyze the causes of fluctuations in national income. The ups-and-downs of national income overtime are known as *business cycles.* Microeconomics does not help us in understanding as to why these cycles occur and what the remedies are.
- *Unemployment:* One of the main economic problems faced by an economy like India is the problem of unemployment. This, again, is one of the areas on which microeconomics does not shed much light. Because, if we are to find a solution to the unemployment problem, we must first understand the causes of this problem. For that, in turn, we must understand how the total employment level in the economy is determined. This is difficult to understand from within the confines of microeconomics.

Macroeconomics

- Macroeconomics is that branch of economics which is concerned with the economic magnitudes relating to the economic system as a whole, rather than to the microeconomic units like individuals or firms. It has, therefore, been called 'aggregative economics'. In the picturesque language of Kenneth Boulding, 'Macroeconomics deals ... not with individual income but with national income, not with individual prices but with the price level, not with individual outputs but with national output'.

Importance of Macroeconomics

- *Income and employment determination:* The determination of national income and of total employment in the country is vital concerns of macroeconomics. Since the volume of unemployment is simply population minus the number of people employed, unemployment is determined as soon as the employment level is known.
- *Price level:* The determination of the general price level is discussed in macroeconomic theories. Upward movement of the general price level is known as *inflation.* Thus, if we want to understand the process of inflation and find ways of controlling it, we must resort to the study of macroeconomics.
- *Business cycles:* The economic booms and depressions in the levels of income and employment follow one another in a cyclical fashion. While income rises and employment expands during boom periods, they shrink during depressions. Since depressions bring business failures and unemployment in their wake, economists have sought remedies to depressions. Discussion of business cycles in general and antidepression policies in particular, falls within the scope of macroeconomics.
- *Balance of payments:* The balance of payments theory is also a part of macroeconomics. The difference between the total inflow and the total outflow of foreign exchange is known as the balance of payments of a country. When this balance is negative (*i.e.* outflow exceeds inflow), the country faces a lot of economic hardships. The causes and remedies of such balance of payments problems are discussed in macroeconomics.
- *Government policies:* The effects of various government policies on the economic variables like national income or the general price level are also studied in macroeconomics. Since, the government occupies an important position in any modern economic system; the analysis of these effects is of obvious importance.
- *Interrelations between markets:* Probably, the most important contribution of macroeconomic theories is to show that different markets of the economic system (for example, the commodity market, the labor market, the bond market, the money market, etc.) are interrelated. Any disturbance in one of these markets affects all the others. (Again, it should be noted that, it is the interrelation between the macroeconomic markets that we are talking about here. The relationship between the markets of the individual commodities is the subject matter of 'general equilibrium theory', which is a part of microeconomics).

Thus, we see that the study of microeconomics and that of macroeconomics are complementary to each other. The limitations of microeconomics are covered by macroeconomics. On the other hand, macroeconomics does not make a detailed study of the individual consumer or producer. This is taken care of by microeconomics. One can hope to form a comprehensive notion of what economics is all about only when one is acquainted with both microeconomics and macroeconomics.

Differences between Microeconomics and Macroeconomics

Microeconomics	Macroeconomics
• It is that branch of economics which deals with the economic decision-making of individual economic agents such as the producer, the consumer, etc.	• It is that branch of economics which deals with aggregates and averages of the entire economy, e.g. aggregate output, national income, aggregate, savings and investment, etc.
• It takes into account small components of the whole economy.	• It takes into consideration the economy of any country as a whole.
• It deals with the process of price determination in case of individual products and factors of production.	• It deals with general price-level in any economy.
• It is known as price theory (since it explains the process of allocation of economic resources along alternative lines of production on the basis of relative prices of various goods and services.)	• It is also known as the income theory (since it explains the changing levels of national income in any economy during any particular time period.)
• It is concerned with the optimization goals of individual consumers and producers (e.g. individual consumers are utility-maximizers, while individual producers are profit maximizers.)	• It is concerned with the optimization of the growth process of the entire economy.
• It studies the flow of economic resources or factors of production from any individual owner of such resources to any individual user of these resources, etc.	• It studies the circular flow of income and expenditure between different sectors of the economy (say, between the firm sector and the household sector.)
• Microeconomic theories help us in formulating appropriate policies for resource allocation at the firm level.	• Macroeconomic theories help us in formulating appropriate policies for controlling inflation (i.e. rising price-level), unemployment, etc.
• It takes into account the aggregates over heterogeneous or similar products (e.g. the supply of steel in an economy.)	• It takes into account the aggregates over heterogeneous or dissimilar products (say, the Gross Domestic Product of any country during any year.)

NATURE OF ECONOMICS

Under this, we generally discuss whether economics is science or art or both and if it is a science whether it is a positive science or a normative science or both.

- *Economics is a science:* A subject is considered science if it is a systematized body of knowledge which studies the relationship between cause and effect.
- It is capable of measurement.
- It has its own methodological apparatus.
- It should have the ability to forecast.

  If we analyze economics, we find that it has all the features of science. Like science it studies cause and effect relationship between economic phenomena. To understand, let us take the law of demand. It explains the cause and effect relationship between price and demand for a commodity. It says, given other things constant, as price rises, the demand for a commodity falls and vice versa. Here the cause is price and the effect is fall in quantity demanded. Similarly like science it is capable of being measured, the measurement is in terms of money. It has its own methodology of study (induction and deduction) and it forecasts the future market condition with the help of various statistical and nonstatistical tools. But it is to be noted that economics is not a perfect science. This is because economists do not have uniform opinion about a particular event. The subject matter of economics is the economic behavior of man which is highly unpredictable.
- *Economics is an art:* Art is nothing but practice of knowledge. Whereas science teaches us to know art teaches us to do. Unlike science which is theoretical, art is practical. If we analyze economics, we find that it has the features of an art also. Its various branches, consumption, production, public finance, etc. provide practical solutions to various economic problems. It helps in solving various economic problems which we face in our day-to-day life.
- Thus, Economics is both a science and an art. It is science in its methodology and art in its application. Study of unemployment problem is science but framing suitable policies for reducing the extent of unemployment is an art.
- *Positive Science:* As stated above, economics is a science. But the question arises whether it is a positive science or a normative science. A positive or pure science analyzes cause and effect relationship between variables but it does not pass value judgment. In other words, it states what is and not what ought to be. Professor Robbins emphasized the positive aspects of science but Marshall and Pigou have considered the ethical aspects of science which obviously are normative.

According to Robbins, economics is concerned only with the study of the economic decisions of individuals and the society as positive facts but not with the ethics of these decisions. Economics should be neutral between ends. It is not for economists to pass value judgments and make pronouncements on the goodness or otherwise of human decisions. An individual with a limited amount of money may use it for buying liquor and not milk, but that is entirely his business. A community may use its limited resources for making guns rather than butter, but it is no concern of the economists to condemn or appreciate this policy. Economics only studies facts and makes generalizations from them. It is a pure and positive science, which excludes from its scope the normative aspect of human behavior.

Complete neutrality between ends is, however, neither feasible nor desirable. It is because in many matters the economist has to suggest measures for achieving certain socially desirable ends. For example, when he suggests the adoption of certain policies for increasing employment and raising the rates of wages, he is making value judgments; or that the exploitation of labor and the state of unemployment are bad and steps should be taken to remove them. Similarly, when he states that the limited resources of the economy should not be used in the way they are being used and should be used in a different way; that the choice between ends is wrong and should be altered, etc. he is making value judgments.

- *Normative science:* As normative science, economics involves value judgments. It is prescriptive in nature and described 'what should be the things'. For example, the questions like what should be the level of national income, what should be the wage rate, how the fruits of national product be distributed among people—all fall within the scope of normative science. Thus, normative economics is concerned with welfare propositions. Some economists are of the view that value judgments by different individuals will be different and thus for deriving laws or theories, it should not be used.

SUMMARY

In this unit we have studied the meaning and different definitions of economics given by noted economists of different time period. Also we discussed the dimensions and nature of economics and concluded that economics is both a science and art.

Introduction to Health Economics

21 unit

INTRODUCTION

Health economics is an applied field of study that allows for the systematic and rigorous examination of the problems faced in promoting health for all. By applying economic theories of consumer, producer and social choice, health economics aims to understand the behavior of individuals, health care providers, public and private organizations, and governments in decision-making. Health economics is used to promote health through the study of health care providers, hospitals and clinics, managed care and public health promotion activities. Health economists apply the theories of production, efficiency, disparities, competition, and regulation to better inform the public and private sector on the most efficient, or cost-effective, and equitable course of action. Such research can include the economic evaluation of new technologies, as well as the study of appropriate prices, anti-trust policy, optimal public and private investment, and strategic behavior. Health economics can also be used to evaluate how certain social problems, such as market failure and inequitable allocation of resources, can impact on the health of a community or population.

Definition of Health Economic

- Health economics is the discipline that determines the quantity and price of scarce resources devoted for the care of the sick and promotion of health. It encompasses the medical' industry as a whole and extends to such fields as the economic analysis of the cost of diseases, benefit of health programs, returns from investments in medical education, training and research.
- Health economics is a field in the study of economics that is generally concerned with the problems that are related to the scarcity of health care within a country.

- According to WHO, defined that health economics is the seeks inter alia-to quantify overtimes, the resources used in health service delivery, their organization functioning and the efficiency with which the resources allocated and used for health purposes and the effect of preventive curative and rehabilitative health services on individual and national productivity.

CONCEPTS OF HEALTH ECONOMICS

The concepts of health economics is discussed under two headings:

Health Concepts

Health

How healthy is a given individual or community? Health has been defined by WHO as 'a state of complete physical, mental and social well-being and not merely the absence of disease or infirmity. This definition although well accepted does not lend itself to direct measurement of health of a given individual or community. It is argued that health cannot be defined 'as a state (but a process) and there is no satisfactory definition of the term 'well-being'. Unless we are able to measure (in some quantitative terms or indices) the health status of the people, we cannot assess the benefits of health services. However, to measure the level of health, some comprehensive and some specific indicators have been advocated by a WHO study group and many more indices have since been developed. There is also no satisfactory definition of disease. It has been well conceptualized that multiple factors e.g. biologic, genetic, nutritional, physical, chemical, mechanical environmental, social, cultural human behavior, psychological and economic play a role in the health or disease status of the individuals and the community.

Further health and socioeconomic progress are very much interdependent and health has been accepted as one of the component welfare. These imply that other developmental sectors have a role to play in determining the health status of the people. This makes the task more difficult to identify and quantify the impact of each developmental sector on the health status and *vice versa*.

Health Services

In all civilized societies the state has assumed the responsibility for the health and welfare of the citizen. Provision has been made in the constitution of most of the governments including India about the health services. Consequently the concept of health services has come into being. For better health care of the people, concepts of comprehensive health care, primary health care, health care for all by the year 2000 AD, health insurance, etc. have been developed and implemented.

- The purpose of health service is to promote health, to prevent, diagnose and treat disease and rehabilitate people incapacitated by disease and injury. This general statement does not indicate precisely what the term health services include. The field of health services is a continuous spectrum and it is extremely difficult not only to define the field of health services but also to break it down into clearly defined categories. But for the purpose of economic analysis it must be identified that what activities should be considered as health service activities. According to Abel Smith activities with primary intention to improve health of the people should be considered as health services. For example, programs like water supply and environmental sanitation are primarily public utility activities and they should not be considered totally as health services. Only supervisory and regulating activities like disinfection, etc. should be considered as part of health services.
- *Medical care:* Includes all services for diagnosis, treatment and medical rehabilitation wherever provided and can be further classified into ambulatory, inpatient and domiciliary care.
- *Public health services:* Personal public health services: nutritional, antenatal, postnatal and other such personal health services, health examination of preschool and school children and of workers, immunization and vaccinations services provided to individuals is personal public health services.
- *Environmental public health services:* Services like disinfection, spraying, oiling, etc. are carried out primarily to protect human health and benefit the community in general and can be grouped as environmental public health services. Collection and notification of health statistics are considered as public health services.
- *Medical education, training, and research:* While computing the cost of health services it is suggested that the cost of training in medical and nursing schools and similar other training institutions directly involved in the training of health manpower should only be included. Similarly, research expenditure which is financed by specifically allocated funds or which can be separately identified should only be included.

Economic Concepts

Concept of Cost

The concept of cost 'of providing health services arises from the fact that goods and manpower are absorbed in the health services which could be used to meet other needs. In case of health and health services, costs are incurred both by the producers of health services, through their use of staff, buildings, equipments, materials and supplies, etc. and by the consumers who use transport to the health centers, drugs and special foods, etc. Overall health service costs should include opportunity costs on both sides'.

Concept of Capital and Recurring Expenditure

In all accounting work it would be useful to distinguish between capital and current costs. The general principle of distinction is that current costs are incurred for benefits immediately obtained while capital costs are incurred for benefits which go on accruing after the end of the accounting period. In theory, any goods with a life of more than a year could be regarded as a capital goods though in practice such strict definition is seldom applied.

Concept of Depreciation

As the capital goods have economic life for more than a year; their economic value diminishes with passage of time. Therefore, the concept of depreciation has come into being. Depreciation rate is the rate of diminution in the value of a fixed asset due to use and/or lapse of time. Whether depreciation should be based on original cost to replacement cost of asset is still a matter of controversy. Further, there is no agreement amongst economists as to the depreciation rate to be used for calculating the annual depreciation cost of capital establishment.

Cost of Sickness

In calculating cost of sickness, a distinction must be drawn between the cost of health care which may or may not be borne directly by the patient and other costs including loss of earning by the patient and his family and additional costs of special foods, clothes and other articles which usually do fall on the patient and his family. To these may have to be added the disability or rehabilitation costs for such items, e.g. appliances or equipments or repairing for more suitable employment. Various conceptual problems have been brought forward by different workers in calculating cost of sickness. All the health economists have differentiated the direct and indirect cost of the disease. Direct costs include cost of prevention, detection, treatment, rehabilitation, research, training and capital investments, whereas loss of output to the economy because of illness, disability and premature death forms the indirect cost.

Measurement of Health Service Benefits

Although some health programs require no economic justification, there is need to quantify the benefits of health programs, so as to enable a fair appropriation of financial resources to be obtained for them. The problems associated with the quantification of the benefits of health services are:

- Health problems are often strongly influenced by the general socioeconomic conditions prevailing.
- The impact of health services depends on their utilization and maintenance by the population and cooperation of the patient. It is, therefore, hardly surprising that only in a few and highly specific cases estimation of the impact of health services on the reduction of health risks and problems have been possible.
- There has been no successful and agreed index of population health status in any country.
- Medical specialists and others value a given health impairment differently.

The WHO Seminar on health economics has opined that although certain types of benefits are measurable directly in terms of money or incomes but most of the benefits of health programs, however, cannot or should not be measured in monetary yardstick. Putting a monetary value on human lives is not considered as a satisfactory procedure.

Cost trends: It is generally believed that better health services would reduce the total volume of sickness in the nation and consequently the need for health services would decline. The state of health service is, thus, seen not only as a wealth producing service, but also as a partially self-liquidating service. It has been, however, observed that expenditure on health is consuming the national income at an increasing rate and if, this trend continues several countries maybe spending some 10 percent of their national income on health services before the year 2000 AD.

FOCUS OF HEALTH ECONOMICS

In every country (and many sub national structures, such as states and provinces), health economics plays, or should play, an important role in policy and operational decisions regarding, among others:

- The appropriate role of government, markets and the private sector in the health sector
- Resource allocation and mobilization that affect the equity and efficiency of public spending on health
- Resource transfer mechanisms to hospitals and health care providers and the incentive systems that underlie them
- Health system organizational structures and linkages between the levels
- Health facility organizational structures

- Mechanisms to change behaviors of the population and health system providers in order to achieve better health.

Health economists can contribute to better decision-making. While most economists train through university degree programs, short- and medium-term training is also required. Furthermore, health economists, even when they do exist and are well trained, are not always part of decision-making in health ministries. A clear need exists to train and empower policy and operational decision makers on how health economics can help make health systems more effective, efficient and equitable.

AREA/SCOPE OF HEALTH ECONOMICS

The economics of health is by no means trivial but has a wider scope. The health care sector is not just another sector as agriculture, industry or financial services. Its output is somewhat elusive but it certainly goes beyond what can reasonably be measured in terms of money. It is primarily due to the fact that here the final output is individual health, or to be more specific, improvements in individual health conditions, the quantities which are not readily comparable between individuals and not measurable in terms of money. This special nature of the sector gives rise to many fundamental problems, which by themselves represent challenges to economic theory. There are several other peculiar difficulties that may arise in the application of economic concepts in the field of health.

- *Box A* contains the conceptual foundation health. It contains a multidisciplinary literature in which one finds economists, epidemiologists, operational researchers, psychologists and sociologists all working and sometimes even working together! The central issues in this box relate to the meaning of 'health', its relationship with 'welfare', and the development of valid and reliable measures of it for a variety of purposes, specific and general. It is impossible for these matters to be addressed without careful attention to the value assumptions that are to be made (and where they should come from).
- *Box B* is concerned with the determinants of health, broadly genetic and environmental, as human capital, not just in the sense of a stream of discounted benefits over an expected lifetime but as a distinctive way of treating health itself—a capital stock that can be invested in, which depreciates, for the demand influences and is influenced by the demand for other human investments. It concerns the interaction between a health production function and a health demand function and has been a highly distinctive research area within health economics.

Flow chart 21.1: Structure of discipline

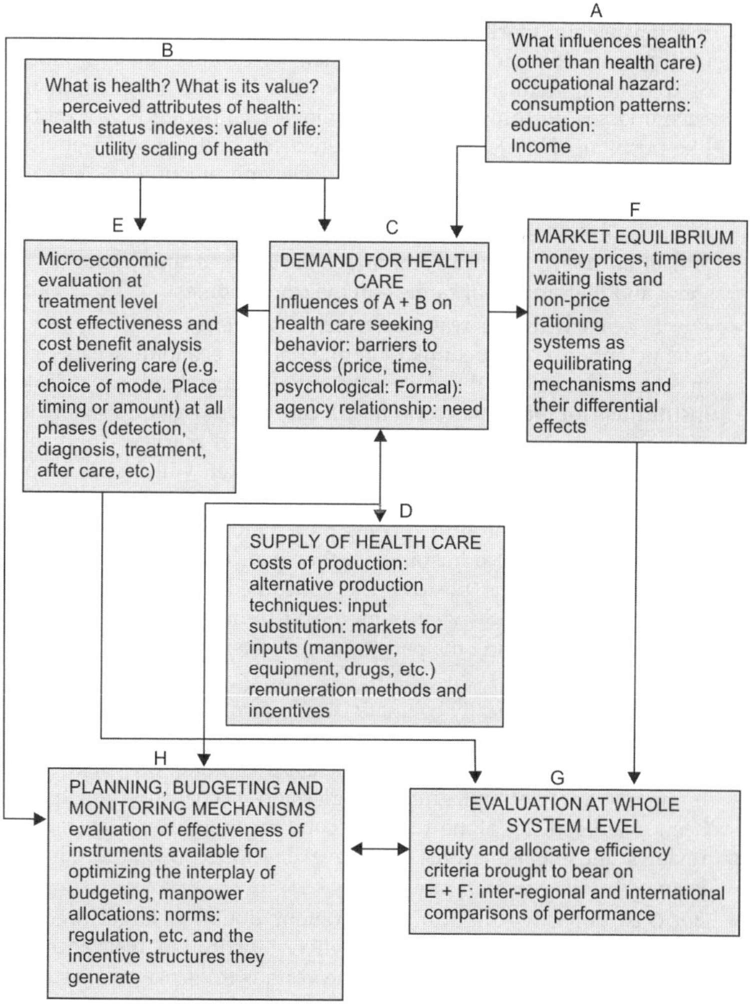

- *Box C* concerns the demand for health care. This demand is a derived demand (from the demand for health) and comes logically after boxes A and B. This is also where utility interdependencies come in (externalities), where the tensions between 'need' and 'demand' (and the advocates of each) are addressed, and where important questions related to the normative significance of revealed demand have been extensively discussed.

- *Box D* contains the material to be expected in supply-side economics: hospital production functions, input substitutions, behavioral relations, labor markets, the responses of institutions and health industry workers to changes in their environments and modes of payment, industrial regulation. The health care 'industry' encompasses not only the more obvious health care organizations like hospitals, HMOs, and general practices, and the again obvious medical supplies sector (pharmaceuticals, equipment, etc.), but also other public and private caring agencies, often dealing with specific client groups like the elderly, the mentally infirm and the disabled, and often doing so on a community basis (for example, caring for them and their informal carers—in their own homes).
- *Box E* deals with the ways in which markets in all these sectors operate and is a major chunk of applied health economics, especially in countries where there is substantial dependence on market institutions for the provision of health care insurance and the delivery of health care. Even where there are no formal markers, the health care system operates as a kind of quasi-market, with, for example, contracts between non-profit public sector agencies, and pseudo-prices (including time prices) being paid. Queuing and waiting lists/times for admission to hospital are thus considered in this box. The material of this box is 'positive' (i.e. concerned with 'what happens', 'what happened' and 'what is predicted to happen' if...) as well as 'normative': evaluating the performance of markets using the tools of welfare economics.
- *Box F* is more specifically evaluative and normative. It is the home of applied cost effectiveness and cost-utility analysis. The literature in this genre is now vast and a book such as this cannot do justice to the immense variety of topics, technologies and mechanisms which have been evaluated, let alone to the secondary literature of systematic reviews and meta-analyzes that have developed over the past ten years.
- *Box G* is primarily American in its content, doubtless largely because of the great variety of health care delivery institution, insurance and reimbursement mechanisms, and the various roles played by federal and state agencies. The evolution of new forms of organization, financing and monitoring/control has flourished apace in the US.
- *Box H* is concerned with the highest level of evaluation and appraisal across systems and countries. The internationally observed differences between the mechanisms, expenditure rates, objectives and outcomes are phenomena needing explanation but they also raise difficult questions of how best to make comparisons (and for what purpose) and how best to infer 'lessons' from one system for another.

ECONOMICS OF HEALTH AND HEALTH CARE SERVICE

There are different understandings of health—each with different implications for the roles of government. It is important to recognize, first, the difference between health and 'health care'. The term health refers to a state either of an individual or of a community. A number of factors including 'health care' may influence this state of health. However, other factors that affect health are poverty, level of education, food intake, access to clean water and sanitary and housing conditions.

The narrowest concept of health sees it as a measure of the state of the physical body organs. An individual is unhealthy if there is a malfunctioning of part of the body. A broader, but related, definition sees health just in terms of the mechanics of the different bodily organs, but in the ability of the body as a whole to function.

In contrast, the WHO definition of health as "a state of physical, mental and social well-being and not merely the absence of disease or infirmity" indicates a clear shift away from earlier narrow organic or functionally-based definitions of health to a more holistic view, it sees the health of an individual or community as being concerned not only with physical (and mental) status, but also with social and economic relationships.

How one views health will affect the type of intervention and planning that is possible. The narrowest definitions are closely associated with a medical model of health in which the role of health services is seen as paramount in restoring the functioning of the unhealthy body. Wider primary health care concepts suggest that broader interventions, including community empowerment and anti-poverty measures, are necessary to promote health. We turn now to different perspectives on the importance of health and on to possible roles of the state in promoting it.

Perspectives of Health

Health as a Right

- Health is viewed by some as a right analogous to justice or political freedom. Indeed, the WHO constitution states that '... the enjoyment of the highest attainable standard of health is one of the fundamental rights of every human being without distinction of race, religion, political belief, economic or social condition'. Although it is difficult to believe that equal health status is attainable in the same way that equal political freedom maybe, health is seen as so fundamental that constraints to its full attainment must be minimized. In part, this involves ensuring access to health care. The government is seen as having a responsibility to ensure this, comparable with its role in ensuring equal justice. According to such a view, a government will be particularly concerned with issues of equity in health and health care.

Health as Consumption Good

For others, health is seen as an important individual objective that is not comparable with justice, but rather with material aspects of life. Such a view often refers to health as consumption good. The government here has no special responsibilities in the promotion of health, but leaves decisions as to its comparative importance to individual consumers. The role of the state under such a view might be limited to ensuring that the health care provided is of an adequate quality (such as ensuring professional standards in the same way that it would monitor the quality of any good or service, such as food).

Health as an Investment

A third view of health is that it is important, but largely it affects the productive ability of the workforce. Illness may affect overall production, either through absenteeism or by lowering productivity through its debilitating effects.

Health Care Services

As most observers agree that consumers demand are affected by various factors such as more ignorant, taste and uncertain in their role as consumers of health services than as purchasers of most other commodities. They cannot assess the quality and character of the health services they consume and are generally unaware of the variety of health care alternatives available for treating a given illness. Ethical standards adopted by the health professions preclude advertising, so consumers are denied access to this form of information concerning the relative merits and costs of various forms of care and treatment.

Moreover, the reluctance of some physicians to discuss illness in non-ethical terms also tends to keep consumers ignorant of feasible treatment alternatives and makes it nearly impossible for them to exercise rational choice. While individuals can choose their physicians, doctors usually determine the kind and quantity of health services individuals consume. While doctors may have some knowledge of the individual's financial resources, these considerations are unlikely to have much influence on the type of care prescribed. The demand and need for medical care is not always the same. For instance, an individual may demand more care than is required medically. Conversely, he may need medical care, but may not be aware of its value. Need is generated by the incidence of illness, while demand is generated by the interrelationship of illness with other factors. To plan for future use of facilities and personnel, demand rather than need for such resources must be projected.

Demand analysis can be applied with appropriate modifications to explain variations in expenditures on medical care services. From the patient's viewpoint, the need for medical care is not always clear-cut. For example, the distinction between a severe cold and pneumonia may not be noticeable to the consumer. Chest pains may indicate either bronchitis or a serious heart condition. In such instances, a high-income family would be expected to take greater precautions and thus incur higher medical care expenditures than a low-income family. Moreover, even after treatment is begun economic factors may influence its duration. A poor family may decide to forego the possible benefit from an extra day in hospital or an additional visit to the physician.

Medical care is characterized by a low degree of substitutability, most medical needs are highly specific and alternative goods are not able to supply the same level of satisfaction. Moreover, medical care is generally wanted for its own sake, most medical care and treatment are unpleasant and generally are not wanted until it becomes a preferable alternative to the pain and other consequences of illness. This implies that the price elasticity of demand for medical care would tend to be low. Grover C Wirick has identified five fundamental factors that can have an impact on the demand for health care services.

- The first is need, when a person suffers from a condition that requires attention, or he/she has some other reason for seeking medical care or examination.
- Secondly, there must be a realization of the need. Either the individual or someone acting in his/her behalf must know that the need exists. A number of psychological processes maybe involved including awareness of the existence and availability of medical skills as well as the benefit likely to be gained through health services. In addition to these, the hopes, fears and beliefs of the individual, as well as the other personal factors such as his/her previous experiences, customers and religion play a significant role. For example, a person with a strong religious conviction against a particular kind of medical treatment may have a different realization of need for care from that of someone with other religious beliefs.
- Third financial resources must be available to implement the care. This capability may take many forms, including the income and assets possessed by the individual or his/her family, insurance coverage, eligibility for free care under a group or government program and availability of care through welfare programs.
- Fourth, there must be a specific motivation to obtain the needed care even with the availability of the other forces such as need, realization and resources, something must initiate the action.
- Fifth is availability of service.

HEALTH AND ECONOMIC DEVELOPMENT

Development is the concern of all developing countries. The health planner, manager, etc. is equally charged with that concern and must be knowledgeable about what development implies and the role health should play in the development of a given country. The following questions are of paramount importance for the health worker in a developing country such as: what is development? How does it differ from economic growth? How can development be measured? What role does health play in development? What role should the health worker play in facilitating development?

Meaning of Economic Development

Development has been variously defined. The modern view of development perceives it as both a physical reality and state of mind in which society has, through some combination of social, economic and institutional processes, secured the means for obtaining a better life.

The definition of 'a better life' may vary from one society to another. Development in all societies, however, must consist of at least the following three objectives:

a. To increase the availability, distribution and accessibility of life-sustaining goods such as food, shelter, health, security and protection to all members of society.
b. To raise standards of living, including higher incomes, the provision of more jobs, better education and better health, and more attention to cultural and humanistic values so as to enhance not only material well-being, but also to generate greater individual community and national esteem.
c. To expand the range of economic and social opportunities and services to individuals and communities by freeing them from servitude and dependence on other people and communities and from ignorance and human misery.

Growth and Development

For a long time, development and economic growth were used interchangeably. Although the two are closely related they are, however, different. Economic growth can be defined as an increase in a country's productive capacity, identifiable by a sustained rise in real national income over a period of years.

The main differences between growth and development can be outlined as follows:

- Development encompasses the total well-being of the individual, a community or a nation, while economic growth is concerned with the increase in per capita earnings of the people making-up the nation.

- Economic growth is one characteristic of development, yet development must not be measured by the rate of economic growth. It is possible for a country to experience economic growth without becoming developed. A country, for example, may acquire a great wealth from its mineral deposits, but have a low level of health services. This is due to the fact that the wealth goes into the hands of a very small minority who might squander it on luxury goods instead of establishing a viable infrastructure.
- Development is concerned with the total person, his economic, social, political, physiological, psychic and environmental requirements. If one of these is not fully cater for, development has not been achieved.

Measurement of Economic Development

The measurement of development has presented social scientists with a problem of finding the suitable tools and techniques to do so and of interpreting the results of such measurements. Several suggestions have been presented for measuring development. One line of research has suggested the use of so-called social indicators. The purpose of these is to measure the well-being of the population by examining factors such as health and nutritional status, level of education, housing conditions and so forth. However, it is easier to calculate GNP, per capita incomes and growth rates.

As a result, in most reports these variables are used as indicators of development. Economic development, in addition to a rise in per capita income, implies fundamental changes in the structure of the economy characterized by:

- Rising share of industry, along with the failing share of agriculture in GNP and increasing percentage of people who live in cities rather than the countryside.
- Passing through periods of accelerating, then decelerating population growth, during which the age structure of the country changes dramatically.
- Changes in consumption patterns as people no longer spend all their income on necessities, but instead move on to consume durables and eventually to leisure-time products and services.
- Meeting the needs of the present without compromising the ability of future generations to meets their own needs (sustainability).
- Participation (mainly) by the citizens of the country in the process as well as the benefit, while economic development and modern economic growth involve much more than arise in per capita income, there can be no development without economic growth.

Health Implications of Economic Development

The associations between health and national development are complex. The interaction is a two-way phenomenon with health being both influenced by and influencing economic development. Improved health has been considered solely a result of economic growth, a part of the product of growth rather than one of its causes.

Some development experts have maintained that health should have low priority in development funding and have tried to justify their opinions with comments such as 'only a rich nation can afford the programs to assure its population's health', or 'a poor nation cannot afford improved health'. The concern of development planners is accentuated by the fact that during the demographic transition, lower death rates are often associated with sustained high birth rates which results in rapid population growth.

While the supply of labor may increase as a result of improved health and reduced death rates, there maybe no corresponding gain in per capita output. Thus, if economic growth is too slow to absorb the additions to the labor force associated with expanded health programs, greater unemployment, both open and disgusted, may result. Thus, improved health in poor societies can be postulated to produce larger populations, greater poverty and ultimately deterioration in health.

However, other development planners and economists are more optimistic regarding the impact of health and nutrition programs on economic growth. There are three different ways by which improved health programs can accelerate development.

- Improved health may increase productivity or efficiency of the labor force leading to greater output and reduced cost per unit of output.
- Better health conditions may serve to open new regions of a country of settlement and subsequent development.
- Attitudinal changes towards achievement and entrepreneurship maybe lined to health and nutrition programs. This linkage has a significant importance to stimulate entrepreneur ship in poor countries.

It has been apparent that where conditions are worst, relatively simple and low cost health programs can produce dramatic reductions of debility and disability of the labor force. In these situations major increments in productivity are most readily apparent. For instance, in the Philippines at one time a survey of major enterprises indicated a daily absenteeism rate of 35 percent, attributed largely to malaria.

Major Determinants of Poor Health

The following are some of the main determinants of poor health which have direct or indirect interdependence with economic development:

- *Population growth:* Rapid population growth implies an increased need for medical and other social services
- Malnutrition
- Sanitary conditions and inadequate shelter
- Education.

There remains a debate on the relation between health status improvements and economic growth. It is argued that health status improvements are attained at the expense of fixed capital entailing a smaller economic growth. That is, the investment funds that could have been used for the growth of the economy at large are to be used for investments in the health service sector which has in part a consumption character. Some argue, however, that investment in basic needs, such as in the health service sector, are investments in the health service sector which has in part a consumption character. Some argue, however, that investment in basic needs, such as in the health service sector, are investments in human capital which in turn is growth promoting. Although some tend to conclude that there is a positive relationship between health and economic development, this does not prove that improvement of the health service sector is a sufficient condition for economic development. On the other hand, a better health status does not guarantee a faster economic growth.

COMMON HEALTH PROBLEMS IN INDIA

In the post-independence period, the growth rate of the urban population in India has always remained higher than the growth rate of the rural population. The size of the country's urban population is projected to increase to nearly 586 million by 2030. By 2015, more than 50 cities in India are expected to have a population of more than one million. It is estimated that urban population growth will account for over two-thirds of total population growth in India in the first quarter of the 21st Century. As elsewhere in the world, the growth rate of the slum population in most cities has been much higher than the growth rate of the non-slum population.

Serious concerns have been raised about increasing disparities in health condition of the population between cities and among different groups of the population in the same city. Using data from India's National Family Health Surveys, a group of researchers at the Urban Health Resource Centre, a technical consultant group to the Ministry of Health and Family Welfare, Government of India, has brought into focus the sharp disparities that exist in health conditions between the urban poor and the better-off population in urban areas of several states.

Diabetes

Diabetes, commonly known as 'sugar' illness, is often related to a sedentary lifestyle, obesity, and stress. It is fast emerging as an important health problem in urban areas. A person has diabetes when the body fails to produce or properly use insulin to convert sugar, starch, etc. into energy. In general, the prevalence of diabetes in the eight cities is higher than the national average both among women age 15–49 (881 per 100,000) and men age 15–49 (1,051 per 100,000). In these cities, the prevalence of diabetes among women varies from 1,124 per 100,000 in Meerut to 3,874 per 100,000 in Chennai. Kolkata and Hyderabad are the other cities where more than 2 percent of women suffer from diabetes. The prevalence of diabetes among men ranges from 430 per 100,000 in Indore to 2,815 per 100,000 in Hyderabad.

Asthma

Asthma, a chronic respiratory disease, is often mistaken for tuberculosis because the symptoms are similar. The prevalence of asthma among women varies from 591 per 100,000 in Delhi to 3,133 per 100,000 in Kolkata, followed by Nagpur (2,845 per 100,000). Among men, the prevalence of asthma is also very high in Kolkata and Nagpur (3,269 and 3,275 per 100,000, respectively). The slum/non-slum situation with respect to prevalence of asthma is mixed in these cities. In Delhi and Kolkata, the prevalence of asthma among both women and men is higher in non-slum areas than in slum areas, whereas the reverse is true in Mumbai, Hyderabad, and Chennai. The prevalence of asthma among the poor in these cities does not show a consistent pattern.

Goiter or Other Thyroid Disorders

- Goiter is usually caused by an iodine deficiency, which leads to an enlargement of the thyroid gland. The only symptom in many cases is a swelling in the neck. Among men, the prevalence of Goiter or other thyroid disorders is highest in Kolkata (730 per 100,000). The prevalence of Goiter among women ranges from 482 per 100,000 in Indore to as high as 4,199 per 100,000 in Kolkata. In Chennai, almost 3 percent of women suffer from Goiter or other thyroid disorders. There are far greater differences in the prevalence of Goiter or other thyroid disorders between slum and non-slum areas among women than men. The prevalence of Goiter or other thyroid disorders is exceptionally high among women in non-slum areas of Kolkata (5,139 per 100,000). In almost every case, poor men and women are less likely than other men and women to have Goiter or other thyroid disorders.

Tuberculosis

- The extreme crowding conditions, lack of proper sanitation, and environmental pollution in very large cities exposes residents, particularly slum dwellers, to a high-risk of contracting tuberculosis, which is a highly contagious disease. In recent years, tuberculosis has re-emerged as a major public health problem in many parts of the world, often as an opportunistic illness related to HIV/AIDS. The disease spreads through droplets that can travel through the air when a person with the infection coughs, talks, or sneezes. In Meerut, Hyderabad, and Chennai, the prevalence of TB is higher among males than females, but the reverse is true in Delhi, Kolkata, Indore, Mumbai, and Nagpur. In every city except Hyderabad, the prevalence of medically treated TB among males is higher in slum areas than in non-slum areas.

HIV/AIDS

The Government of India has been making extensive use of mass media, especially electronic media, to increase awareness of AIDS and methods of avoiding HIV/AIDS. Men's knowledge of AIDS is nearly universal in every city. In every city except Meerut, 89–99 percent of women have heard about AIDS. Slum/non-slum differentials in the knowledge of AIDS among men are small in every city. Among women, knowledge of AIDS is consistency lower in slum areas than in non-slum areas, although the differences are small in many cities. Poor people, particularly poor women, are least aware of AIDS in these cities. In Meerut, less than 50 percent of poor women have heard about AIDS.

Fertility and Family Planning

- Teenage fertility does not vary much across cities (from 5–8 percent). Teenage fertility is generally much higher among slum women than non-slum women, and highest among poor women. In the eight cities, 59–77 percent of currently married women are using a method of family planning. In seven of the cities, the contraceptive prevalence rate is lower in slum areas than in non-slum areas. The contraceptive method mix differs substantially between slum and non-slum areas of these cities. Women in slum areas are much less likely to use modern spacing methods but are generally more likely to use permanent methods. The use of modern methods of contraception is generally lowest among poor women.

Infant and Child Mortality

The infant mortality rate (IMR) varies widely across these cities, ranging from 28 per 1,000 live births in Chennai to 63 per 1,000 live births in Meerut. Differentials by slum/non-slum residence do not show a consistent pattern.

Child Health

In every city, at least 90 percent of children of age 12–23 months have received some vaccinations. However, the proportion of children who have received all basic vaccinations is not very high in any of the cities, ranging from 43 percent in Meerut to 78 percent in Chennai. In every city except Chennai, vaccination coverage is higher for children in non-slum areas than in slum areas for almost every vaccination. In Delhi, Kolkata, and Nagpur, the coverage of each vaccination is much lower for poor children than it is for other children. In Chennai, however, vaccination coverage is slightly higher among poor children than among non-poor children for each vaccination.

Maternal Care

Although the utilization of antenatal care services differs substantially among the cities and between their slum and non-slum areas, in almost all cases poor women are the least likely to receive antenatal care services. At least 60 percent of deliveries took place in health facilities, except in Meerut where only 46 percent of deliveries were conducted in health facilities. Institutional deliveries were nearly universal in Chennai, and were almost as high (92 percent) in Hyderabad. All indicators of delivery and postnatal care were consistently better in non-slum areas than in slum areas in all cities except Indore and Chennai.

Nutritional Status and Anemia among Children

The proportion of children who are underweight ranges from 20–23 percent in Hyderabad, Kolkata, and Chennai to 39 percent in Indore. Slum children generally have poorer nutritional status than non-slum children. Anemia is widespread among children in these cities (49–68 percent of children ages 6–59 months). Except in Kolkata, anemia among children is more widespread in slum areas than in non-slum areas, but even in non-slum areas, anemia is very high, ranging from 47 percent in Mumbai to 67 percent in Meerut. Anemia is higher among poor children than non-poor children in every city.

Nutritional Status and Anemia Among Adults

- In every city, poor women and men are more likely to be abnormally thin than non-poor women and men. At least one out of four poor women and men are undernourished. Overweight and obesity are notable problems among adults in all eight cities. Women and men in non-slum areas are much more likely to be overweight or obese than those in slums. Even in slum areas of Hyderabad and Chennai, about one-third of women are overweight or obese. At least 4 in 10 women are anemic in both slum and non-slum areas in every city.

Tobacco and Alcohol Consumption

- A wide range of serious diseases, including several types of cancers and heart and lung diseases are associated with tobacco use. Tobacco use among women can cause a variety of reproductive health problems, such as difficulty in becoming pregnant and an increased risk of infertility, pregnancy complications, premature births, low-birth-weight babies, stillbirths, and infant deaths (United States Department of Health and Human Services, 2004). Similarly, frequent use of alcohol is related to several health and social-psychological problems.

  In India, tobacco is used in several forms, such as smoking of cigarettes or *bidis*, chewing of *paan masala* or *gutkha*, and applying tobacco to the teeth or gums. Smoking and tobacco use, particularly smoking cigarettes or *bidis*, is not common among women. Smoking of cigarettes or *bidis* is almost non-existent among women in every city except Delhi and Meerut, where 1 percent of women smoke. Use of any type of tobacco by women is more evident, but still very low, ranging from 1 percent in Chennai to 6–7 percent in Kolkata, Mumbai, and Nagpur. Tobacco use among men is much more widespread. In every city, more than one-third of men age 15–49 use tobacco in some form.

  The use of tobacco is particularly high among poor women and men in these cities. In every city, at least one out of two poor men uses tobacco. In Kolkata and Indore, the proportion of poor men using tobacco is particularly high (76 and 87 percent, respectively). Ten percent or more of poor women in Mumbai (11 percent), Delhi (12 percent), Kolkata (14 percent), Nagpur (15 percent), and Indore (17 percent) use tobacco in some form.

  Alcohol use among women in these cities is negligible (less than 1 percent in every city except Hyderabad, where it is 3 percent). Alcohol consumption is far greater among men, ranging from 23–24 percent in Indore and Meerut to 45 percent in Chennai. As is the case for tobacco use, among men alcohol drinking is generally more prevalent in slum areas than in non-slum areas. Only in Kolkata is alcohol use among men slightly higher in non-slum areas than in slum areas. Alcohol use is particularly high among poor men in every city, especially Chennai (65 percent) and Indore (56 percent).

SUMMARY

In this unit we discuss about the health economics is concerned with issues related to the allocation of scarce resources to improve health, this includes both resource allocation within the economy to the health sector and within the health care system to different activities and individuals. Health economists can contribute to better decision-making. While most economists train through university degree programs, short- and medium-term training is also required. The health care sector is not just another sector as agriculture, industry or financial services. The health planner, manager, etc. is equally charged with that concern and must be knowledgeable about what development implies and the role health should play in the development of a given country. Health Resource Center, a technical consultant group to the Ministry of Health and Family Welfare, Government of India, has brought into focus the sharp disparities that exist in health conditions between the urban poor and the better-off population in urban areas of several states.

22 unit

Costs of Health Care

INTRODUCTION

Despite numerous attempts by many governments to contain accelerating costs in the health care field during the past two decades, medical expenditures have continued to grow rapidly as a percentage of Gross National Product (GNP) throughout the world. This escalation diverts resources from other important national and international goals, such as job creation, housing, education, economic development, and the environment. Although medical expenses are higher in the US than in any other country, the cost crisis is not limited to one nation; it is a worldwide problem. Moreover, the medical expenditure challenge is noncyclical; it continues to grow worse with time. Consequently, new and innovative interventions in the health care field will be required to slow this growth and, ultimately, to decrease medical spending.

CONCEPT OF COST

- Economists define a cost as the value of resources used to produce a good or services. However, the way these resources are measured can differ. There are two main alternatives with respect to measurement of these resources: financial and economic costing.
- '*Financial cost* represents actual expenditure on goods and services purchased. Costs are thus described in terms of how much money has been paid for the resources used in the project or services. In order to ascertain the financial costs of a project, we need to know the price and quantity of all the resources used or, alternatively, the level of expenditure on these goods and services'.
- '*Economists conceptualize costs* in broader way. They define costs in terms of the alternative uses that have been forgone by using resources

in a particular way. These economic or opportunity costs recognize the cost of using resources as these resources are then unavailable for productive use elsewhere'.

- The basic ideas are that is that things have a value that might not be fully captured in their prices. It is not difficult in many health programs to identify resources inputs for which little or no money is paid: volunteers working without payment; health messages broadcasts without charge; vaccines or other suppliers donated or provided at large discount by organizations or individuals. Thus, the values of these resources to society, regardless of who pays for them, are measured by opportunity cost.
- Economic cost then include the estimated value of goods or services for which there were no financial transaction or when the price of a specific good did not reflect the cost of using it productivity elsewhere. The main ways that financial and economic costs differ is in the way they treat:
  - Donated goods and services.
  - Others inputs whose prices and incorrect or distorted.
  - Valuation of capital items.
- The theory and the concept of cost arise from the fact that economic resources are scarce by nature. Had it not been for the scarcity of resources, the concept and theory of cost may not exist as such. Scarcity has two sides:
  (a) The infinite nature of human wants.
  (b) The finite or limited nature of resources available to produce goods and services.

TYPES OF COSTS

Direct and Indirect Costs

Direct costs refer to the resource consumption in the provision of health care interventions. They encompass the entire current resource use and, depending on the timeframe under consideration, also future resource use attributable to the program. Future costs can span a lifetime in some therapeutic areas.

Direct costs are further split into direct medical and direct nonmedical costs. Direct medical costs refer to the resource consumption in the health care sector associated with the provision of health care interventions. Resource consumption includes for example, the costs of hospital stays, outpatient visits, drugs, medicinal substances and devices. Direct nonmedical costs refer to resources supporting the medical services delivered in the health care sector. Depending on the perspective, these can be, for example, travel costs to medical interventions or the valuated time spent by patients and their family caregivers in relation to their illness.

Indirect costs denote the production losses due to incapacity for work (in the case of illness), occupational disability (in the case of long-term illness or disability), and premature death.

Opportunity Costs

Opportunity costs, too, are a basic theoretical cost concept in health economic evaluation. They define the value of scarce resources in the production of health care interventions. Opportunity costs refer to the benefit of resources regarding the next best alternative use of the resources. As is shown in microeconomic theory, opportunity costs are reflected in the market prices of a perfectly competitive market. However, most markets in the health care sector are imperfect: prices are regulated by public institutions, or negotiated between associations of providers and health insurance funds, or do not even exist, which means that prices often are no adequate indicators of opportunity costs. Thus, for example, the prices of drugs, consisting of patented and off-patent drugs grouped together in jumbo groups, differ from the "actual" social opportunity costs.

Total Cost

Total cost refers to the total outlays of money expenditure, both explicit and implicit on the resources used to produce a given output.

Fixed Cost

Fixed costs are the expenditure incurred on the factors such as capital, equipment, plant; factory building which remains fixed in the short run and cannot be changed. Therefore, fixed costs are independent of output in the short run, i.e. they do not vary with output in the short run. Even if no output is produced in the short run, these costs will have to be incurred.

Variable Cost

Variable costs are costs incurred by the firms on the employment of variable factors such as labor, raw materials, etc. whose amount can be easily increased or decreased in the short run. Variable costs vary with the level of output in the short run. If the firm decided not to produce any output, variable costs will not be incurred.

Marginal Versus Average Costs

A basic decision in cost estimation is the choice of average costs or marginal costs. Average costs are the costs per unit of output, marginal costs are the extra costs of producing one extra unit of output, i.e. one additional patient treated or one additional unit of intervention produced. One difference between the assessment of average costs and marginal costs is that fixed costs (such as buildings and equipment) are included in average costs, but are not considered in marginal costs. In health care there are scenarios where costs often increase more than proportionally when production output is expanded, and marginal costs will exceed average costs.

Which cost concept should be applied in cost estimation—average cost or marginal cost—depends on the specific research question. In general, health economic evaluation supports decision-making on investment decisions (adoption of new technologies, licensing or coverage decision), which means that long-term costs (and effects) are relevant (in which all costs, including the short-term fixed costs, are variable). Moreover, the basic question in health economic evaluation concerns the additional costs (and effects) when output is slightly increased or decreased. Accordingly, the concept of long-term marginal cost is favored in health economic evaluation.

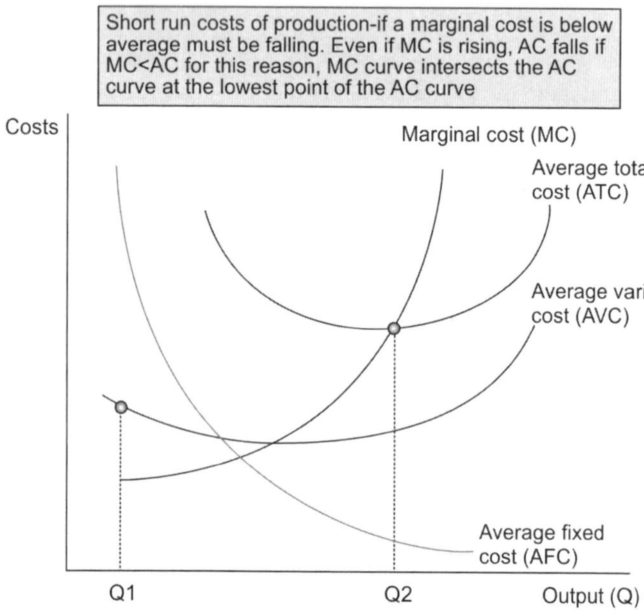

Fig. 22.1: Graphically curve of costs

Average cost is the cost per unit of output. It is obtained by dividing the total cost (TC) by the total quantity produced (Q)

$$\text{Average} = \frac{Q}{TC}$$

Marginal cost is the additional cost incurred to produce an additional unit of output. Or it is the cost of the marginal unit produced.

Example:

A company produces 1000 typewriters per annum. Total fixed cost is ₹ 1,00,000 per annum. Direct material cost per typewriter is ₹ 200 and direct labor cost ₹ 100.

Variable cost per typewriter = direct material + direct labor

= 200 + 100 = ₹ 300

Total variable cost (1000 x 300) = ₹ 300000

Fixed Cost = ₹ 100000

Total cost = ₹ 400000

TC = ₹ 400000

Average Cost = *Q*

TC = ₹ 400

If output is increased by one typewriter, the cost will appear as follows:

Total variable cost (1001 x 300) = 300300

Fixed cost = 100000

Total = 400300

Here the additional cost incurred to produce the 1001th typewriter is ₹ 300 (400300–400000). Therefore, the marginal cost per typewriter is ₹ 300.

Sunk Costs

Sunk costs are those cannot altered by any change. They are the costs incurred in the past. This cost is the result of past decision, and cannot be changed by future decisions. Once an asset has been bought or an investment made, the funds locked up represent sunk costs. As these costs do not alter when any change in activity is made they are sunk and are irrelevant to a decision being taken now. Investments in fixed assets are examples of sunk costs. As soon as fixed assets have been installed, their cost is sunk. The amount of cost cannot be changed.

COST-BENEFIT ANALYSIS

Cost-benefit analysis is the most comprehensive and theoretically sound form of economic evaluation and it has been used as an aid to decision making in many different areas of economic and social policy in the public sector for more than fifty years.

Cost-Benefit analysis (CBA) estimates and totals up the equivalent money value of the benefits and costs to the community of projects to establish whether they are worthwhile. These projects maybe dams and highways or can be training programs and health care systems. The main difference between cost-benefit analysis and other methods of economic evaluation that were discussed earlier in this series is that it seeks to place monetary values on both the inputs (costs) and outcomes (benefits) of health care.

Among other things, this enables the monetary returns on investments in health to be compared with the returns obtainable from investments in other areas of the economy.

Within the health sector itself; the attachment of monetary values to outcomes makes it possible to say whether a particular procedure or program offers an overall net gain to society in the sense that its total benefits exceed its total costs. Cost-effectiveness and cost-utility analysis do not do this because they measure costs and benefits in different units. CBA requires program consequences to be valued in monetary units, thus, enabling the analyst to make a direct comparison of the programs incremental cost with its incremental consequences in commensurate units of measurement, be they Birr, dollars, or pounds.

CBA compares the discounted future streams of incremental program benefits with incremental programs costs; the difference between these two streams being the net social benefit of the program. In simple terms, the goal of analysis is to identify whether a program's benefits exceed its costs, a positive net social benefit indicating that a program is worthwhile. CBA is a full economic evaluation because program outputs must be measured and valued. In many respects CBA is broader in scope than CEA/CUA. Because CBA converts all costs and benefits to money, it is not restricted to comparing programs within health care, but can be used (although not without problems) to inform resource allocation decisions both within and between sectors of the economy. CBA is broader in scope and able to inform questions of allocative efficiency, because it assigns relative values to health and non-health related goals to determine which goals are worth achieving, given the alternative uses of resources, and thereby determining which programs are worthwhile.

- Both costs and benefits are assigned a monetary value. The benefits of any intervention can then be compared directly with any costs incurred.
- If the value of benefits exceeds the costs of any intervention, then it is potentially worthwhile to carry that intervention out.
- If society funds projects for a given budget, then it can maximize the benefits generated by social spending.

- It is concerned with allocative efficiency.
- It is concerned with the question, is a particular goal worthwhile. Potentially it can answer questions such as should extra money be used for heart transplants or improving housing.
- Method requires that all resources and benefit generated by an intervention need to be assigned a monetary value. Therefore, needs to cost things which have no market value, i.e. changes in health, quality of life, length of life, pain, etc.
- Methods of valuing.
- Willingness to pay (WTP).
- Human capital approach.
- The net welfare gain or net value of a project X (NVX) is equal to

$$NVX = WTPX - WTY$$

- Where y refers to the next best alternative project. If the latter is not or cannot be defined.

$$NVX = WTPX - WTPXi$$

- Where WTPXi refers to society while WTP is for the inputs used alternatively in the economy at large.

If NVX is positive then, project X maybe undertaken. When several projects compete with each other, it is evident that the one with the highest NV needs to be selected in order to maximize welfare.

This shows the CBA for projects that have benefits or costs in the current period. It is evident that projects may also entail future benefits and future costs.

Making use of the social discount rate r, we can calculate the net present value (NPV) of a project.

$$NPV = [(Bt - Ct) / (1 + r) - 1]$$

Where 'B' and 'C' refer to benefits and costs respectively, with 't' is the time index. In fact, 'Bt' is equal to the WTP for the nth project at time 't', while 'Ct' has to be understood as the benefits forgone in period 't'. Note that if NPV > 0 society's welfare will increase; hence, the project can be adopted. If several projects are competing with each other the one with the highest NPV should be chosen.

COST-EFFECTIVENESS ANALYSIS

When different health care interventions are not expected to produce the same outcomes both the costs and consequences of the options need to be assessed. This can be done by cost effectiveness analysis, whereby the costs are compared with outcomes measured in natural units for example, per life saved, per life year gained, and pain or symptom free day. Many cost-effective analyzes rely on existing published studies for effectiveness data, as it is often too costly or time consuming to collect data on costs and effectiveness during a clinical trial. Where there is uncertainty about the costs and effectiveness of procedures sensitivity analysis can be used, which examines the sensitivity of the results to alternative assumptions about key variables. In what follows these methods of analysis are described and the possibilities how the benefits of alternative interventions should be valued are discussed.

CEA is concerned with technical efficiency issues, such as: what is the best way of achieving a given goal or what is the best way of spending a given budget. Comparisons can be made between different health programs in terms of their cost effectiveness ratios: cost per unit of effect. Under CEA effects are measured in terms of the most appropriate unidimensional natural unit. So, if the question to be addressed was: what is the best way of treating renal failure? Then the most appropriate ratio with which to compare programs might be 'cost per life saved'. Similarly, if we wanted to compare the cost-effectiveness of programs of screening for Down's syndrome the most appropriate ratio might be 'cost per Down's syndrome fetus detected'. In deciding whether long-term care for the elderly should be provided in nursing homes or the community the 'cost per disability day avoided' might be the most appropriate measure.

- The advantage of the CEA approach is that it is relatively straight-forward to carry-out.
- It is often sufficient for addressing many questions in health care. However, it is not comprehensive. The outcome is unidimensional under this analysis, but often health programs generate multiple outcomes.
- For example, in Downs' syndrome screening, fetus detected is one outcome, but miscarriages avoided might be another very relevant outcome measure, especially if, say, blood testing is being compared to amniocentesis. But this cannot be incorporated into this form of analysis. So, CEA not only assumes that the outcome of the health program is worthwhile per se, but also that it is the most appropriate measure. A further problem with CEA is comparability between very different health programs. Cost per fetus detected maybe a useful way to compare the efficiency of blood testing versus amniocentesis, but how would these be compared to, say, drugs aimed at reducing cholesterol. Health programs with different aims cannot be compared with one another using CEA: cost per unit reduction in cholesterol cannot meaningfully be compared with fetus detected. Hence, CEA is useful when comparing programs within like areas, where common 'currencies' can be used.

If the outcomes of alternative procedures or programs under review are the same, or very similar, then attention can focus upon the costs in order to identify the least cost option the method of evaluation will be cost-minimization analysis. If, however, the outcomes are not expected to be the same, then both the costs and consequences of alternative options need to be considered. Cost-effectiveness analysis is one method of economic evaluation that allows this to be done.

Measures of Effectiveness

In order to carry-out a cost effectiveness analysis it is necessary to have suitable measures of effectiveness. These will depend on the objectives of the particular interventions under review. In all cost effectiveness analysis, however, measures of effectiveness should be defined in appropriate natural units and, ideally, expressed in a single dimension.

Common measures used in several studies have been "lives saved" and 'life years gained'. Thus, Boyle and colleagues, in their study of neonatal intensive care of very low birth weight babies, measured effectiveness in terms of mortality rates at the time of discharge of newborn infants from hospital. Their study compared two periods-one before the introduction of neonatal intensive care, and another after its introduction and measured cost effectiveness in terms of additional costs per life saved.

Several other measures of effectiveness have been used by different researchers (see the box below), these have included the number of pain or symptom free days resulting from alternative drug regimens in the treatment of duodenal ulcers; and the number of episodes of fever cured and deaths prevented in the treatment of chloroquine resistant malaria in African children.

Most of the above mentioned studies express effectiveness in terms of a single dimension and thereby permit direct comparison between alternative procedures in terms of their marginal cost per unit of outcome. Sometimes, however, the alternatives under examination have multiple outcomes. Nonetheless, many of these choices can be dealt within the cost-effectiveness analysis framework. Thus, if one procedure emerges as less costly and of equal or greater effectiveness than all the other options on each dimension of effectiveness, it is clearly the most cost effective option.

For example, the comparison of day surgery with overnight inpatient care for cataract surgery, measured outcomes in terms of the number of both operative and postoperative complications, and in terms of visual acuity of patients three to six days and 10 weeks to six months after surgery. Patient satisfaction was also elicited through a questionnaire. As day surgery emerged as the more effective option on practically all of these effectiveness measures, and was subsequently less costly, the evidence suggests that it is the preferred option.

One argument for carrying out analysis in this way, i.e. not always seeking to combine outcome measures into a single unit, is that the variations across a number of dimensions are made clear to decision makers rather than being concealed within an aggregate measure. This can sometimes permit more informed decision-making, although it can also result in tortuous attempts to compare apples and oranges.

Examples of Measures of Effectiveness:

- Cases treated appropriately
- Lives saved
- Life years gained
- Pain or symptom free days
- Cases successfully diagnosed
- Complications avoided.

Costs-minimisation Analysis

Cost-minimization analysis is an appropriate evaluation method to use when the case for an intervention has been established and the programs and procedures under consideration are expected to have the same or similar outcomes. In these circumstances, attention may focus on the cost side of the equation to identify the least costly option.

Advantages

- It is simple to carry-out, requires costs to be measured, but only that outcomes can be shown to be equivalent
- It avoids needlessly quantifying data

Disadvantages

- It can only be used in narrow range of situations
- It requires that outcomes be equivalent.

Example 1: Cost-Minimization Analysis suppose we are comparing two programs involving minor surgery for adults. Both accomplish the outcome of interest, and from an examination of effectiveness data differ in no# other significant respects except that one requires hospital admission for at least one night, while the other (a day surgery program) does not. If we identified the common outcome of interest—operations successfully completed—we would find that it could be achieved to the same degree (i.e. identical number of surgeries) in either program, though presumably at different costs. The economic evaluation is then essentially a search for the least cost alternative. Analysis such as this is often called cost-minimization analysis. We might also be interested in the distribution of costs (e.g. in this case to what extent does the day-surgery program shift costs to the patient), but our principal efficiency comparison will be made on the basis of cost per surgical procedure.

CMA is really a special form of cost-effectiveness analysis, where the consequences of the alternative treatments being compared turn out to be equivalent. It can be seen from the box below that there are nine possible outcomes when one therapy is being compared with another. In three of the nine cases the analysis reduces to a CMA.

Example: 2. Cost-Effectiveness Analysis suppose that our interest is now the prolongation of life after renal failure and that we are comparing the costs and consequences of hospital dialysis versus kidney transplantation. In this case, the outcome of interest—life years gained—is common to both programs; however, the programs may have differential success in achieving this outcome, as well as differential costs. Consequently, we would not automatically lean toward the least cost program unless, of course, it also resulted in a greater prolongation of life. In comparing these alternatives we would normally calculate this prolongation and compare cost per unit of effect (i.e. cost per life-year gained). Such analyses, in which costs are related to a single, common effect, which may differ in magnitude between the alternative programs, are usually referred to as cost-effectiveness analysis. Note that the results of such comparisons maybe stated either in terms of cost per unit of effect, as in this example, or in terms of effects per unit of cost (life-years gained per dollar spent). The latter is a particularly useful approach when working within a given budget constraint, as long as the alternatives under consideration are not of radically different scale.

Furthermore, although the alternatives used in this example are similar in that both could be considered variants of an overall renal program, it should be noted that cost effectiveness analysis could be performed on any alternatives, which have a common effect. Thus, kidney transplantation could be compared to heart surgery if the common effect of interest was life-years saved. Similarly, an influenza immunization program could be compared to a home care program if a common effect of interest, perhaps disability days avoided, could be identified.

Discounting Benefits (in cost-effectiveness analysis)

Costs incurred at different points in time need to be "weighted" or discounted to reflect the fact that those that occur in the immediate future are of more importance than those that accrue in the distant future. This raises the question: should the benefits or effects of alternative procedures also be discounted? (For details about discounting refer to section three of this material).

In answering this issue there is a difference among economists. If a zero discounting (no discounting applied) were adopted, the main consequence would be to change the relative cost effectiveness of different procedures. Using a positive discount rate means that projects with long lasting effects receive lower priority. If a positive rate is replaced by a zero rate, procedures such as neonatal care-which lead to benefits over the recipient's entire future lifetime-will, become relatively more cost effective. In practical terms, it is probably true to say that while the case for using a zero discount rate for benefits has powerful intellectual and may gain empirical support in the future, it will be too hasty to recommend that positive rates be discarded in economic evaluations.

- Cost-effectiveness analysis is a form of economic evaluation in which the costs of alternative procedures or programs are compared with outcomes measured in natural units for example, cost per life year saved, cost per case cured, cost per symptom free day.
- Effectiveness data are ideally collected from economic evaluations built in alongside clinical trials. In the absence of dedicated trials researchers need to draw on the existing published work.
- Sensitivity analysis should be applied when there is uncertainty about the costs and effectiveness of different procedures. This investigates the extent to which results are sensitive to alternative assumptions about key variables.
- There is debate among economists about whether benefit measures should be 'time discounted' in the same way as costs. If they are not, projects with long lasting effects will become relatively more cost effective for example, maternity services and health promotion. But it will be probably wrong to recommend this as a standard practice.

SUMMARY

In health economic evaluations, a mere comparison of technology costs between new and existing health technologies is not sufficient. New technologies are frequently more cost-intensive than existing health technologies, which is particularly true for drugs. However, in general, health interventions not only differ in mere technology costs, but also in their impact on (follow-up) costs for other health care services (and, of course, on benefit effects). Thus, the increased cost of a new technology maybe offset by savings in other health care sectors. Cost offsets will be achieved when the new technology (e.g. new drug) results in a cost reduction for other health care services (e.g. hospital stays and outpatient visits) compared to the alternative technology.

Demand and Supply in Health Care

23 unit

INTRODUCTION

Economics is the science that deals with the production, distribution, and consumption of goods and services, or the material welfare of mankind. There are several different reasons that healthcare economics have changed but the most substantial reason would be the supply and demand of care. Supply and demand is the relation between things that cause the price of something to be set. There are millions of people in the world who are in need of care and the more care people need the more equipment and treatments are needed. There is new technologies coming out every year and new treatments causing prices to go up, this is where supply and demand comes in. Health care is one of the largest items that are going to have a supply and demand because of the needs of its patients. The more that people get sick the greater the need for health care, this may not be the best thing for certain patients because with the greater demand for health care the higher the costs may go. During the 1900's the American Medical Association (AMA) started to become a force that was found nationwide. During the 1900's surgery was becoming the common thing for doctors to do, thus leading to patients having to pay money for their care. This has lead to the change in how people pay for their care and therefore making the way for funding of health care.

CONCEPT OF DEMAND

The economic demand is derive from the human needs and wants based on the capacity to purchase certain goods and services in the societal market. In this sense, there are two conditions to meet the economic demand: (1) the willingness to buy the products; and (2) the capacity of paying the amount for that particularly products.

The creation of economic demand through the willingness to buy the products may follow the needs and wants of the individual. The existence of human beings is condition to satisfy the physiological or survival needs in order to bring stable physical, social and mental state. This kind of need is best describes in the 'Maslows Hierarchy of Needs'. Likewise, the common basic survival needs are food, clothing, shelter, and others. While, the economic wants are derive from need. However, they are the preference and choice of the consumer on particular product to satisfy the needs of the individual.

The economic demand of the health sector primarily focuses the ability to cure and care the sick or ill patients in the hospitals, clinics and medical care. As a service-oriented business on health care are supported by the medical personnel such as physicians, nurses, attendants, caregivers and midwives. The demand on health care is also presents the medical inputs in curing illness or disease of the patient such as medicines, laboratory facilities and equipment and other tangible medical products.

If an individual decides to be confined in hospital he must consider his ability to pay for the medical bills in the hospital. The usual demand for the confinement for the individual with low income is always in government hospitals. Those with higher income bracket who has enough money to pay their medical bill they usually confine themselves with private hospital. The preference to stay in the private hospital even do it is very expensive they are assured of better health care service than the government hospital.

In health economics, it follows the general rule of economics in the principle of demand that when the price of good or service is high the tendency is the demand is also low. There is a direct relation of the level of price and demand for the goods and services in the societal market. However, these are the factors that affect the demand curve for the demand of medical products and services:

- The increasing average income of people tend to prefer the services of private medical hospital because of the better health services they offered in their air conditioned room, fully equip medical facilities and better medical services. Although, the private medical hospitals are quite expensive in their confinement they are willing to pay for such services because of higher income.
- The increasing population of a locality may result to the increasing medical care services particularly in the urban areas. The increase of commercial activities may result to migration in the urban areas. The hospital is strategically located in the urban areas provided more opportunity to get patients in the urban areas.
- The substitute products can be done from the lowering rates of hospital has become more competitive and can get more patients to be confined in this hospital. The quality health services given in

this hospital can substitute their affordable service for physician fee, medical services and other service they are providing to the patient. The complementary products are usually done in the promotional activities of the hospital. However, it is rarely done to attract the stakeholders the improvement of their services and better quality of care given to the patients.

- The influence of the stakeholder confine themselves in the hospital is also reflected from the added medical service such as X-ray radiographic equipment, sterilizing equipment, operating room instrumentation, fetal monitors, infant incubators, ECG instruments, operating table lights, ct scans, other medical instruments, and operating room equipment. The competent physicians are the most important factor why stakeholders are attracted to be confined or for their medical check in the hospital.

Reasons for the Increase Demand

- The affordable and low cost charges of medical services such as laboratory fees, private room rates, physician fees, medicine charges and other similar charge expenses upon confinement
- The modest income received by the stakeholders provides them to go for medical check and confinement with tertiary hospitals who are fully equip to give quality service to their patients
- The increasing population and mobility of labor to the urban areas where hospital is strategically located to give service to the stakeholders
- The presence of modern and technologically advanced gadgets to monitor patient's health. Likewise, the presence of competent physicians to correctly diagnose the illness of the patient.

These are the economic demand for health care market in relation to hospitalization, illness because of age and gender, self-medication, diagnosis of the doctor, and income of the patient.

- In Illness, the hospitalization of individual is a health care market that needs to pay the services of the hospital such as physician fee, medical fee, drugs and medicine expenses, hospital room fees and other expenses in the process of healing the patient's illness. The economic demand is the payment of hospitalization fee such physician fee, medical fee, drugs and medicine expenses, and hospital room fees.
- In case of age, there are health conditions that maybe present to the elderly people. The degree of demand is the treatment of certain diseases, which they are very prone to diabetes, stroke, heart attacks, cancer, tuberculosis, influenza and other diseases. The economic demand is the payment of medical fees for

confinement and check-up of elderly people on illnesses such as diabetes, stroke, heart attacks, cancer, tuberculosis, influenza and other diseases.

- In self-medication, the personal treatment of illness has its own prescription based on previous diagnosis or consultation with their friends or relatives. The individual may now prescribes drugs as part of self-medication which going to buy paracetamol, antibiotic, pain reliever and other generic drugs that can be bought in the pharmaceutical or drugstores such as paracetamol, antibiotic drugs, pain relieving medicine which they believe through consultation with their friends and relatives will cure the illness of the individual. The economic demand is the individual buys paracetamol, antibiotic drugs, and pain relieving medicine in pharmaceutical or drugstores.
- The diagnosis of the physician may follow the ultimate economic demand of the patient. We always follow the advice of the healthcare provider as the result the medical diagnosis in the hospital, clinic and medical centers.
- The ultimate decisions to take the medicine are dependent to you whether you want self-medication or simply follow the order of your physician. The demand here when individual is willing to buy medicine as prescribe by the doctor such as case of life threatening illness such as dengue, typhoid fever, influenza, pneumonia and other related diseases.
- The income of the patient is the main measure of demand. The high income patient has the tendency to be confine in the more expensive hospital. The private hospitals have high fees in the use of hospital private room, physician fees, laboratory fees, medicine expenses and other hospital fees. The poor patients prefer to be confined in district or provincial government hospitals because it is less expensive than private hospital.

Types of Demand

There are three types of demand. They are:

1. *Price Demand:* It refers to the various quantities of the good which consumers will purchase at a given time and at certain hypothetical prices assuming that other conditions remain the same. We are generally concerned with price demand only. In the explanation of the law of demand given above, we dealt in detail with price demand only.

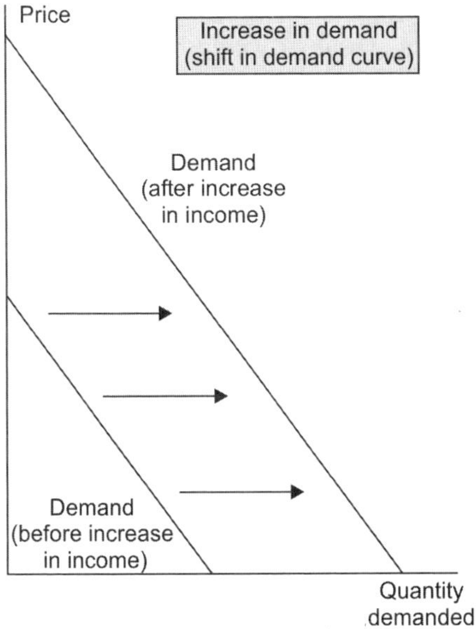

Fig. 23.1: Demand curve

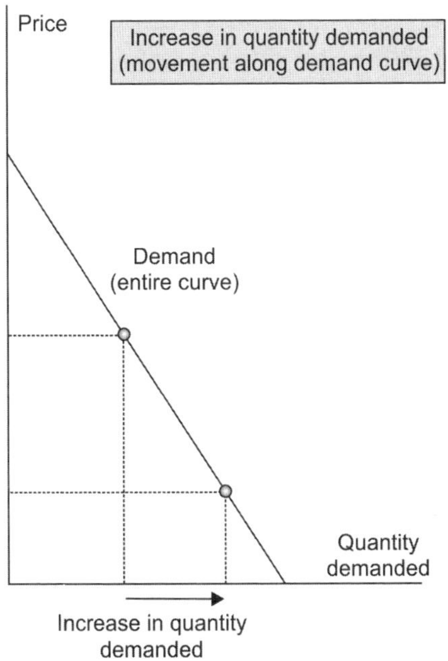

Fig. 23.2: Quantity demand curve

2. *Income demand:* Income demand refers to the various quantities of a commodity that a consumer would buy at a given time at various levels of income. Generally, when the income increases, demand increases and vice versa.
3. *Cross demand:* When the demand of one commodity is related with the price of other commodity is called cross demand. The commodity maybe substitute or complementary. Substitute goods are those goods which can be used in case of each other for example, food items. In such case demand and price are positively related. This means if the price of one increased then the demand for other also increases and vise versa. Complementary goods are those goods which are jointly used to satisfy a want. In other words, complementary goods are those which are incomplete without each other. These are things that go together, often used simultaneously. For example, pen and ink.

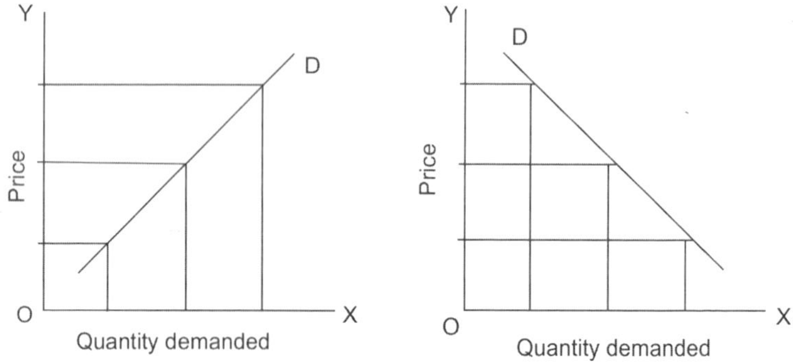

Fig. 23.3: Cross demand curve

SUPPLY

In economics, supply is used in a sense symmetrical with demand. The quantity of a good that producers offer for consumption is seen as determined by certain economic variables, of which the most important is the price at which the good can be offered.

The sellers (supplier) are the producers of goods and services at an acceptable price in the market. Always remember that producers and sellers (businesses) produce and sell to make profits. They prefer a scenario where they can sell their products at higher price-simply because it will give them higher profits. The economic law of supply and demand provides the basis on the price mechanism system that is now acceptable the market. As general rule in the law of economic supply: If the supply of the product is high, it follows that the price is low. If the supply of the products is low, it follows that the price is high. Therefore, the supply of the product has inverse relationships to the price in the market.

The economic supply provides information about the 'quantity supplied' which is determined by the amount of commodity sold in the market. These are major factors that influence the quantity supplied of the economic goods in the market.

- The input prices in the production of certain goods such as the wages/ salary compensation, raw materials, capital investments and other production costs may possibly reduce the quantity supplied in the market. The increase of the input prices decreases the production of goods because this may reduce the profit of the firm.
- The mass production of economic goods through the use of modern technologies may reduce the cost of the production at the same time produce more goods in the market. It is more profitable to use technology as can easily produce higher level in the transformation of economic goods.
- The expectations on the rise on the prices of the economic products in the future. The rise of the economic supply depends so much on the rise of the prices of products in the market.

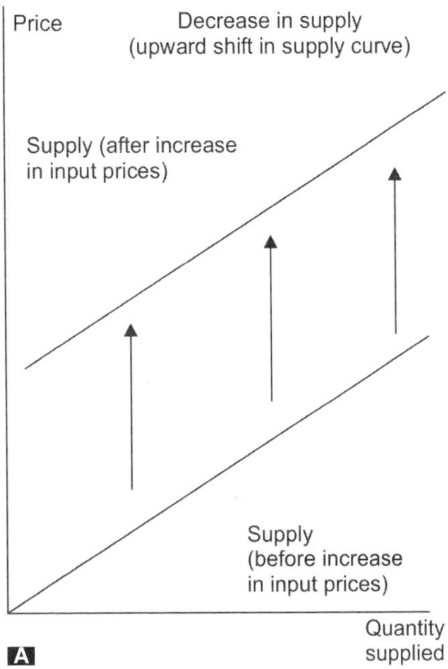

A

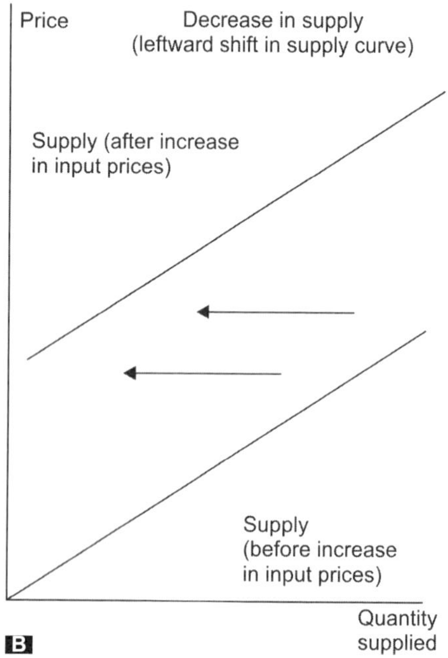

Figs 23.4A and B: Supply curve

In the case of supply of medical care the producer is the hospital that provides health care service for the patient. In hospital, the health care services consist of the primary, secondary and tertiary prevention. The primary prevention provides in the promotion and illness prevention of health. Secondly, the secondary prevention provides the diagnosis and treatment of illness. While the tertiary prevention provides the health care services for the rehabilitation, restoration and palliative health care.

The economic supplies for the medical cares are the hospitals, clinics, medical centers, drug stores and pharmaceutical companies. It should be noted that the term 'goods' in health economics are those needed medicine and medical diagnosis of patients. These are pharmaceutical companies, drug stores and medical supplies who are considered as the 'producers and suppliers' of medicines, drugs, medical equipment and facilities. While 'services' which still in the category of 'supply' is the professional service given by a physician, likewise the consultation fees, medical fees, laboratory fees, and other related hospitalization fees of patients.

PRODUCTION FUNCTION

It is a technical relationship between inputs and the maximum outputs or outcomes of any procedure or process. Thus a production function may relate the maximum number of patients that can be treated in a hospital over a period of time to a variety of input flows like doctor- and nurse-hours, and beds. For econometric purposes the relationship is usually postulated to be in a particular mathematical form, of which one is the so-called Cobb-Douglas production function, X = kA a Bb where X is the rate of output (or throughput of clients), k, a and b are positive constants, and A and B are rates of use of two inputs. The production function specifies efficient combinations of inputs required at each rate of output, viz. the fewest of each needed to produce that output. Depending on the values of parameters like a and b an equal proportional increase in all inputs may entail either a larger, smaller or equal increase in output. This corresponds to increasing, decreasing or constant returns to scale

HEALTH CARE INDUSTRY IN INDIA

The healthcare sector is facing unparalleled challenges in an increasingly customer oriented environment. A lot of health problems need intensive medical treatment and personal care. Treatment cannot be given in a patient's house or in the clinic. This is possible only in a hospital, for it consists of large number of professionally and technically skilled people who apply their knowledge and skill with the help of world-class expertise, advanced sophisticated equipments and appliances. Hospital management performs its duties in the organizational setting of the hospital. It utilizes resources, people and technology to perform organizational goals, of which the most important is patient care. In the past, the hospitals were considered alms houses. They were set-up as charity institutions specially for the poor and weaker sections of the society. The healthcare industry in recent years has restructured its service delivery system in order to survive in an unforgiving environment resulting from maturation of the industry, reduced funding and increased competition. The restructuring has focused on finding effective ways to satisfy the needs and desires of the patients. Consumer satisfaction is a basic requirement for healthcare provider because, the satisfaction related to quality of healthcare is provided by hospitals. Satisfaction is important when patients themselves and institutional healthcare service buyers make selection decisions. The health care services in the hospital vary from one hospital to another. Basically, there are three categories of service, e.g. line services, staff services and auxiliary services. The line services include emergency services, out-patient services, in-patient services, intensive care unit and operation theaters. The staff services are central sterile supply, diet, laundry, laboratory, radiology and nursing. The auxiliary services include registration and indoor care records, stores, transport, mortuary, security and engineering. In the case of patients admitted in the hospital, many groups get involved, i.e. the personnel at the admission counter, the junior/senior residents taking the history of patients and examining patients, the nurses giving patients care and doctors examining patients. There are six stages that are involved in the hospital for treatment of patients, viz.

a. Admission
b. Diagnosis
c. Treatment
d. Inspection
e. Control
f. Discharge

The technology vision 2020 for healthcare was evolved by a panel of healthcare specialists drawn from various parts of the country 1. The team studied the strength of the present healthcare system, problems and the methods for improving healthcare to entire cross-section of the Indian society. The team has identified the imperatives for eradication of three major diseases – tuberculosis, HIV/AIDS and waterborne diseases by the next decade. Every year more than ₹ 5000 crore is spent on importing medical devices and equipments 2.

The Government of Tamil Nadu is also totally committed in building healthy people, not only by making available quality medicare facilities at the door step of every citizen in the remotest corner of the state, but also by providing medical facilities of the highest order, keeping pace with rapid technological developments in the field of medicine. At present 14 Government Medical Colleges 3 have been functioning in 12 districts to improve tertiary care in the state of Tamil Nadu. Now the government is seized of the problem of providing quality health care service to the common man.

Health Care in India

Health care is a big concern in India, Since India is a developing country where a large section of population is below poverty line, health and hygiene are not up to the mark. It is reported that in India, annually, 22 lakh infants and children die from preventable illnesses, 1 lakh mothers die during the child birth and 5 lakh people die of tuberculosis. Also around 5 million people suffer from HIV/AIDS and numerous others die of diarrhea and malaria. The plight of the least advantaged is increased because of the poor public health systems. The government hospitals and health care centers do not completely address to the needs of the poor. On the other hand, the private health care institutions charge exorbitant amount of money, which automatically renders them beyond the reach of many. However, the private health care sector in India is flourishing at the cost of the public. According to some critics, the national policy of the country lacks specific measures to achieve the stated goals. For instance, there is no proper integration of the health care services with the wider socioeconomic and social development. There is lack of nutritional support and sanitation and there is poor participation of the people and government officials at the local level. The central government adopts the strategy of improving the health systems through five-year plans. It cooperates with the state government for that purpose and for sponsoring major health programs. The central and state Governments share the expenditure they meet in providing health care to the people. In mid 1990s, the government spent 6% of the GDP6 on health, which is one of the highest levels of expenditure in the developing nations. The central and state governments set the goals and strategies in consultation with the Central Council of Health and Family Welfare. The Ministry of Health and Family Welfare monitors the workings of the Central Government and provides technical and administrative services along with medical education. According to a World Bank study the per capita spending on health in India is around ₹ 320 per year with a significant input of 75% from private households. The state governments contribute 15.2%, the central government 5.2%, third party employers 3.3% and the municipal government and foreign donors provide about 1.3% to the total spending, of which 58.7% goes to primary health care (curative, preventive and promotional) and 38.8% is spent on the secondary and tertiary ones. Despite the efforts of the state and central governments efforts, the health care in India is in a bad condition because of several factors—the rapidly increasing population of the country, high level of corruption in government and nongovernment health care organizations and lack of awareness amongst people.

In India, the hospitals are run by government, charitable trusts and by private organizations. The government hospitals in rural areas are called the Primary Health Center (PHCs). Major hospitals are located in district head quarters or major cities. Apart from the modern system of medicine, traditional and indigenous medicinal systems like Ayurvedic and Unani systems are in practice throughout the country.

The Indian Health Service provides public funded care for indigenous people. Employer benefit based health insurance remains quite common with larger employers. Workers injured on the job are covered by government mandated worker compensation insurance and wage replacement benefits. These benefits vary considerably state-to-state and employers bear the cost of this insurance. Businesses with considerable risks, such as bridge-building, mining, or meat processing face far higher worker compensation insurance costs than do office based clerical businesses. Although the medical colleges and research institutes form a backbone structure for providing healthcare, the private hospitals and nursing homes also are becoming an increasingly necessary part of the healthcare structure in the country. India is an under developed country and 50% of the population live in urban areas in an extremely below the poverty condition. As they are lured by massive industrialization, economic and educational opportunities in cities like Chennai, Mumbai, Kolkata and Delhi are over crowded and the statistics says about one fifth live in slums. Most of the health problems in India are generated from these slums only. Many are exposed to new types of risks associated with industrial pollution, road accidents, air pollution, poisonings, threat to child adolescent health, etc. Drainage system is poor in Cities like Chennai, Kolkata, and Mumbai, etc. which cause high incidence of infections, disease and epidemics. High densities of dwellings and lack of internal roads cause poor accessibility for emergency and life-saving services. New squatter settlements come-up on the periphery often on inhabitable lands because of their low values and cause environmental hazards. In the recent Bhopal gas tragedy, around 3000 persons mostly from the peripheral slums were killed and it clearly revealed the vulnerability of squatters. Urban malaria, tuberculosis and pneumonia, leprosy, meningitis, preventable infections in children such as measles, whooping cough and polio, diarrhea diseases and intestinal worm infections are some of the most common health problems apart from higher morbidity and mortality due to accidents.

Failure of Urban Health Care System

Health Care System in India in the last 45 years has focused on increasing coverage in the rural areas. There has been little or no development of organized health care services for the vast urban areas. The 3,600 odd cities and towns of India with some 40 million people living in slums have to depend largely on private practitioners (mostly quacks) for their health care needs. Out of the 3,000 plus urban local bodies in India only about 100 have some semblance to a Health Care System service while the rest have only a sanitary inspector or even a lower functionary to look after the Health Care System. It is not uncommon to see medical colleges and hospitals belonging to various medical systems such as modern, ayurveda and homeopathy in one Indian city. India provides an excellent example of medical pluralism. People follow home remedies, spiritual remedies and treatment from various medical systems simultaneously or one after another. Metropolitan urban areas provide medical facilities, which are available in developing countries such as cardiac surgery, treatment of all kinds of cancers, or in brief, for the diseases which are associated with affluence. The major diseases identified in South—East Asia Region under WHO are malaria, filarial and other mosquito–borne diseases, diarrhea diseases, leprosy, tuberculosis, sexually transmitted diseases, poliomyelitis and other children diseases, tetanus, nasopharyngeal and cervical cancers, visual impairment and blindness, etc.

The organized sectors in urban areas such as employees of government and public undertakings bargain for medical benefits like Employees State Insurance Scheme and Government Health Schemes. In some cases, medical expenses are reimbursable if treated at recognized hospitals. At the same time, there is a lot of overlap and even the private medical practitioners seem to thrive well simultaneously. However, the unorganized sector such as domestic workers, self-employed, porters, cart-pullers, load-carriers and urban poor mostly living in slums do not get these benefits. They are also deprived of piped water and modern sanitation, or in any case, the facilities are woefully inadequate. Urban poor, whose hallmark in expenditure is cheapness, get adulterated food and drugs. On an average, milk, milk-products, edible oils, wheat flour, spices and even tea leaves are adulterated to the tune of 50 percent. Mental health has yet to receive due attention in India. While westernized urban elite requires the services of psychiatrists in increasing number, for others family continues to provide psychic treatment. If crime rate, suicide, divorce, riots and indiscipline are considered as parameters of mental health, then urban area needs urgent attention. It is often said that a large proportion of population suffers from protein calorie malnutrition. However, the range of nutrition in which people can function efficiently without getting nutritional deficiencies is wide and what are commonly given, as recommended quantities for intake of nutrients are much higher than what are required. Urban poor unfortunately use bottle feeding and baby feeds under the influence of commercial advertising on radio, television, and through other popular media like films. The revolution in drugs coincides with freedom from colonial rule. The drug industry has developed out of proportion in comparison with basic amenities like potable water and sanitation. Pharmaceutical industry measures developed out of proportion of country in terms of intakes of per capita consumption of drugs. In India, drugs are only consumed among 20 percent urban people. The per capita consumption is perhaps the lowest in the world. However, this code does not represent the correct picture in view of the fact that about 75 percent population in rural areas and urban poor has yet to have access to drugs. Major share of these drugs are taken away by vitamins, tonics, and antibiotics. It is estimated that out of the total production 25 percent is taken away by vitamins and tonics, and 20 percent by antibiotics. Diseases like dengue fever, hepatitis, tuberculosis, malaria and pneumonia continue to plague India due to increased resistance to drugs. In 2011; India finally developed a

Totally drug-resistant form of tuberculosis 10. India is ranked 3rd among the countries with the most number of HIV-infected. Diarrheal diseases are the primary causes of early childhood mortality. Approximately 1.72 million children die each year before turning one. These diseases can be attributed to poor sanitation and inadequate safe drinking water in India.

Causes for Poor Health

Always health maintenance has been a problem in India. Health services have been a problem due to lack of education and poverty. Another reason is inadequate in health services due to insufficient health facilities offered to the common men. Funds allotted by the government for medical facilities are not used for this purpose properly. There are many governments owned and operated hospitals but the doctors are not available in time. Even the people do not know when the doctors will be available in the hospitals. Most of the doctors who serve in the government hospitals have own clinics and spend most of time in their own clinics. In case of an emergency, many hospitals are asked to deposit money first before patient can be admitted. Sometimes the poor do not have money to deposit immediately. Sometimes the poor have been given low quality medicines which leads to many problems. Moreover, the reasons for health care are as follows:

- *Poor sanitation:* As more than 122 million households have no toilets and 33% lack access to latrines, over 50% of the population (638 million) defecates in the open. This is relatively higher than Bangladesh and Brazil (7%) and China (4%). Although 211 million people gained access to improved sanitation from 1990–2008, only 31% uses them. 11% of the Indian rural families dispose of child stools safely whereas 80% of the population leave their stools in the open or throw them into the garbage. Open air defecation leads to the spreading of diseases and malnutrition through parasitic and bacterial infections.
- *Inadequate safe drinking water:* Access to protected sources of drinking water has improved from 68% of the population in 1990 to 88% in 2008 However, only 26% of the slum population has access to safe drinking water 17 and 25% of the total population has drinking water on their premises. This problem is exacerbated by falling levels of groundwater, caused mainly by increasing extraction for irrigation. Insufficient maintenance of the environment around water sources, groundwater pollution, excessive arsenic and fluoride in drinking water pose a major threat to India's health.
- *Government takes steps to improve healthcare system in india* Union Minister of Health and Welfare takes steps to improve the healthcare delivery system and several medical facilities. Under the plan the Center has launched for control of cardiovascular diseases, cancer, diabetes, stroke, sports injury and health of the senior citizens.

CHARACTERISTICS OF HEALTH CARE (OR MEDICAL SERVICE

Health care services have some unique characteristics. Its own which are distinctly different from other services. Some of the characteristics of health care service are given below:

- Other than preventive care, the demand for health care services arises when normal functioning of human organism fails due to the presence of diseases. This kind of unpredictability of demand cannot be observed in other services except public welfare services like, police services, national defense services, and fire services. It is unpredictable when an individual will be attacked by a disease. Hence, the demand for health care service is sporadic and irregular.
- The outcome of health care service is not deterministic. Risk of disability, patient's survival treatment and health recovery remains, to a greater extent, always be uncertain. Hence, consumption of this service never implies that the consumer (patient) will get desired utility or satisfaction from the service.
- The service is guided by the objective of customer's welfare but the customer (patient) cannot test the product before consuming it. Here doctors or physicians act as a main intermediate agent of the service producing units. The quality of medical product and physician's efficiency is affected by the producer-customer relation.
- Asymmetric information are more than that of other services because in the health service a patient is not always aware exactly what disease happened to him/her or the degree of severity he/she is facing and the kind of treatment is required for that.
- The market for health care service is not perfectly competitive. Here the entry to the profession is restricted by licensing. So the supply is limited, and that makes in some cases, its market as monopoly in nature.
- The price of the goods and other services are determined by the market mechanism and/or profit maximization motive but medical-service-prices are in many cases influenced by the modalities of social welfare, as a result, extentisive price discrimination is observed in this service.

DEMAND SIDE AND SUPPLY SIDE

As we know, central to the workings of any market economy are the laws of supply and demand. When the supply, price, quality and demand for a product or service are aligned the market can and does work to its optimum. The laws of supply and demand that underlie the nation's economy in general also apply to the provision of health care services. Yet, the health care market is significantly distorted. One reason for this distortion is a disconnect between the supply and demand of services. This, in turn, is driven in part by the fact that consumers are not actively engaged and appropriately educated as partners in their utilization of health care services.

Demand Side

- 'Demand side' strategies are focused on just that issue: altering how health care services and products are utilized by consumers, with the ultimate goals of achieving the triple Aim objectives of improved population health, reduced per capita cost of care and enhanced consumer experience of care. A key demand side strategy is insurance benefit design: that is, structuring both the benefits provided and the consumer's use of those benefits in such a way as to manage utilization of health care services by heightening patients' awareness of costs. Altering a benefit package by changing the scope, amount and cost of services provides the opportunity to both incent and discourage utilization of a variety of health care services. Evidence-based and well-implemented demand side strategies can help to make consumers partners with providers in fostering positive changes in health care delivery.

Supply Side

- Demand side strategies alone cannot solve the health care system's woes. They must be coupled with supply side strategies in order to achieve the triple aim objectives of improved population health, reduced per capita cost of care and enhanced consumer experience of care. Payment and delivery reforms have the ability to impact the supply side of the equation. Examples of supply side interventions are numerous: Physician training programs and specialty societies make decisions on residency class sizes as a way to affect supply of providers into the market; drug pricing negotiations between health plans and pharmaceutical companies allow health plans to limit the cost and types of pharmaceuticals available in a given formulary; and health plans use network tiring, access and in network/out of network policies to control access to the supply side of the delivery system.

SUMMARY

In this unit we discuss about the demand and supply of health care services in that an individual 'produces' his or her own health, employing combinations of personal health services and health behaviors. The relationship between these inputs and health outcomes is given by a health production function. Given the product technology and prices of input and such exogenous factors as the person's genetic make-up, revealed as one ages, individuals make decisions about their health and the levels of the health inputs they 'employ'. Typically, the relationship between inputs and health outcomes for an individual is uncertain. Decision analysts have developed decision trees, which are a useful tool for analyzing decisions made under conditions of uncertainty.

Financing of Health Care in India

24 unit

INTRODUCTION

Most health systems in the developing world are characterized by mixed public and private financing and delivery of care. For a health system to perform well–that is, to provide needed, good-quality health services to all who need the services–public and private financing agents need to generate an appropriate amount of revenue from all sources relative to what is possible in the country; pool risk effectively; create appropriate incentives for quality service provision from all providers including public, private, and not-for-profit; and allocate resources to the most effective, efficient, and equitable interventions and services irrespective of the sector. These functions should be managed efficiently, minimizing administrative costs.

Definition of Health Financing

According to WHO defined health financing as the 'function of a health system concerned with the mobilization, accumulation and allocation of money to cover the health needs of the people, individually and collectively, in the health system'; the 'purpose of health financing is to make funding available, as well as to set the right financial incentives to providers, to ensure that all individuals have access to effective public health and personal health care'.

SOURCES OF FINANCING OF HEALTH CARE SERVICES

The major sources of financing health care are as follows:

- *Fees for service and insurance:* The most essential mode of health care financing is the fees for service. Fees are charged to cover the cost of the provided services. This is commonly found in many government health care facilities in developing countries. It is done so as to raise funds and to possibly discourage 'unnecessary demand'. The World Bank suggested this type of health care financing but in differential manner, i.e. community preventive services should be rendered free, curative primary care by user charges and potential personalised preventive care at a reduced cost.

Disadvantages:

- Collection may be difficult or complex.
- It may not encourage equity.
- It discourages the real users (because price is a determining factor).
- It is regressive because the poor are greatly affected.
- Waged labourers who are not paid during the course of sickness will be affected.
- Peasant farmers with highly seasonal income will face difficulties in paying for the health bills especially during pre-harvest period (which is also time they become more sick).

Exemption schemes have been advocated to get around equity problems in health care financing but it has its own problems as well. The question of 'who should be exempted' is a major obstacle. 'Is it based on income level?' 'If on income level at what level should be?' 'What is the process of selecting exempts and who determine the exemption?' ('The beauty is in the eyes of the beholder'). Exemption process can also discourage utilization of services due stigmatizing of holders of such.

- Insurance coverage is another means of health care financing. Here the risk of illness is pooled among the insured group. There are various alternative combinations of coverage are available within the insurance schemes. Various combinations can be: in-patient or out-patient cover, with/out obstetric cover, exclusion of chronic diseases cover etc. Premium (monthly payment to the insurance company) depends on some factors.

  These factors are:

  - *Type of care required:* This is to know what type of medical conditions will be paid for; will it include preventive services?
  - *Health status of the insuree:* This can be determined by health indicators such as Age, Occupation (high-risk?), life habits (smoking, alcoholism) and by conducting a medical test. This is done to possibly select high-risk insurees that would consume more and afterwards make exorbitant claims from the insurance. Potentially high-risk insuree may require paying high premiums or not covered for some services consumed.

- *Co-payment agreement:* This will determine the amount of premium to be paid. Insuree agreeing to part-payment of some procedures maybe required to pay lower premium. A reimbursement method may also be put in place-where the insuree pay for the consumed services and afterwards make claims from the insurance.

Disadvantages:

- It encourages stratification of health care system. Within the same community different people holds different insurance cover for their health as a result of their ability to pay varied amount of premiums.
- Spreading of risk rarely occurs because the higher the risk the higher the premium to be paid.
- Administrative costs may make it inefficient as a revenue generator (paperwork for claims, advertisement, medical tests, etc).
- They tend to emphasize curative over the preventive care (5) difficulty in controlling overall medical costs—there can be abuse by demanding more than needed.
- Tendency towards poor remuneration for the doctors (paying less for some difficult procedures, etc).
- It encourages changing of jobs- in that insurance policies are tied to employment.

• *Health Maintenance Organization (HMO):* This is a variant of general insurance scheme. The members pay an annual amount of money to a health care provider to keep them healthy. The provider in turn provides services required directly or through a third party (i.e. pay other person/other health care provider services not available in their center). The practice here acts as the insurance company. It has the tendency to reduce its own costs through preventive care and hence minimizing unnecessary sophisticated medical procedures. It has been proposed to be a regime to the escalating health care costs in USA.

  Disadvantage:

  They may discriminate against members of the HMO schemes (those with lower educational background and cannot push for their rights) e.g. referring them to higher hospitals where a higher costs maybe paid by the referring HMO.

• *Tax revenue and national insurance:* National Insurance Scheme (NIS): This widens the base of private schemes with payments tied to wage levels. It differs from private insurance scheme in that the cover is identical and premiums are based on the level of income (not on health status).

Health care is often part of social security schemes. Contributions to the scheme are from the employees, employers and in some instances the State (government). Collection of premiums is better done among salaried individuals rather than the artisan, peasant farmers, etc. (no regular employment). Equity maybe a big question here because stratification of care may be obvious (due to level of premium). Where services are not available carriers of social insurance scheme may only have 'paper rights'.

In some countries where social security schemes have being the method of caring for the health of the people. The government care for the populace from her own sources of revenue. The services are provided at minimal or no direct cost to all the citizens in cases of most comprehensive schemes. Equity, here depend on means of raising finance and the means of rationing and distributing the health care resultant from the 'free service'. Raising finance can be from PAYE tax (Pay as you earn) which is progressive and regressive if from indirect tax (also depending on goods and services taxed). It is believed that Tax revenue and national insurance encourages equity and coverage (relative). Also, have potential to reduce unit costs through economics of scale and coordination of services.

- *Disadvantages:* Systems financed by tax revenue or national insurance are generally regarded as inefficient because there are no incentives to cut costs and addition of administrative costs.
- *Community financing:* UNICEF under the Bamako initiative suggested community fund raising to finance health care. One of these is service-use (e.g. Drug Revolving Funds (DRF)) and others which are community based (e.g. pre-paid community taxes). This has the advantage of community participation. The amount of money arising from such community in the overall that will be available for health will limit its uses not to think of if it has to be re-distributed to other communities
- *Loans and grants:* Loans and grants maybe used to provide resources for health care financing. This can be through technical assistance or provision of free drugs. Loans are mostly used for capital financing while grants have the subsidizing effect on the cost of provision of services. Loans are to be re-paid back at a later time. Loans are to be properly looking into so as to avoid noosing your neck in to difficult, concealed, stringent economic conditions. The World Bank usually give soft loans with little interest and longer period of payment but it should be noted that such loans can actually compound the economic recovery of a developing nation. Loans and grants are sometimes tied to a particular project or the way and where the money is to be spent e.g. donor may require that equipment and personnel must be purchased from their market. This may lead to purchase of spare parts

and technical staff from abroad for maintenance purposes. Sources of loans and grants come from World Bank, Non-governmental organizations, foreign countries and organizations (EEC, EU, ECOWAS), etc.

ROLE OF STATE AND CENTRAL GOVERNMENT ON FINANCING OF HEALTH CARE SERVICES

Role of Government within the Health Sector

- *Health system strengthening:* Important issues that the health systems must confront are lack of financial and material resources, health workforce issues and the stewardship challenge of implementing pro-equity health policies in a pluralistic environment. The National Rural Health Mission (NRHM) launched by the Government of India is a leap forward in establishing effective integration and convergence of health services and affecting architectural correction in the health care delivery system in India.
- *Health information system:* The Integrated Disease Surveillance Project was set up to establish a dedicated highway of information relating to disease occurrence required for prevention and containment at the community level, but the slow pace of implementation is due to poor efforts in involving critical actors outside the public sector. Health profiles published by the government should be used to help communities prioritize their health problems and to inform local decision making. Public health laboratories have a good capacity to support the government's diagnostic and research activities on health risks and threats, but are not being utilized efficiently. Mechanisms to monitor epidemiological challenges like mental health, occupational health and other environment risks are yet to be put in place.
- *Health research system:* There is a need for strengthening research infrastructure in the departments of community medicine in various institutes and to foster their partnerships with state health services.
- *Regulation and enforcement in public health:* A good system of regulation is fundamental to successful public health outcomes. It reduces exposure to disease through enforcement of sanitary codes, e.g. water quality monitoring, slaughterhouse hygiene and food safety. Wide gaps exist in the enforcement, monitoring and evaluation, resulting in a weak public health system. This is partly due to poor financing for public health, lack of leadership and commitment of public health functionaries and lack of community involvement. Revival of public health regulation through concerted efforts by the government is possible through

updating and implementation of public health laws, consulting stakeholders and increasing public awareness of existing laws and their enforcement procedures.

- *Health promotion:* Stopping the spread of STDs and HIV/AIDS, helping youth recognize the dangers of tobacco smoking and promoting physical activity. These are a few examples of behavior change communication that focus on ways that encourage people to make healthy choices. Development of community-wide education programs and other health promotion activities need to be strengthened. Much can be done to improve the effectiveness of health promotion by extending it to rural areas as well; observing days like 'Diabetes day' and 'Heart day' even in villages will help create awareness at the grassroots level.
- *Human resource development and capacity building:* There are several shortfalls that need to be addressed in the development of human resources for public health services. There is a dire need to establish training facilities for public health specialists along with identifying the scope for their contribution in the field. The Public Health Foundation of India is a positive step to redress the limited institutional capacity in India by strengthening training, research and policy development in public health. Pre-service training is essential to train the medical workforce in public health leadership and to impart skills required for the practice of public health. Changes in the undergraduate curriculum are vital for capacity building in emerging issues like geriatric care, adolescent health and mental health. In-service training for medical officers is essential for imparting management skills and leadership qualities. Equally important is the need to increase the number of paramedical workers and training institutes in India.
- *Public health policy:* Identification of health objectives and targets is one of the more visible strategies to direct the activities of the health sector, e.g. in the United States, the 'Healthy People 2010' offers a simple but powerful idea by providing health objectives in a format that enables diverse groups to combine their efforts and work as a team. Similarly, in India, we need a road map to 'better health for all' that can be used by states, communities, professional organizations and all sectors. It will also facilitate changes in resource allocation for public health interventions and a platform for concerted intersectoral action, thereby enabling policy coherence.

Role of Government in Enabling Intersectoral

The Ministry of Health needs to form stronger partnerships with other agents involved in public health, because many factors influencing the health outcomes are outside their direct jurisdiction. Making public health a shared value across the various sectors is a politically challenging strategy, but such collective action is crucial.

- *Social determinants of health:* Kerala is often quoted as an example in international forums for achieving a good status of public health by addressing the fundamental determinants of health: Investments in basic education, public health and primary care.
- *Living conditions:* Safe drinking water and sanitation are critical determinants of health, which would directly contribute to 70—80% reduction in the burden of communicable diseases. Full coverage of drinking water supply and sanitation through existing programs, in both rural and urban areas, is achievable and affordable.
- *Urban planning:* Provision of urban basic services like water supply, sewerage and solid waste management needs special attention. The Jawaharlal Nehru National Urban Renewal Mission in 35 cities works to develop financially sustainable cities in line with the Millenium Development Goals, which needs to be expanded to cover the entire country. Other issues to be addressed are housing and urban poverty alleviation.
- *Revival of rural infrastructure and livelihood:* Action is required in the following areas: Promotion of agricultural mechanization, improving efficiency of investments, rationalizing subsidies and diversifying and providing better access to land, credit and skills.
- *Education:* Elementary education has received a major push through the Sarva Siksha Abhayan. In order to consolidate the gains achieved, a mission for secondary education is essential. "Right of children to Free and Compulsory education Bill 2009" seeks to provide education to children aged between 6 and 14 years, and is a right step forward in improving the literacy of the Indian population.
- *Nutrition and early child development:* Recent innovations like universalization of Integrated Child Development Services (ICDS) and setting up of mini-Anganwadi centers in deprived areas are examples of inclusive growth under the eleventh 5-year plan. The government needs to strengthen ICDS in poor-performing states based on experiences from other successful models, e.g., Tamil Nadu (upgrading kitchens with LPG connection, stove and pressure cooker and electrification; use of iron-fortified salt to address the burden of anemia). Micronutrient deficiency control measures like dietary diversification, horticultural intervention, food fortification, nutritional supplementation and other public health measures need intersectoral coordination with various departments, e.g. Women and Child Development, Health, Agriculture, Rural and Urban development.

- *Social security measures:* The social and economic spinoff of the Mahatma Gandhi Rural Employment Guarantee Scheme (MREGS) has the potential to change the complexion of rural India. It differs from other poverty-alleviation projects in the concept of citizenship and entitlement. However, employment opportunities and wages have taken the center stage, while development of infrastructure and community assets is neglected. This scheme has the necessary manpower to implement intersectoral projects, e.g. laying roads, water pipelines, social forestry, horticulture, anti-erosion projects and rain water harvesting. The unlimited potential of social capital has to be effectively tapped by the government.
- *Food security measures:* Innovations are required to strengthen the public distribution system to curb the inclusion and exclusion errors and increase the range of commodities for people living in very poor conditions. It is essential that the government puts forth action plans to increase domestic food grain production, raise consumer incomes to buy food and make agriculture remunerative.
- *Population stabilization:* There is all round realization that population stabilization is a must for ensuring quality of life for all citizens. Formulation of a National Policy and setting up of a National Commission on Population and Janasankhya Sthiratha Kosh reflect the deep commitment of the government. However, parallel developments in women empowerment, increasing institutional deliveries and strengthening health services and infrastructure hold the key to population control in the future.
- *Gender mainstreaming and empowerment:* Women-specific interventions in all policies, programs and systems need to be launched. The government should take steps to sensitize service providers in various departments to issues of women. The Department of Women and Child Development must take necessary steps to implement the provisions of 'Protection of Women from Domestic Violence Act, 2005.' Training for protection officers, establishment of counselling centers for women affected by violence and creating awareness in the community are vital steps. Poverty eradication programs and microcredit schemes need to be strengthened for economic and social empowerment of women.
- *Reducing the impact of climate change and disasters on health:* Thermal extremes and weather disasters spread of vector-borne, food-borne and waterborne infections, food security and malnutrition and air quality with associated human health risks are the public health risks associated with climate change. Depletion of

non-renewable sources of energy and water, deterioration of soil and water quality and the potential extinction of innumerable habitats and species are other effects. India's 'National Action Plan on Climate Change' identifies eight core 'national missions' through various ministries, focused on understanding climate change, energy efficiency, renewable energy and natural resource conservation. Although there are several issues concerning India's position under UNFCCC, it has agreed not to allow its per capita Greenhouse gas emissions to exceed the average per capita emissions of the developed countries, even as it pursues its social and economic development objectives.

The Ministry of Health, in coordination with other ministries, provides technical assistance in implementing disaster management and emergency preparedness measures. Deficient areas include carrying out rapid needs assessment, disseminating health information, food safety and environmental health after disasters and ensuring transparency and efficiency in the administration of aid after disasters. Implementation of Disaster Management Act, 2005 is essential for establishing institutional mechanisms for disaster management, ensuring an intersectoral approach to mitigation and undertaking holistic, coordinated and prompt response to disaster situations.

- *Community participation:* Community participation builds public support for policies and programs, generates compliance with regulations and helps alter personal health behaviors. One of the major strategic interventions under NRHM is the system of ensuring accountability and transparency through people's participation – the Rogi Kalyan Samitis. The Ministry of Health needs to define a clear policy on social participation and operational methods in facilitating community health projects. Potential areas of community participation could be in lifestyle modification in chronic diseases through physical activity and diet modification, and primary prevention of alcohol dependence through active community-based methods like awareness creation and behavioral interventions.

FACTORS INFLUENCING THE STATE'S ABILITY TO FINANCE HEALTH CARE SERVICES

- *Demography data:* These have three major influences on health care financing and provision.
  (a) *The population growth rates:* Sharp growth rate or population doubling time are very high in most developing nations. These will in no doubt strain the meagre available resources. This

will affect not only the financing of health care but other social amenities such as roads, water, electricity, etc.

(b) The composition of the population maybe such that there are increased number of children and elderly in the population. This is the usual scenario in developing country's population with high growth rates. The children and elderly are known to consume a lot of health care resources. The antenatal, obstetric, under 5 children are heavy users of health facilities. This is also true of the elderly with chronic diseases such as diabetes, cancer, hypertensive heart diseases, musculoskeletal disorders, etc.

(c) The ratio of dependents to economically productive individuals in the population will also have a major effect on funding of health. In a population with more than 45% children (<15 years) and say 30% elderly (>60 years) will increase the economic burden on the producers. This scenario is very common among many developing countries- with high growth rates where there are more children (dependants) than the producers.

- *Economic recession:* The global recession of 1970s and 1980s have rendered a devastating effect on the economy of many developing countries with high debt burdens and debt servicing, high inflation rates, Structural Adjustment Programme (SAP) etc. These led to many governments of the developing countries not to been able to maintain not to talk of expanding the existing health care system. The SAP has in its package economic measures such as devaluation, increased import prices and decreased funding on health and education.
- *Expectations from health care:* There are increasing pressures from the population on the expectations on health care. Majority will like to enjoy the health care facilities similarly available in the first world countries. This is usually associated with the use of high-Tech equipment which most of the time are imported.
- *Drive for equity:* Many segments/regions of most developing countries are under served with health care facilities. Also, majority have access only to basic but limited health care. One of the principles of primary health care is to improve coverage; this is contrary to the sophisticated health care facilities needed by the middle class in the urban areas.
- *Changing disease pattern:* As the income of an individual rises there is a change in the pattern of the disease to be observed. The diseases associated with poverty are rapidly disappearing leaving the room for those of the affluence. Major health problems in developing countries are preventable and are relatively cheap to deal with when compared with that of the advanced countries (Heart diseases, Cancer, Diabetes etc). The change in disease pattern associated with change in social status will invariably lead to an increasing cost for health care of those diseases. Also, when new diseases are being discovered (e.g.

HIV/AIDS, SAS, Bird flu) or that previous diseases that are not medically diagnosable based on the available knowledge then, are now possible through the use of high sophisticated and expensive medical equipments.

Increase Effective Resource Level in Health Care Financing

As a result of the afore-mentioned factors affecting health care funding, there is a need to look into what areas and measures that can be introduced to improve health care financing. The followings are areas to look into with the hope of improving resources to finance health care:

Efficiency

The existing services should be look into with the hope of improving them. This can best be done by:

- *Appraisal:* Cost-effectiveness analysis may suggest alternative approaches to specific health problems that are better or more effective.
- *Contracting out:* Some of the services can be contracted out to individuals and companies to improve effectiveness, e.g. catering, cleaning, security services etc.
- *An internal market:* This is selling of services to one another within the same organisation, e.g. X-rays. There is an assumption that this will improve efficiency.
- *Information dissemination:* Comparative information about various segments of the establishment can be disseminated to enhance peer group pressure to change practice that will bring about better efficiency.
- *Management team composition:* The clinicians are to be involved in decision-making body because they have more influence on the way resources are used. Their involvement in management team will invariably improve their level of awareness to cost and better efficiency.

Reallocation of Resources (Within the Health Sector)

This is allocation of resources to priority areas. This is better observed in changing pattern of disease, e.g. eradication of smallpox. Allocation should be based on planning—say based on the proportion of various groups in a population (% of children, elderly, etc.). Currently, most countries are allocating huge amount resources on the prevention, control and management of HIV/AIDS as compared to some other diseases.

Reallocation of Resources to Health Sector (from other sectors)

- This done by the government by allocating more resources to health by reducing allocation to other sectors such as defense. It should be noted here that what reallocation of such funds would achieve in health sector might equally be achieved through education and agriculture. Similar result can also be observed through provision of social infrastructure.

Criteria for Choosing a Financing System

The choice of funding system involves a major policy decision. The followings are clear criteria for selection of the best method. The first 3 deals with any financing system while the last 3 hold true for primary health care system:

Viability and Simplicity of Use

Any financing system must possess the ability to be made to work. Careful consideration of technical feasibility is very important. Complex, bureaucratic and costly mechanism must be avoided. Say paying stations remote from places of consumption of services (use of banks, etc). Cultural acceptability of the financing system must be considered in a community.

Revenue-generating Ability

A system is said to be generating revenue when the cost of production is much less than the revenue earnings or when the sale of goods and services are greater than that of the resources inputted, i.e. output/income greater than input/expenditure.

Effects on Service Provision

The mode of financing health care can be non-incentive to the users. You can create non-incentive to urban dwellers to use a secondary level of care (Hospital) as a primary care center by introducing heavy out of pocket charges into the outpatient department. The contrary will be done to those patients referred from the primary health care center to the secondary centres. Also, in third party health care financing, some services such as preventive services may carry more remuneration for the practitioner than extraction of wisdom tooth. Some other treatment maybe discouraged such esthetic care (orthodontic)—payment of such may not cover the entire practitioner's bill.

Effects on Equity

Equity here means 'equal access to care for those in equal need'. There are two types of equity: Horizontal and Vertical equity. Horizontal means equal treatment of equals: those with similar health needs be given equal opportunity to access and treatment. Vertical equity means unequal treatment for unequal's those with greater needs would obtain concessional access, e.g. more resources for TB prevention and control in endemic areas or lower income groups may have treatment and transport fare subsidized. This must be considered before a choice of financing system is chosen. User charges may discourage lower income earners from using/consuming a particular service(s). Social insurance may favor services utilization by urban high income earners. Fund raising can be regressive or progressive depending on the relative income of the users. It is regressive if it takes a greater percentage of income from the lower income earners; it could be progressive if it takes a greater percentage of income from the higher income earners. The tax system of a country can be regressive if tax is placed on essential goods or progressive if placed on luxury goods. 'Under tax based system, collective financing of health care is carried out in such a way that there is a transfer of resources from the richer elements of society to the poor and sick group'. In user charges, the sick will pay for the services she/he consumes without any cross-subsidy from others in the community (rich, healthy individuals).

Community Participation

User charges allow the individual consumer to get involved in decision making. This is done by direct strengthening of direct relationship between the consumer and the provider.

Multi-sectorialism

This describes the involvement of other sectors of life to play key role in health care system (Engineers, Sociologists, etc). A financing system may allow or disallow the involvement of other sectors of the society. User charges may not encourage fees collected for clinical services to be used for the provision of water for a particular community. This is contrary with the use of tax-based system.

SUMMARY

In this unit we discuss about there are rising interest of many on escalating health care costs globally and how it should be financed. Many developing countries inherited heavy dependence on tax revenues from the colonial rule to finance health care. Many countries of the world have undergone reforms since late 1970s. The World Bank advocated the use of direct user-charge finance system. Loans and grants maybe used to provide resources for health care financing. The form and level of health care financing are now a major policy for most developing country governments. Community participation builds public support for policies and programs, generates compliance with regulations and helps alter personal health behaviors.

Index

Page numbers followed by *f* refer to figure.

D

M

N

O

P

Q

R

S

W